D1562542

Oxford American Handbook of
Clinical Diagnosis

Oxford American
Handbook of
Clinical
Diagnosis

Gregg Y. Lipschik

Joan M. Von Feldt

Lawrence Frame

Scott Akers
University of Pennsylvania School of Medicine
Philadelphia, Pennsylvania

Salvatore Mangione
Thomas Jefferson School of Medicine
Philadelphia, Pennsylvania

Huw Llewelyn
Kettering General Hospital
Kettering, Northamptonshire
England

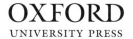

OXFORD
UNIVERSITY PRESS

OXFORD
UNIVERSITY PRESS

Oxford University Press, Inc., publishes works that further
Oxford University's objective of excellence
in research, scholarship, and education.

Oxford   New York
Auckland Cape Town Dar es Salaam Hong Kong Karachi
Kuala Lumpur Madrid Melbourne Mexico City Nairobi
New Delhi Shanghai Taipei Toronto

With offices in
Argentina Austria Brazil Chile Czech Republic France Greece
Guatemala Hungary Italy Japan Poland Portugal Singapore
South Korea Switzerland Thailand Turkey Ukraine Vietnam

Published by Oxford University Press, Inc.
198 Madison Avenue, New York, New York 10016

www.oup.com

Oxford is a registered trademark of Oxford University Press

Library of Congress Cataloging-in-Publication Data

Oxford American handbook of clinical diagnosis/Gregg Lipschik ... [et al.].
p. ; cm. —(Oxford American handbooks)
Adapted from: Oxford handbook of clinical diagnosis/Huw Llewelyn ... [et al.].
2nd ed. 2008.
Includes bibliographical references and index.
ISBN 978-0-19-536947-2 (flexicover : alk. paper)

1. Diagnosis—Handbooks, manuals, etc. 2. Physical diagnosis—Handbooks,
manuals, etc. 3. Medical history taking—Handbooks, manuals, etc. I. Lipschik,
Gregg, 1954- II. Oxford handbook of clinical diagnosis. III. Title: Handbook of clinical
diagnosis. IV. Series: Oxford American handbooks.
[DNLM: 1. Diagnosis, Differential—Handbooks. 2. Medical History Taking—
Handbooks. 3. Physical Examination—Handbooks. WB 39 O973 2009]
RC71.3.O938 2008
616.07'5—dc22   2008054687

10 9 8 7 6 5 4 3 2 1

Printed in China
on acid-free paper

For Angela

and

for Debra

Preface

This book explains how to use a history, examination, and preliminary tests to arrive at a diagnosis. This helps us as clinicians to anticipate what may happen next and how interventions may influence the disease process. We are also better equipped to share with our patients and colleagues what we are thinking and doing.

The approach used here enables clinicians to focus on symptoms, physical signs, and initial test results that are likely to lead to a diagnosis. This is based on the principle that diagnostic leads with short differential diagnoses will be more informative than those features with long lists of causes.

Each sign or symptom on a page is followed by a list of diagnoses with associated suggestive and confirmatory clinical and laboratory features. The reader may scan down the page to see which entries are compatible with the patient's findings thus far. The compatible findings can then be used as evidence for the diagnosis.

In the spirit of the Oxford American Handbooks, readers are encouraged to be critical about the contents of the book, to make changes, and to let us know of any significant differences in opinion or errors.

GL & HL

Acknowledgments

This book is based on ideas and teaching methods developed originally by Dr. Huw Llewelyn at King's College Hospital, London. Dr. Llewelyn also designed and wrote this book with the assistance of his colleagues Drs. Hock Ang, Anees Al-Abdullah, and Keir Lewis. It was edited for the U.S. market by Drs. Gregg Lipschik, Joan Von Feldt, Lawrence Frame, Salvatore Mangione, and Scott Akers.

Contents

Some important questions and answers about this book

1. How is this book different from other textbooks?

Most medical books describe a disease process and give physiological, biochemical, and other explanations for the causes and complications and how these processes can be treated. They also describe what symptoms, signs, and test results occur. When a patient presents with new symptoms and other findings, readers must somehow work out which, of all the conditions they have read about, the patient has.

This book is different. It lists the causes of findings that are the best clues (or "leads") and then outlines some findings, which, when used in combination with the lead, suggest the diagnosis with a reasonably high probability, or confirm it.

The number of findings is usually small, for two reasons. The first is that many findings occur often in many other diseases and are therefore nonspecific; it is only a few that form powerful predictors. The second reason is practical—it is only possible to build up experience of small combinations of findings because it is difficult to find many patients with the same large combination of findings.

The diagnostic findings given in this book are based mostly on an impression of what other doctors expect in the form of evidence for a diagnosis during clinical discussions (or in an evidence-based past medical history). Ideally, these findings should have been shown to form the best combinations that identify patients who respond well to treatment compared to placebo in clinical trials. Failing this, they should be the combinations recognized by convention as being the best (known as "diagnostic criteria"). In the absence of both these situations, one has to resort to impressions of what most physicians would think reasonable.

The usefulness of suggestive findings would also require more studies on their frequency of occurrence in association with different diagnostic criteria in various clinical settings.

2. Does this book claim to reveal all the mysteries of diagnosis?

No—the way in which our minds work is a mystery, as is much of the diagnostic process. *Diagnosis* is based on the Greek "to know through." In the context of medicine, it is to see through the patient's symptoms and other findings to imagine and understand what may be happening in terms of current theories applied to medicine. The decision of what to do is made by using the diagnosis to infer what will probably happen next and how the process can be changed by various available interventions.

Physicians learn to do this by experience, so that as they take a history and examine a patient, it "dawns" on them what may be going on, what may happen next, and what they should do. In essence, their diagnosis is a title or label for what they are imagining in terms of current processes and future events.

The process is uncertain. Philosophically, we can only show that other diagnoses or hypotheses are improbable and that the patient's findings are probably explained by only one known diagnosis. However, there may be some other processes not yet discovered by basic medical research, with which the patient's findings are also compatible. Therefore, the outcomes of actions based on a presumed diagnosis have to be monitored and the diagnosis and decision revised, if necessary. The process is often cyclical, so that the physician is supplementing the patient's own reparative and homeostatic feedback processes.

The diagnostician has to be alert to new concerns, symptoms, and other findings and must be able to interpret them to arrive at new diagnoses and decisions. Surgeons may have to do this as they are operating on a patient; what may appear to be a simple, routine procedure may produce surprises and require a quick, innovative, and skilled response. Diagnosis is thus bound up with clinical management. Physicians depend on such rapid intuitive processes to get through their day with the speed and efficiency required of them.

In some cases a doctor will listen to the patient, conduct an examination, and decide what to do (e.g., giving a pain-relieving drug, pressing on a bleeding wound, or sending the patient quickly to the hospital) without consciously thinking of a diagnosis. It is only on reflection that he or she will offer an explanation and describe what was imagined subconsciously at the time the decision was made. This is often described as "empirical" medicine.

3. What approach to diagnosis does this book describe?

In addition to our private inner thoughts and diagnoses, we have to use transparent thought processes to explain to others what we are doing. This is how we explain to patients what we think is wrong and what should be done. It is also central to teamwork involving members of other disciplines who have to help to provide the medical care arising from the various diagnoses that apply to a patient. It is also essential when handing over care to other teams, which is an increasingly prominent feature of modern medicine.

So, however mysteriously the mind works, the decisions, diagnoses, and evidence must also be communicated very clearly to doctors, nurses, and others in the team, the patients, and their supporters. The diagnosis may also have to be coded for clinical audit, activity analysis, and payment. The evidence and reasoning must be communicated in order that others can understand and, if necessary, continue the thought processes. This is the public, explicit form of diagnosis and decision making, in contrast to the private, rapid, intuitive process that often leads to diagnoses and decisions in the first place.

The explicit diagnostic thought process can also be used to arrive at the diagnosis in the first place. This has to be done very often by those with little experience but not infrequently by those with wide experience when they inevitably meet new situations. This book describes how this is done.

4. Is there is a simple concept on which transparent diagnosis is based?

Yes—it based on the idea of small, predictive combinations of information. If a group of patients with a combination of features turns out to have some diagnosis with a known frequency, then if more features are added, the frequency of the outcome in the new combination will increase, decrease, or remain the same. However, the original frequency will represent the average of the new frequencies in the groups formed by subdividing the original group. Thus, a small combination of features that predicts an outcome with a very high frequency can be very useful.

This book outlines findings that form useful combinations for diagnosis and thus predict the outcome of treatment. It does not specify the detailed, logical structure of the combinations. Before this can be done, it would be necessary to conduct systematic studies during day-to-day care at the same time as data are collected for analysis.

Thus, all of the *total evidence* of positive and negative findings is taken into account, but *central evidence* is identified within it, which is used to summarize the total evidence.[1] If different combinations of central evidence point to different diagnoses, then these may be simultaneous or differential diagnoses.

5. What are "leads," and how are they used?

A *lead* is a finding associated with a limited number of conditions and that is thus easier to investigate. The titles of the pages of this book represent such leads. An unusual or disturbing symptom or physical sign may well be a good lead. In the same way, extreme results of measurement are often good leads.

If the reader discovers a good lead when taking the history or examining the patient, then in turning to the appropriate page, he or she will be able to scan down the page to see if the patient has other features that form a combination that point to one of the diagnoses.

If the patient's findings are compatible with a number of different predictive combinations, then these will represent the differential diagnoses (provided that they are also capable of causing the presenting complaint). The approach of assembling a combination of findings by selecting items of information that occur commonly in one cause, but rarely in others rarely, is the probabilistic version of logic by elimination.[1,2,3] Leads have also been referred to as "pivots."[4]

6. At what point in a medical career is this book useful?

This book, along with its approach, can be used throughout a medical career. It can be used by students beginning their medical studies, to learn the principles of interpreting clinical information. It can be referred to at any time during clinical clerkships, internship, or residency, when assessing patients or when tackling diagnostic exercises on paper.

This handbook is also designed to help physicians deal with problems clearly by using a logical and flexible approach when they are on strange territory. More importantly, it helps students and doctors to defend

1. Llewelyn DEH (1975). A concept of diagnosis: a relationship between logic and limits of probability. *Clin Sci Mol Med* **49**;7.

2. Llewelyn DEH (1979). Mathematical analysis of the diagnostic relevance of clinical findings. *Clin Sci* **57**(5);477–479.

3. Llewelyn DEH (1981). Applying the principle of logical elimination to probabilistic diagnosis. *Med Informatics* **6**(1);25.

4. Eddy DM, Clanton CH (1982). The art of diagnosis: solving the clinicopathological conference. *Engl J Med* **306**;1263–1268.

their diagnoses and decisions, and if necessary, to help them to explain their reasoning to patients, nurses, and other doctors verbally or in evidence-based past medical histories.

A traditional past medical history that summarizes diagnostic evidence for others would be very helpful when handing over a patient's care to another team, especially when transferring a patient between specialties with mutually unfamiliar conventions of diagnostic evidence. Such an approach would also reduce unnecessary duplication and wasting of resources, and might be used on computer systems for health care.

7. In what situations can this book be used?

The book can be used in a number of situations. It can be read after taking a history, examining a patient, and arriving at diagnoses and a management plan. The latter will include a positive finding summary or problem list, proposed investigations, and initial treatments. The positive findings can then be looked up in this book, beginning with those most striking or severe, to see if you have considered important causes and ways of confirming them.

This book can be used for problem-based learning. Thus, after trying to solve a problem without the aid of this book, use it for a second attempt. Make your own notes on the blank pages if you find that a cause or important finding has not been mentioned. As with other Oxford Handbooks, we would welcome suggestions. Some diseases are only common in examinations (partly because they provide physical signs that are reliably stable over many years). They are often rare in clinical practice except in specialized departments.

8. How does the structure of the book work?

The main part of the book describes the findings that can emerge at each step of the history and examination and as a result of doing the preliminary tests. Each page will describe the list of the main differential diagnoses to be considered for a lead that is starting point for the diagnostic reasoning process. Alongside each diagnosis there is an outline of the typical evidence that suggests the diagnosis with sufficient probability to justify doing confirmatory tests. It may then outline the typical results of doing these tests to provide reasonable evidence to confirm the diagnosis. There will be some duplication in that these details will be repeated for the reader's convenience each time the diagnosis is listed as a cause of a symptom or sign.

9. How can the book be used as a learning tool?

When you read the book, imagine that you have come across a patient with the finding(s) forming the title for that page. Cover the differential diagnoses on the left-hand side of the page with your hand or a book-mark to see if you can predict the diagnosis from reading the findings on the right-hand side of the page. This is the direction in which your mind should be working when trying to think about diagnosis and solve diagnostic dilemmas. You can then read the whole page for an overview. You should always try to recall what you know already about something before reading about it, in order to learn in an integrated way.

10. Can a transparent diagnostic approach improve the diagnostic accuracy of an experienced physician?

It is a common experience that if we try to give a carefully reasoned justification for an intuitive opinion, especially by writing it down, we may find that we cannot justify it easily and will reconsider our opinion. Conversely, if our explicitly reasoned justification confirms our intuitive opinion, then we will feel more confident in its success.

This is illustrated by what happened when data assembled by the late Professor Tim de Dombal were analyzed. The surgeon was correct in his intuitive diagnosis 235/300 = 78.3% of the time, and a transparent, logical approach using small combinations of findings was correct 230/300 = 76.6% of the time. However, the surgeon and transparent, logical approach agreed about the diagnosis in 221/300 of cases. When there was agreement in these 221 instances, the diagnosis was correct in 200/221 = 90.5% of cases.[1]

11. How does this approach relate to diagnostic algorithms?

The suggestive and confirmatory evidence under each diagnosis represents the findings that would have been chosen by following the path down a diagnostic algorithm in order to arrive at the diagnosis. However, instead of locking the reader into a fixed sequence, this book allows the reader to scan the different diagnoses and recognize which findings on the page best fit those of the patient.

In a sense, each page provides a form of pattern-recognition table. The confirmatory evidence should be compatible with only one diagnosis.

1. Llewelyn, DEH, (1988). Assessing the validity of diagnostic tests and clinical decisions. MD thesis. University of London.

12. How comprehensive is the information about each diagnosis?

There is not enough space in a handbook of this kind to describe all the combinations of evidence that might point to a diagnosis. Therefore, each page describes some of the differential diagnoses and, for each of these, an outline of typical findings that are suggestive and confirmatory. This provides a start to which further information can be added by the reader in the Oxford Handbook spirit.

The diagnostic causes of a lead are usually listed in the order of their frequency in those patients with the lead. (Sometimes they are grouped together because of causal similarity, e.g., into cardiac causes and not in an order of frequency.) A major factor in determining this order is the prevalence of those with the diagnosis in the overall study population. Therefore, the order of the diagnoses on the page may vary between clinical settings. Readers should try to insert the order number of the diagnostic causes in terms of probability in their own clinical settings.

13. What is meant by *facts*, *opinions*, and *evidence* in the book?

Evidence is an account of real events that supports what we believe. It is made up of *facts*. Thus, facts are also accounts of real events. Real events are transient and immediately become memories that are easily forgotten or distorted. Evidence is usually shared with others, thus it must be recorded carefully using conventions that other people will accept. One of these conventions is that the record of a fact must bear a time and date so it can be corroborated (e.g., by questioning other witnesses). If such details are omitted, this may arouse suspicion, even if there is no need to seek corroboration. In many cases a listener would judge the probability of corroboration or of replicating the finding to be high.

Most evidence takes the form of contemporaneous notes or printed numerical values from a measuring device. In other cases, a finding is preserved, e.g., an X-ray, a photograph, or a video recording with sound. However, all these methods are subject to error or some other distortion, and the method of detection and recording has to follow appropriate conventions if they are to be accepted by others.

In this book, *evidence* is described as being "suggestive" or "confirmatory" of a diagnosis and when it is applied to a real patient, will have to bear a date or time. Evidence about a single patient may be termed "particular evidence," whereas evidence about a group of patients may be termed "general evidence."

The principle of replication also applies to general evidence. For example, 1/77 (1.3%) of normotensive diabetic patients taking placebo with an albumin excretion rate (AER) starting between 20 and 40 μg/minute had nephropathy within 2 years.[1] This would be general scientific evidence.

If we took the pile of 77 records from the study, we could simulate repeat studies by selecting a set of notes at random from the pile, examining it, returning it, and doing this 77 times. If a large number of such simulated studies were done, then from the binomial distribution there would be a 99.7% chance of finding nephropathy in 0/77 or 1/77 or 2/77 or 3/77 or 4/77 of patients with a controlled BP in different simulated studies (i.e., from 0% [0/77] to 5.2% [4/77]). There is thus a 99.7% chance of replicating the finding of 1/77 by a repeat result being between 0/77 and 4/77 inclusive.

By comparison, the standard 95% confidence interval for 1/77 is 0.03% to 7.02% and the 99% confidence interval for 1/77 is 0.01% to 9.37%. However, the probability of replication between two limits is more similar to the percentage confidence interval if the numbers in the study are high and the observed result is near to 50%.

A *fact* is an account of an observation, but an *opinion* is a prediction about something that has not yet (or even cannot) be seen. If an opinion can be checked by observation, it can be founded on evidence (it is substantiable). If it can never be observed, it cannot be founded on evidence (it is unsubstantiable). An opinion can thus be substantiated if it can be based on past evidence.

For example, if an individual patient's AER is between 20 and 40 μg/minute, then an opinion that such a diabetic patient with a controlled BP is unlikely to develop nephropathy would be well founded or substantiated by the fact that of 77 such past patients, only 1 went on to get nephropathy in a particular study.

14. How do these ideas relate to statistical and other models of diagnosis?

Statistical and other mathematical methods (many based on Bayes theorem) generate a value much like a diagnostic test. These may be calculated estimates of some biological value, e.g., a calculated glomerular filtration rate, a diagnostic score, or an estimated probability. All these numerical outputs of a calculation can be treated in the same way as direct measurements by calibrating them against the frequency of some outcome (e.g., the proportion who progress to requiring dialysis within 2 years—see Fig. 2.3). The numerical outputs could then be incorporated into the suggestive or confirmatory evidence for the diagnosis.

1. Llewelyn DEH, Garcia-Puig J (2004). How different urinary albumin excretion rates can predict progression to nephropathy and the effect of treatment in hypertensive diabetics. *J Renin Angiotensin Aldosterone Syst* 5;141–145.

Decision analysis[1,2] is essentially a process that estimates the result of a detailed therapeutic clinical trial on a hypothetical group of patients in a transparent way when a real detailed trial is not available or impracticable. The analysis is usually applied to an individual patient who thus is identical to all those in the hypothetical group. The approach uses available estimates of outcome frequencies in the medical literature from related studies and also estimates from the patient of the range of personal well-being that should be gained from each outcome.

The analysis involves calculating the average degree of well-being for each treatment outcome in a transparent way. Doctors may do this for an individual patient by estimating the outcome of such a hypothetical trial without making calculations. This approach is not covered in this book.

1. Dowie J, Elstein A (1988). *Professional judgement. A reader in clinical decision making.* Cambridge, UK: Cambridge University Press.

2. Llewelyn H, Hopkins A (1993). *Analysing how we reach clinical decisions.* London: Royal College of Physicians of London.

Symbols and abbreviations

±	with/without
→	imply
↑	increased
↓	decreased
°	degrees
>	greater than
<	less than
5-HIAA	5-hydroxyindole acetic acid
Ab	antibody
ABG(s)	arterial blood gas(es)
ACE	angiotensin-converting enzyme
ACTH	adrenocorticotrophic hormone
ADH	antidiuretic hormone
AER	albumin excretion rate
AFB	acid-fast bacillus
ALS	amyotrophic lateral sclerosis
ALT	alanine transaminase
AML	acute myeloid leukemia
ANA	anti-nuclear antibody
ANCA	anti-neutrophil cytoplasmic antibody
A-P	anterior to posterior
ARDS	acute respiratory distress syndrome
AS	aortic stenosis
ASOT	anti-streptolysin O titer
AST	asparate transaminase
AV	atrioventricular
AXR	abdominal X-ray
β-hCG	β-human chorionic gonadotrophin
BM	bone marrow
BMI	body mass index
BP	blood pressure
bpm	beats per minute
BUN	blood urea nitrogen
cANCA	cytoplasmic anti-neutrophil cytoplasmic antibody
CAPD	continuous ambulatory peritoneal dialysis
CBC	complete blood count
CC	chief complaint
CFS	chronic fatigue syndrome
CHF	congestive heart failure

CIN	cervical intraepithelial neoplasia
CK-MB	creatine kinase MB isoenzyme
CLL	chronic lymphocytic leukemia
CML	chronic myeloid leukemia
CNS	central nervous system
COPD	chronic obstructive pulmonary disease
CPK	creatine phosphokinase
CRF	chronic renal failure
CRP	C-reactive protein
CSF	cerebrospinal fluid
CT	computerized tomography
CTPA	computerized tomographic pulmonary angiogram
CV	cardiovascular
CVA	cerebrovascular accident; costovertebral angle
CVP	central venous pressure
CVS	cardiovascular system
CXR	chest X-ray
DC	direct current
D-dimer	dextrorotatory dimer
DH	drug history
DIC	disseminated intravascular coagulation
DIP	distal interphalangeal (joint)
dL	deciliter
DL_{CO}	carbon monoxide diffusing capacity
DM	diabetes mellitus
DOB	date of birth
DVT	deep vein thrombosis
ECG (EKG)	electrocardiogram
ECT	electroconvulsive therapy
EEG	electroencephalogram
EF	ejection fraction
EGD	esophagogastroduodenoscopy
ELISA	enzyme-linked immunosorbent assay
EMG	electromyography
ENT	ear, nose, throat
ERCP	endoscopic retrograde cholangiopancreatography
ESR	erythrocyte sedimentation rate
FDP(s)	fibrogen degredation product/s
FEV_1	forced expiratory volume (1 second)
FH	family history
FiO_2	fraction of inspiried oxygen
Fl	fluorescein
FSH	follicular stimulating hormone
FT3	free T3
FT4	free T4

FUO	fever of unknown origin
FVC	forced vital capacity
G6PD	glucose-6-phosphate dehydrogenase
GALS	gait, arms, legs, spine
γGTP	γ glutamyl transpeptidase
GBM	glomerular basement membrane
GCS	Glasgow Coma Scale
GH	growth hormone
GI	gastrointestinal
GP	general practitioner
G/g	gram
G/dL	grams/deciliter
GTT	glucose tolerance test
GU	genitourinary
Hb	hemoglobin
HBsAG	hepatitis B surface antigen
hCG	human chorionic gonadotrophin
HCV	hepatitis C virus
Hg	mercury
HIV	human immunodeficiency virus
HLA-B27	human lymphocyte antigen B27
HPI	history of present(ing) illness
HR	heart rate
HR-CT	high resolution computerized tomography
HSV	herpes simplex virus
HUS	hemolytic uremic syndrome
IGF	insulin-like growth factor
IgM	immunoglobin M
IHD	ischemic heart disease
IM	intramuscular
IP	interphalangeal (joint)
IUD	intrauterine contraceptive device
IV	intravenous
IVC	inferior vena cava
JVP	jugular venous pressure
K	potassium
L	liter
LDH	lactate dehydrogenase
LFT	liver function test
LH	luteinizing hormone
LIF	left iliac fossa
LMN	lower motor neuron
LN	lymph node
LP	lumbar puncture
LV	left ventricle (or ventricular)
LVF	left ventricular failure
LVH	left ventricular hypertrophy

MCHC	mean corpuscular hemoglobin concentration
MCHC	mean corpuscular hemoglobin concentration
MCP	metacarpophalangeal (joint)
MCV	mean corpuscular volume
MI	myocardial infarction
mmHg	millimeters of mercury
mmol	millimoles
MP	metatarsophalngeal (joint)
MRA	magnetic resonance angiogram
MRCP	magnetic resonance cholangiopancreatography
MRI	magnetic resonance imaging
MS	multiple sclerosis
MSU	mid-stream urine
Na	sodium
NSAIDs	nonsteroidal anti-inflammatory drugs
NSAP	nonspecific abdominal pain
OAHCD	*Oxford American Handbook of Clinical Diagnosis*
P2	pulmonary component of second heart sound
P-A	posterior to anterior
PA	pernicious anemia
PaO$_2$	arterial oxygen tension
PAS	periodic acid Schiff
PCO$_2$	carbon dioxide tension
PCP	*Pneumocystis* pneumonia
PCR	polymerase chain reaction
PCWP	pulmonary capillary wedge pressure
PE	pulmonary embolism
PEFR	peak expiratory flow rate
PFK	phosphofructokinase
PFT	pulmonary function test
PIP	proximal interphalangeal (joint)
PMH	past medical history
PND	paroxysmal nocturnal dyspnea
po	*per os* (by mouth)
PR	*per rectum* (by the rectum)
PSA	prostate-specific antigen
PT	prothrombin time
PTT	partial thromboplastin time
PUO	pyrexia of unknown origin
qd	*quaque die* (once daily)
qid	*quater in die* (four times daily)
RA	right atrium (or atrial)
RBB	right bundle branch
RHF	right-sided heart failure
RIF	right iliac fossa
RLQ	right lower quadrant
RS	respiratory system

RUQ	right upper quadrant
RV	right ventricle (or ventricular)
SBE	subacute bacterial endocarditis
SH	social history
SHBG	sex hormone-binding globulin
SLE	systemic lupus erythematosus
STEMI	ST-elevation myocardial infarction
SVC	superior vena cava
SVT	supraventricular tachycardia
TB	tuberculosis
TFT	thyroid function test
tid	three times a day
TSH	thyroid-stimulating hormone
TURP	transurethral resection of the prostate
UMN	upper motor neuron
URI	upper respiratory infection
URTI	upper respiratory tract infection
UTI	urinary tract infection
VGCC	voltage-gated calcium channel
VSD	ventricular septal defect
WBC	white blood cell (count)
WHO	World Health Organization

The diagnostic process

Introduction

On the eve of clinical clerkships, at the end of basic science training, the medical student has mastered more information than he or she will ever again know in a lifetime. Yet it is precisely at this time that developing the clinical scenario is most awkward. Simply put, the problem is one of incompatibility of two sets of knowledge.

Medical knowledge comprises millions of facts. It must be organized by disease state and by pathophysiology. Information is easily retrieved, once mastered, if organized by disease state or pathogenesis. Clinical information, obtained from a single patient during the interview and exam, similarly comprises hundreds, if not thousands, of facts.

The patient, however, rarely presents as a disease. More commonly, the patient presents as a loosely constructed chain of complaints, each further from the chief complaint, and each of uncertain relation to the other. A patient may present with a chief complaint, accompanied by an elaborate psychological construct to prevent disclosure of painful events. Occasionally the patient presents with a chief complaint accompanied by a distressingly detailed essay on bodily functions and their manifestations in each of the special senses.

It is the clinician's job to manage the information obtained during the interview in such a way that the patient's problem is accurately assessed. The difficulty lies in the fact that the vast medical information the student commands is not in an accessible format during the clinical situation.

To a certain extent, medical information must be relearned in a clinical format, such as clinical presentations. In other words, the polymerization of deoxyhemoglobin into a gelatinous network that contorts the otherwise supple red cell into an unyielding and obstructive mass can present as fever and shortness of breath in an African-American man (sickle chest syndrome). Relearning the body of information mastered in medical school as presentations is neither efficient nor, in most cases, necessary.

Fortunately, there are techniques that enable the budding clinician to make the two bodies of knowledge—the medical information and the patient data—compatible. These techniques are simply thought processes. They aren't unique to medicine, but they comprise much of the fabric of clinical experience. Paradoxically, many seasoned clinicians cannot explain such thought processes well. They are "second nature," like riding a bike or driving a car, only the skills involved pertain to cognition, rather than movement. Students generally learn them by trial and error, by emulation of their instructors, and simply as a product of experience.

Developing a differential diagnosis

There are two different thought processes involved in the diagnostic and clinical decision-making process. The first is the process of arriving at the diagnosis and the second is explaining and checking the diagnosis. It is very important to recognize this difference. The process of discovering the diagnosis is performed in a systematic way, but the urgency of the situation or disruptive events may frequently result in the planned sequence being abandoned.

Diagnoses are arrived at in the form of imagined processes with different degrees of certainty. These diagnoses, some tentative, others more certain, will suggest relevant tests to clarify the situation and treatments to try and reverse or divert the course of the diagnoses. This first thought process depends on the individual diagnostician's imagination combined with different types of thought processes ranging from rapid pattern recognition for familiar issues to a more tentative approach when in unfamiliar territory.

Students will almost always be in unfamiliar territory at first, and no doctor can become familiar with every situation. Doctors who see many patients will come across unfamiliar problems more often, making medical practice a constant challenge and highlighting the need for a more methodical checking process.

Problem-solving skills

Information processing is a primary goal of the physician–patient interaction. It proceeds in three phases: data processing, hypothesis generation, and creation of a differential diagnosis. The division between these phases is somewhat artificial, but it is practical.

Data processing

Immediately after the patient encounter, and possibly after reviewing some basic labs and radiographic studies, an accounting of all positive and negative findings takes place. During this phase, the clinician undertakes the process of collecting and examining all the "findings," or data, and analyzing them to look for a common relationship between them. By trying to fit these findings together to make a more accurate hypothesis, the top (or most likely) diagnoses will emerge from this process. Toward that end, a positive finding is an abnormal finding in the patient; a negative finding is either a normal finding that was expected to be abnormal, or the absence of a positive finding that was expected to be present.

During early attempts at this type of data analysis, we suggest that you create a table to help you master this process. First, make a list of all positive and negative findings. This step involves the following:

- Listing all positive and negative symptoms
- Listing all positive and negative physical findings
- Listing all positive and negative laboratory findings

For example, a positive finding in a patient with chest pain is that the pain is closely associated with exertion and relieved with rest. A negative finding in such a patient would be the absence of relief of the pain with nitroglycerin (because one would expect such a response with chest pain from coronary artery disease). Data processing is also the first step in generation of a problem list.

Also, consider each of the following attributes of findings:

- Assessment of relevance to the chief complaint. Each finding is examined for its relevance by classifying it as definitely relevant, possibly relevant, or irrelevant (separate problem).
- Assessment of reliability (certainty) of each finding. It is normal for findings to be equivocal. Inexperienced clinicians will have many more equivocal findings than will seasoned clinicians, simply because of their lack of experience. However, not all equivocal findings pertain to experience of the clinician. For example, a heart murmur may be equivocal to the most talented cardiologist, simply because that is the nature of the human body. The important thing is to acknowledge equivocal findings when they occur.
- Hypothesis generation. This process begins during the patient encounter, often within the first few minutes after the interaction has started. While the clinician is still recording factual information (either in written notes or in memory), various pieces of information rise to the surface.

The skills used here are unique in that they are performed while the patient and clinician are speaking or while the clinician is examining the patient. Such skills allow the clinician to process and refine the data as they are obtained. Seasoned clinicians can perform most of their problem-solving skills during this phase, and the student will be increasingly able to do so with experience and practice.

The goal of this phase is to develop a hypothesis or working diagnosis (3–4 diagnoses) that might explain the patient's presentation. This working diagnosis will generate a set of questions that the clinician needs to ask. These questions will depend on the manifestations that the disease is expected to produce in a patient.

Note that hypothesis generation is not answer generation. The process simply allows the clinician to prioritize possibilities. Clinical decision-making is derived from medical knowledge, personal theories, assumptions, experience, traditions, and lore, and this mental strategy is sometimes called medical heuristics, such as "gestalt" and "string along."

Skills used during hypothesis generation include consideration of demographics and chief complaint, the limited survey, and pattern recognition. We will explore the use of each of these tools briefly.

Demographics and the chief complaint

Taking into account what is epidemiologically most likely in a given population, a small amount of information can yield surprisingly accurate hypotheses.

For example:
- 32-year-old woman with polyarthritis → rheumatoid arthritis
- 28-year-old man with thrush → acquired immune deficiency syndrome (AIDS)

Although gender, ethnic, and racial differences are generally de-emphasized to prevent discrimination, in some cases, they are a valid or even necessary consideration:
- 28-year-old African-American woman with hilar adenopathy → sarcoidosis. (In the United States, sarcoidosis affects blacks 10–20 times more commonly than it does whites. In Europe, the disease more commonly affects whites.)
- 22-year-old woman of Mediterranean descent with hemolytic anemia → glucose-6-phosphate dehydrogenase deficiency

It is important to consider, however, that the reason for the racial or gender differences may have been biased in the original observations, as is the case for coronary artery disease in women.

Survey of the possible causes

This is based on only the initial presentation and accompanying symptoms. It can be taken using one of the formats outlined below. All formats should be used when doing a survey because a single format does not cover everything.

Organ system

Though these are somewhat artificially divided, they are easily recalled and understood, allowing access to a comprehensive database.

Anatomy

An anatomy survey is similar to one of an organ system, but concerns the "finer points" of anatomy. An anatomy survey lends itself well to the surgical specialties. For example, when considering the differential diagnosis of nausea and vomiting, consider lesions in the external auditory canal, as the general somatic afferent fibers from this area are carried by the vagus nerve, which also carries parasympathetic fibers to the upper gastrointestinal (GI) tract.

Pathogenesis

The pathological processes that cause disease can be classified, and consideration of this classification is helpful in generating hypotheses and differential diagnoses. "VITAMIN C" is one useful mnemonic for recalling these mechanisms of disease:

V = vascular
I = infectious
T = toxic or traumatic
A = autoimmune
M = metabolic
I = idiopathic (some call it inflammatory)
N = neoplastic or nutritional
C = congenital or genetic

Pattern recognition

The expression "when you hear hoof beats don't think zebras" is a reminder that common diagnoses are common and should be considered first. As clinical skills improve, however, students become able to consider uncommon illnesses and atypical presentations. It may help to think about each diagnosis you consider in the context of whether it is a common or uncommon illness and whether it is a typical or atypical presentation. An example of this process in relation to chest pain and shortness of breath is presented in Table 1.1.

Table 1.1 Pattern recognition in diagnosing chest pain and shortness of breath

Illness or presentation	Typical	Atypical
Common	Pneumonia	Bleeding ulcer
Uncommon	Vasculitis	Metastatic cancer

- Common presentation of common illness—pneumonia
- Uncommon presentation of common illness—bleeding ulcer (with severe anemia)
- Common presentation of uncommon illness—granulomatous ANCA-positive vasculitis (Wegener's)
- Uncommon presentation of uncommon illness—metastatic ovarian cancer

When generating a hypothesis, group the findings together to create patterns. Establish the relationship between findings, which may be inter-dependent or mutually exclusive.

Findings may also be "lumped" instead of "split." Lumping is the most efficient way to begin the problem-solving process and consists of com-bining as many findings as possible into a single category. Splitting the findings into the most appropriate category is a process that "keeps the clinician honest." Specifically, the findings should be attributed to the correct cause. An important rule is that a younger patient will tend to have only one problem explaining all manifestations, whereas an older patient may have multiple problems, each contributing to the presentation.

For example, consider the syndrome of dyspnea, pleuritic chest pain, fever, and leg pain. When initially considering this group of symptoms, many clinicians would propose a pulmonary embolism (PE) as the etiology: dyspnea, pleuritic chest pain, and fever are related to the PE, and the leg pain is from the deep vein thrombosis that caused the PE. However, dyspnea, pleuritic chest pain, fever, and leg pain could also represent pneumococcal pneumonia in a patient, who has leg pain attributed to a basketball injury the day prior to presentation. The choice between these (and other) scenarios might rest on the patient's age or past medical his-tory, or on other features of the history or physical.

Some forms of pattern recognition are described next.

Clusters
This is a group of findings that, when found together, have a relatively high positive predictive value (i.e., they are specific) for a given finding. For example:
- Tremors + tachycardia + weight loss = hyperthyroidism
- Polyuria + polydipsia + polyphagia = hyperglycemia
- Polyuria + constipation + lethargy = hypercalcemia

Syndrome recognition

Syndromes are more specific than clusters—i.e., they are more likely to have only one cause. Often, they are given names or eponyms, For example:

- *Horner's syndrome:* ptosis, miosis, enophthalmos, anhidrosis ipsilaterally
- *Superior vena cava syndrome:* elevated jugular venous pressure, visible anastamotic veins, and reversal of flow of the supraumbilical veins

Gestalt

While this is a form of cluster, the emphasis is on the relative ease of recognition of the whole picture, rather than a more laborious construction of its parts. The suffix "-oid" allows the term to be used with sufficient (lack of) precision. The actual diagnosis of a syndrome or disease depends on the component parts and is associated with greater specificity. For example:

- *Cushingoid habitus* = centripetal obesity
- *Cushing's syndrome* consists of truncal obesity, hypertension, fatigability, amenorrhea, hirsutism, purple abdominal striae, edema, glucosuria, and osteoporosis.
- *Cushing's disease* (as described by Cushing accompanying a basophilic pituitary tumor) refers to this syndrome when the cause is specifically a pituitary tumor. Note the increasing specificity from "Cushingoid" to "Cushing's syndrome" to "Cushing's disease."

Finding a "key clue"

This will be a "maximally" specific clue, almost pathognomonic for a diagnosis in question—for example, the presence of splinter hemorrhages in the proximal nail beds in bacterial endocarditis. If the other findings fit, then you probably have the diagnosis. If they don't, then look further. (Such specific clues are not that common.)

Template matching

In this technique, the clinician knows intimately all of the manifestations of a particular disease. She or he will then try to fit the findings of the patient into the possible presentations of that disease. Think of the disease in question as a blueprint, and the findings are added into the blueprint in such a way that they ultimately fit the template. This technique is the one most used by subspecialists, who perform consults to determine whether a patient has a particular disease or not. It is based on the fact that diseases present in multitudes of ways, for reasons that are not always apparent.

Weight of evidence

When all the findings do not neatly support a diagnosis, one assesses where the "weight of the evidence" lies. In other words, if most of the findings support endocarditis, but the blood cultures are negative, the patient is still considered to have endocarditis. However, diagnostic errors can be made when using this technique. See discussion in Dynamic Diagnoses and the Possibility of Cognitive Error, p. 12.

Timing of findings in relation to each other
The closer in time two findings develop, the more likely it is they are related. Consider, however, that the two clues may be unrelated.

Use of algorithms
Algorithms are specific for the symptom being addressed. Experienced clinicians use these all the time but keep them recorded only in their minds. Such algorithms that are in frequent use are generally too complex to be printed easily (because the branch points are highly detailed). However, simplified versions are very amenable to students' use, and can be sought on a case-by-case basis through each subspecialty.

"String-together technique"
This technique involves linkage of one finding to another, e.g. dyspnea and chest pain in a blind, 56-year-old man who was completely healthy until he developed severe back pain from a ruptured disc. Heavy ibuprofen use for the pain led to gastric ulceration with subsequent blood loss. The blood loss manifested as melena (black stools), but was unapparent to the patient because of his sight impairment. The anemia became so profound (hemoglobin of 4) that he developed dyspnea and chest pain without having a significant degree of coronary atherosclerosis.

Generation of a differential diagnosis

The top diagnoses are prioritized in two ways: the most likely diagnoses and the most important ones (i.e., urgent or life threatening). The primary diagnosis (the one suspected most) is usually presented first, with supporting evidence.

However, occasionally, there is a diagnosis that is urgent and this should be presented first, even though it is less likely than the primary diagnosis. For example, consider a *40-year-old female with abdominal cramping and uterine bleeding*. If the history and exam suggest the possibility of an ectopic pregnancy, this diagnosis should be listed first, even though the more likely diagnosis is uterine fibroadenomas.

Frequently, there are still some discrepant details in the primary diagnosis. Early in the evaluation of a patient, there may be missing data, and the case cannot be made convincingly for the primary diagnosis. Then, other diagnoses should be discussed systematically, as alternative diagnoses.

A seasoned clinician will be able to generate a primary diagnosis quickly, but, as discussed below, cognitive bias may adversely impact the consideration of other diagnoses. It is usually best to consider at least three diagnoses. A good habit is to consider diagnoses broadly enough to include at least three organs or categories of disease.

Consider the patient described in Box 1.1.

Finally, in the generation of a differential diagnosis, occasionally findings "don't fit." Such findings can be explained in four ways:

- The diagnosis being considered is wrong.
- The finding was obtained in error and needs to be confirmed by re-interview or re-examination.
- The finding represents a separate problem.
- It's just "one of those things" that happens often in medicine, and is explained by the saying "the patients don't read the books."

The generation of the differential diagnosis guides management. Your diagnostic plan will be directed by obtaining any missing data necessary to confirm the primary diagnosis (retrieving old records, observation of the patient over time, laboratory results, or imaging studies). Your therapeutic plan will be guided by the most urgent and then the most likely diagnoses.

Box 1.1 Case study

A 49-year-old man, emigrated from India 20 years ago, presents with fever, chronic productive cough, and weight loss. Physical exam is significant for a temperature of 99.0°F, otherwise unremarkable vital signs, and rales in the upper left posterior lung field. He has a left upper lobe infiltrate on chest X-ray.

Differential diagnosis

Infection

This is most consistent with pulmonary tuberculosis. In support of this diagnosis (a) the patient has an uncle who had tuberculosis, and (b) the timing of exposure is most consistent with the diagnosis of tuberculosis. However, problems with this diagnosis include the following: until 3 months ago, he was healthy without known immunocompromise, and tuberculosis is unusual without an underlying debilitated state.

Alternatively, the presentation could be explained by fungal pneumonia, for example, with histoplasmosis, blastomycosis, or coccidioidomycosis. However, he has not been in areas endemic for these organisms and, again, he is not known to be immunocompromised.

Malignancy

Primary pulmonary malignancy is another possibility. In support of this diagnosis, the patient has constitutional symptoms, including weight loss. However, problems with this diagnosis are that he has been a nonsmoker all his life and has no other known risk factors for primary lung carcinoma. The isolated left upper lobe infiltrate is less likely to be metastatic malignancy, although an obstructive endobronchial lesion with pneumonia as a consequence is still a possibility.

Vasculitis

Other less common possibilities include granulomatous anti-neutrophil cytoplasmic antibody (ANCA)-positive vasculitis (Wegener's). In support of this diagnosis, the patient has constitutional symptoms and a history of recurrent sinus infections. However, problems with this diagnosis include the fact that his sinus symptoms seem fairly minimal currently, and there is no evidence of renal disease by exam.

Dynamic diagnoses and the possibility of cognitive error

Clinical diagnosis is not a static classification system based on diagnostic criteria or their probable presence. It is a dynamic process. It is important to realize that the techniques described above, including pattern recognition, "gestalt," and template matching, are critical to the efficient function of busy clinicians and are developed over time. These methods can be regarded as a diagnostic snapshot of what is happening at a particular point in time. However, the patient's illness is a dynamic process that changes with time. Changes in the patient's status and new laboratory and imaging data provide more information that needs to be accounted for in the evolving diagnosis and care process.

Diagnosis reflects the clinician's knowledge, clinical acumen, and problem-solving skills. In everyday practice, clinicians use expert skills to arrive at a diagnosis, often taking advantage of various mental shortcuts known as heuristics. Although the final "working diagnosis" (usually the primary diagnosis) expedites the management plan, it is a temporary diagnosis with much missing data.

The heuristics described above, such as the "string-along" method and "gestalt," also lend themselves to cognitive errors, i.e., failures of perception and cognitive bias. Interestingly, cognitive errors are only rarely due to lack of medical knowledge.

Graber et al. studied 100 cases of diagnostic error identified through autopsy discrepancies, quality assurance activities, and voluntary reports.[1] They found that the underlying contributions to error fell into three natural categories: "no fault" (no identified process), system related (related to health system–based processes), and cognitive. In their study, the most common cognitive errors involved defective synthesis. Premature closure, i.e., the failure to continue considering reasonable alternatives after a primary diagnosis is reached, was the single most common cause.

This highlights the importance of recognizing that diagnosis is a dynamic process. One example given in the study was a wrong diagnosis of musculoskeletal pain after a motor vehicle accident; a ruptured spleen was eventually found. Other common causes of cognitive error in Graber et al.'s study included faulty context generation, misjudging the salience of findings, faulty perception, and errors arising from the use of heuristics. Overall, inadequate knowledge was least common.

Faulty context generation, or failure to consider aspects of the patient's situation that are relevant to the diagnosis, can be devastating.

1 Graber ML, Franklin N, Gordon R (2005). Diagnostic error in internal medicine. *Arch Intern Med* **165**:1493–1499.

For example:

A 65-year-old woman with hypertension presented with chest pain and electrocardiogram (ECG) evidence of an acute coronary syndrome. She was sent home with the diagnosis of myocardial infarction. However, mild anemia was missed at initial diagnosis, and the patient died at home 2 days later from a perforated gastric ulcer.

Patient encounters with initial care providers in internal medicine, family practice, and emergency medicine have the greatest likelihood of diagnostic uncertainty and the greatest possibility of delayed or missed diagnoses. However, all specialties are vulnerable to cognitive error. This was discovered in findings from several benchmark studies of medical error.[2–4]

An important example of cognitive error is *anchoring bias*, the tendency to lock onto salient features in the patient's initial presentation too early in the diagnostic process, then failing to adjust the initial impression in light of later information. This cognitive error can be made worse by *confirmation bias*, the tendency to look for confirming evidence to support the working diagnosis rather than looking for evidence to refute it, despite the latter being more persuasive and definitive.

Another common type of cognitive bias is *gender bias*, the tendency to believe that gender is a determining factor in the probability of diagnosis or a particular disease when no such predisposition basis exists. Generally, this results in overdiagnosis in the favored gender and underdiagnosis of the neglected gender.[5]

Understanding that we are all susceptible to cognitive errors, it is important to consider and record more than one diagnosis from the very beginning of the patient encounter. We suggest an organized data processing of the accumulated information, and documentation of not only the features of the history and physical that support the primary and secondary diagnoses but also the features that refute them. It is probably wise to consider at least three diagnoses, preferably involving more than one organ system. For example, if a 37-year-old woman presents with irregular, heavy, vaginal bleeding, three organs or systems that might be considered include 1) uterine, 2) hematological (low platelets), and 3) endocrine (thyroid disease).

2 Brennan TA, Leape LL, Laird NM, et al. (1991). Incidence of adverse events and negligence in hospitalized patients: results of the Harvard Medical Practice Study 1. *N Eng J Med* **324**:370–376.
3 Wilson RM, Runciman WB, Gibberd RW, et al. (1995). The Quality in Australian Health Care Study. *Med J Australia* **163**:458–471.
4 Thomas EJ, Studdert DM, Burstin HR, et al. (2000). Incidence and types of adverse events and negligent care in Utah and Colorado. *Med Care* **38**:261–262.
5 Croskerry P (2003). The importance of cognitive errors in diagnosis and strategies to minimize them. *Acad Med* **78**:775–780.

Summary

In summary, the differential diagnosis is constructed only after all the data (history, physical, laboratory findings, and imaging) are collected and organized. Information processing is an important goal of the physician–patient interaction. It proceeds in three phases: data processing, hypothesis generation, and, finally, generation of a differential diagnosis.

Data processing is a simple process of collecting all the "findings" and then trying to fit those findings together to make a more accurate hypothesis. Data processing is not only critical to the development of a diagnosis but also helps the development of a problem list.

Hypothesis generation requires the use of multiple methods of aggregating information. These include pattern recognition techniques, such as "string-along" methods and "gestalt."

Generation of a diagnosis is a dynamic process that depends on pattern recognition and experience. The primary diagnosis (the one most suspected or most life threatening) is presented first, with supporting evidence. Other diagnoses should be routinely considered and discussed systematically as alternative diagnoses.

Clinicians use a complex method of clinical decision-making that includes medical knowledge, experience, assumptions, and traditions as hypothesis-generating shortcuts. These shortcuts allow for efficient information management in a time-limited encounter; however, they may lend themselves to diagnostic error. Diagnostic errors occur, even with experienced clinicians. Therefore, broad differentials can mitigate some of these cognitive biases that may lead to medical errors.

Transparent diagnosis

Transparent diagnosis

The introductory chapter discussed the thought processes used when arriving at a diagnosis. Many of these are subconscious and poorly understood, for example, pattern recognition.

There is also a tradition in medicine of discussing and justifying diagnoses openly. This happens during conferences on morbidity and mortality and on management, for example, the clinicopathological conferences (CPCs) at the Massachusetts General Hospital, which have been published for many years in the *New England Journal of Medicine*.

Eddy and Clanton studied the thought processes of doctors when they were analyzing symptoms, signs, and test results at these CPCs. The authors concluded that they were searching for single items or aggregates of information that were associated with as small a number of differential diagnoses as possible. Any diagnosis chosen from this list became a "hypothesis." Eddy and Clanton referred to these hypothesis-generating items as "pivots."[1] They were called "diagnostic leads" in articles describing the mathematical basis of this reasoning process,[2,3,4,5] and this is what they are called in this book, which is based on the detailed understanding described in these studies. If such a lead was only associated with one diagnosis, then it would be "pathognomonic" (i.e., a necessary condition for that diagnosis) and, thus, a part of the definition of the diagnosis.

In the absence of definitive diagnostic evidence, the pivot, or diagnostic lead, is used to suggest a differential diagnosis and to generate hypotheses. Eddy and Clanton described how experienced diagnosticians looked for further information to try to "prune" (or rule out) some of these hypothetical possibilities until only one was confirmed. If the remaining diagnosis was confirmed by the combination of pivot and pruner, then the items of information used to do this would be sufficient diagnostic criteria and thus form a part of the diagnostic definition.

Such reasoning with definitive information can be represented easily with algorithms. However, in many cases the combination would not confirm the diagnosis but only point to it with a high probability, thus suggesting it on the basis of weight of evidence.[2,3,4,5]

1 Eddy DM, Clanton CH (1982). The art of diagnosis: solving the clinicopathological conference. *N Engl J Med* **306**; 1263–1268.
2 Llewelyn DEH (1975). A concept of diagnosis: A relationship between logic and limits of probability. *Clin Sci Mol Med* **49**; 7.
3 Llewelyn DEH (1979). Mathematical analysis of the diagnostic relevance of clinical findings. *Clin Sci* **57**(5); 477–479.
4 Llewelyn DEH (1981). Applying the principle of logical elimination to probabilistic diagnosis. *Med Informatics* **6**(1); 25.
5 Llewelyn DEH (1988). Assessing the validity of diagnostic tests and clinical decisions. MD thesis. University of London.

The problem is that students and inexperienced doctors may not have the knowledge to identify diagnostic leads and to chase up a diagnostic possibility by ruling out its rivals or showing that they are improbable. These combinations are sometimes recognized without assembling them logically when they are referred to as "key clues," "clusters," or "syndromes" that are pathognomonic or have short differential diagnoses.

This handbook provides its readers with this information to allow them to recognize the best diagnostic leads and to follow them by generating diagnostic hypotheses. Each page heading represents a diagnostic lead, and the page contains its differential diagnoses. Alongside each of these diagnoses are the clinical findings that *suggest* that the diagnosis is probable, and the findings that *confirm* it by ruling out its rival diagnoses from the group of patients with that combination.

It is important to understand why the information needed to suggest or confirm diagnoses is usually small. Many templates of disease have much in common; e.g., many of the symptoms and physical signs of pneumonia, pulmonary embolus, and heart failure are the same. It is the *differences* that allow the diagnostician to differentiate between them. These differences are described in the pages of this book as findings that suggest or confirm diagnoses. Negative findings are also important in this role of suggesting or confirming diagnoses (but negative findings are not helpful as diagnostic leads, because people with most other diseases and those who are healthy also have them).

The descriptions alongside each diagnosis on a page are often brief because the differences between diagnoses may be few. This is why the diagnostic process may be difficult for the novice to master quickly but look simple in the hands of the expert, who knows what to focus on.

Unlike textbooks that concentrate on describing diseases processes, often in vivid and elegant detail, this book focuses on findings that are useful during the diagnostic process, to speed up the reader's acquisition of diagnostic skills. The reader is encouraged to add to this information or modify it. However, little if any evidence has been collected yet to substantiate the performance of leads and differentiators.

How to use this book

The book can be used in two ways.
1. You may browse its pages and try to guess from your knowledge of anatomy or physiology the possible diagnoses linked to it. You should keep covering the column of diagnoses and test to see whether you can guess each diagnosis by reading the findings that suggest or confirm it. By doing this, you will begin to acquire the type of knowledge used by experienced doctors at the CPCs.
2. The book can also be used when solving diagnostic problems. Write down your differential diagnoses and put in brackets after each diagnosis the positive and negative findings that you think support each diagnosis. Look up the patient's positive findings in this book: they will be represented by page headings. If you see a diagnosis on the page that you have not considered, consider it. As you view the differential diagnoses you have considered, look at the suggesting and confirming findings to see if you have already looked for them; if not, do so.

The diagnostic lead

Unless a finding happens to be a pathognomonic diagnostic criterion that already confirms a diagnosis, it will be associated with more than one diagnosis. It will therefore have to be interpreted in combination with other findings before a single diagnosis becomes more probable or can be confirmed. These combinations may be recognized immediately as highly predictive clusters or syndromes. If not, the combination may have to be assembled logically by using one of the component findings as a "lead" and using the others to make up a combination that identifies a group of patients within which all but one diagnosis is improbable or eliminated.

Each page in Chapters 3–18 of this book is based on the concept of a lead that is predictive of a list of differential diagnoses. The *suggesting* findings on each page can be used to make a diagnosis more probable; the *confirming* findings will make that diagnosis certain. The principle of using logic to assemble patterns or syndromes is as follows.

If a 24-year-old man presents with acute abdominal pain localized to the right lower quadrant (RLQ) and is accompanied by guarding, then this cluster of findings suggests appendicitis. This working diagnosis might be confirmed during a laparotomy by seeing the definitive finding of a red, swollen appendix and treated with appendectomy with resolution of the pain so that the diagnosis becomes final.

Logic based on proportions

The same combination of findings can also be assembled logically because RLQ pain would be a good short lead due to appendicitis (e.g., in 40/100 of hypothetical patients with the lead), nonspecific abdominal pain (NSAP) (e.g., in 60/100). Guarding occurs commonly in appendicitis but rarely in those with NSAP, which means that the probable diagnosis is appendicitis.

Note that NSAP is an example of a group of very important diagnoses. These are self-limiting conditions that resolve spontaneously before any treatment other than relief of symptoms is required. These nonspecific (NS) diagnoses (e.g., NS headache, NS chest pain) are the most common diagnoses in medicine. They are confirmed by careful follow-up but typically present with a small number of symptoms and signs that are mild and of recent onset. Learning to deal with these safely using appropriate follow-up is one of the most important diagnostic skills to be acquired.

Diagnostic logic using proportions is helped by choosing a lead with a small number of diagnostic possibilities that account for a high proportion of patients (e.g., over 95%—ideally 100% as in the above example).

Another important principle is that the low frequency of a single finding gives an upper limit for the frequency of occurrence of a combination that includes that finding. Thus, if guarding occurs in 5% × 60 = 3 of those with NSAP, then guarding with RLQ pain must occur in 3 patients or fewer (as the presence or absence of RLQ pain will further subdivide the group of 3 who have guarding).

Care must be taken with the rest of the logic, however. If guarding occurs in 50% and RLQ pain also occurs in 50% of those with appendicitis, it is possible that each finding occurs in different halves of the group with appendicitis and that these findings never occur together in those with appendicitis. Under these circumstances, it would be wrong to assume that most patients with RLQ pain and guarding had appendicitis. However, if guarding occurred in 95% and RLQ pain occurred in 85% of those with appendicitis, then even if they occur together as infrequently as possible (i.e., there was maximum negative statistical dependency), both have to occur in at least 80% (i.e., $0.95 + 0.85 - 1 = 0.80$). In terms of patient numbers, this would be at least 80% $\times$ 40 = 32 of the original 100 patients. Therefore, appendicitis must occur in at least 32/(32+3) = 91% of those with RLQ pain and guarding.

Assumptions and estimates

It is commonly assumed that findings such as guarding and RLQ pain occur together by chance in conditions such as appendicitis. This can be used to give an estimate of the likelihood of discovering a combination of findings in patients who have a diagnostic criterion. Thus the likelihood of getting the combination of RLQ pain with guarding in those with appendicitis would be assumed to be 95% $\times$ 85% = 80.75%. This is called the statistical independence assumption.

However, if RLQ pain and guarding were assumed to occur as often as possible in the same patients with appendicitis (i.e., there was positive statistical dependency), then the combination would occur in 85% of those with appendicitis.

Central evidence

Once a diagnostic criterion is discovered (e.g., a red, swollen appendix), as this does not occur in the other conditions by definition, it rules them out completely. The probability of the diagnosis (e.g., of appendicitis) then becomes 100%, irrespective of the nature of the preceding findings.

Thus, many findings discovered in the early part of the diagnostic process are often not mentioned when better evidence becomes available later (even if the better evidence does not give 100% certainty). Better evidence is often assumed to give a good estimate of the probability for the total evidence. This small combination of powerful evidence is often called the "relevant" or "central" evidence. However, the patient's original presenting complaint is always relevant because, unless it resolves, the diagnosis does not become final. An alternative or additional diagnosis may have to be considered to explain the patient's findings.

Evidence-based differential diagnosis

In practice, this reasoning process is done informally and little thought is given to the underlying rigorous, logical principles, frequencies, or simplifying assumptions. However, if we wish to practice evidence-based medicine and evidence-based diagnosis, it is important that careful thought be given to the underlying logical principles of diagnosis.

It will be necessary to collect data on the frequency in diagnostic leads or pivots of various diagnoses. This will include clinical findings and test results (including numerical test results) in different clinical settings. It will also be important to determine the frequencies of symptoms, signs, and distributions of numerical test results in patients with various differential diagnoses and in patients with diagnoses of different degrees of severity.

Differential diagnosis and diagnostic screening

The arithmetic used to represent the screening of populations for diagnoses is different from the arithmetic of differential diagnosis. It might be helpful to an epidemiologist to know the proportion of times a particular diagnosis will be confirmed in due course after the positive screening test has been investigated to determine its cause. One can measure this proportion directly in a study—e.g., of 12 patients who are dipstick positive for micro-albumin, 8 turn out eventually to have incipient nephropathy.

However, instead of measuring the proportion of 8/12 directly, this frequency of 8/12 = 0.75 is usually calculated by epidemiologists and statisticians indirectly by applying Bayes theorem to 1) an estimate of the prevalence or incidence of the diagnosis, 2) the prevalence or incidence of the screening test result in the population to be studied, and 3) an estimate of the frequency of the test result in those confirmed to have the diagnosis.

Screening in the diagnostic setting

It is not only epidemiologists who perform screening tests. These tests are also performed by primary care physicians and specialists who look after populations of patients who are asymptomatic but who have a high risk of developing some condition, e.g., diabetic nephropathy. If such a patient is asked *open* questions, e.g., "Do you have any symptoms that you wish to tell me about?" severe symptoms may be remembered but minor ones may be forgotten. If the patient is asked *closed* questions, e.g., "Does your urine froth sometimes?" then fewer symptoms may be missed but spurious positive responses may be given, perhaps to agree with the doctor.

Similarly, if a detection process is made more biochemically sensitive, e.g., by calling a smaller color change on the urine dipstick paper positive, then it may result in more spurious false-positive results. However, if the process is modified by calling only a larger color test change on the urine dipstick positive, it may be less biochemically (and statistically) sensitive.

If a sensitive screening test is negative, the patient is usually reassured that no further tests are necessary. However, if, for example, a preliminary urine test for microalbuminuria is positive, then the confirmatory tests of three 24-hour urine collections together with urine microscopy and culture may have to be done to see if early diabetic nephropathy is present.

Waiting rooms and Venn diagrams

The accompanying Venn diagram (Fig. 2.1) represents 20 diabetic patients in a waiting room, of whom 9 are known to have incipient nephropathy. Twelve patients have a positive dipstick test. There are 8 patients with incipient nephropathy who are dipstick positive; these are enclosed in the overlapping circles. There are 7 patients who have no incipient nephropathy and are dipstick negative, and they fall outside both circles. There are 4 patients who are dipstick positive with no incipient nephropathy and a single patient who is dipstick negative with nephropathy.

These numbers are also represented in the usual 2 × 2 table (see Table 2.1), which also show the totals with and without incipient nephropathy and those who are dipstick positive and dipstick negative.

The different meanings of "sensitivity"

The term *sensitive* is used for not only a detection process but also the proportion of positive test results when the gold-standard test result is positive. In the above example, the sensitivity was 8/9 and is shown near the top of the probability map (Fig. 2.2). This probability map shows the relationship between the 8 logical propositions that can be based on a Venn diagram. Read the line representing sensitivity from right to left as follows: if there is incipient nephropathy, then 8/9 are dipstick positive.

The obverse of this is the false-negative rate: if there is nephropathy, then 1/9 are dipstick negative. The converse to the sensitivity is the positive predictive value, which is read from left to right as follows: if the dipstick is positive, then 8/12 have nephropathy.

The negative predictive value is at the bottom of the map and may be read as follows: if the dipstick is negative, then 7/8 have no nephropathy. The converse is read in the reverse direction and is called the "specificity": if there is no nephropathy, then 7/11 are dipstick negative.

Finally, the obverse of the specificity is the false positive rate: if there is no nephropathy then 4/11 are dipstick positive. The prevalence of incipient nephropathy in the population studied is 9/20 and the prevalence of dipstick-positive patients is 12/20 (note that there are 4 prevalences).

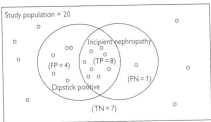

TP = true positives, FP = false positives, FN = false negatives, TN = true negatives

Figure 2.1 Venn diagram.

	Nephropathy	No nephropathy	Totals
Dipstick positive	8(TP)	4(FP)	12
Dipstick negative	1(FN)	7(TN)	8
Totals	9	11	20

Sensitivity = TP/(TP + FN) = 8/9   Specificity = TN/(TN + FP) = 7/11
Positive predictive value= TP/(TP + FP) = 8/12   Negative predictive value= TN/(TN + FN) = 7/8

Table 2.1 2 × 2 table.

The arithmetic representation of the converse relationship is called *Bayes theorem*:

Prevalence of nephropathy	×	Sensitivity	÷	Prevalence of dipstick positive)	=	Positive predictive value
9/20	×	8/9	÷	12/20	=	**8/12**

Effect of clinical setting on diagnostic probabilities

The nature of the clinical setting can affect the predictive probabilities of the differential diagnoses of diagnostic leads. The group discussed previously was patients in a diabetic follow-up clinic waiting room.

The data might be different in another setting such as a primary care waiting room for asymptomatic patients having annual checkups or an antenatal clinic. For example, if another waiting room contained many new diabetic patients, the prevalence of incipient nephropathy might be lower (e.g., 4/20) because the nephropathy in newly diagnosed diabetics was at an earlier stage, so that fewer would test positive with a dipstick (e.g., the sensitivity might be 2/4). If the incidence of a newly dipstick-positive result was 8/20, the positive predictive value in this new setting would be less at 2/8:

$$4/20 \times 2/4 \div 8/20 = \textbf{2/8}$$

Probability map

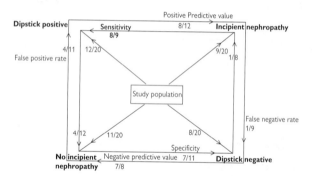

Figure 2.2 Probability map.

Diagnostic leads again

If the predictive value of a positive dipstick was 2/8, this begs the question: what was producing the positive result in the other 6/8, or 75%, of patients? In this new clinic we might find that 2/8 had a urinary tract infection and 4/8 had had nonspecific microalbuminuria (which means that when another urine specimen was taken, the test was negative). This might mean that new patients were less expert at producing an uncontaminated specimen.

In the diabetic follow-up clinic, the positive predictive value was 8/12, so that only 4/12 = 33.3% had some other diagnosis, e.g., 3/12 had a urinary tract infection (UTI) and only 1/12 of these patients had nonspecific microalbuminuria.

What is important here is that the differential diagnosis of a positive dipstick is the same in both clinical settings, but the proportions of the three different diagnoses are different. However, the tests used to investigate the finding in this situation are definitive, e.g., the urinalysis result is assumed to confirm or exclude a UTI. A negative urinalysis is also a necessary condition for diagnosing diabetic nephropathy, together with three 24-hour urine collections to confirm or exclude the diagnosis. Repeating the dipstick test is assumed to confirm or exclude nonspecific microalbuminuria.

In other words, building these test results into the definitions means that the probabilities of the diagnoses rise to 100% or drop to 0%. This result is not affected in this situation by the initial predictive value of a positive dipstick result in the different settings. This means that the information in this book can be used in any clinical setting, provided that confirmatory tests are used eventually.

In the current absence of data on diagnostic leads and differentiators, the reader has to rely on common sense and experience to estimate the initial probabilities given by the lead and the provisional probabilities given by the suggesting findings of each differential diagnosis.

Usefulness of findings in differential diagnoses

1. In order for a symptom, signs, or test result to be useful as a diagnostic lead, as small a number of differential diagnoses as possible should account for as high a proportion of patients as possible (e.g., 95% but ideally 100%) of patients with that finding.
2. In order for a finding to be a strong differentiator between the postulated diagnosis associated with a diagnostic lead and the rival possibilities, it must occur as often as possible in the postulated diagnosis being chased and as rarely as possible (ideally never) in at least one of the rival differential diagnoses.

It should be noted that (2) refers to the ratio of two sensitivities and not the likelihood ratio, which is the sensitivity divided by the false-positive rate (the false-positive rate being 1—the specificity). The mathematical basis of this is described elsewhere.[1,2,3,4]

Research needs to be done to establish which test results provide powerful diagnostic leads and differentiators. Where such tests are lacking, new ones can be designed on the basis of scientific understanding of disease processes and therapeutics.

1 Llewelyn DEH (1975). A concept of diagnosis: a relationship between logic and limits of probability. *Clin Sci Mol Med* **49**;7.
2 Llewelyn DEH (1979). Mathematical analysis of the diagnostic relevance of clinical findings. *Clin Sci* **57**(5):477–479.
3 Llewelyn DEH (1981). Applying the principle of logical elimination to probabilistic diagnosis. *Med Informatics* **6**(1);25.
4 Llewelyn DEH (1988). Assessing the validity of diagnostic tests and clinical decisions. MD thesis. University of London.

"Gold-standard" diagnostic criteria: are they valid?

Pay careful attention to the patient's diagnosis when considering if a treatment is expected to be of benefit. It does not matter how powerful a treatment might be; it will not work if it is given to the wrong patients and may indeed do more harm than good by causing adverse effects with no prospect of benefit.

The role of a physician is to decide which patients will benefit from a specific treatment or advice, and this is done by arriving at a diagnosis. For this reason, the explanation given for a treatment is bound up with the diagnosis. This applies to the explanation for how the treatment changes the imagined underlying process and to the pragmatic result of a clinical trial comparing the response to treatment with that of something else. So, a perfectly valid diagnostic criterion will help to identify all those and only those patients who will respond to a treatment.

If only a proportion of patients respond to a treatment, then it is better to subdivide the diagnosis to identify those who do and those who do not respond. For example, only a proportion of patients suffering from a myocardial infarction (MI) benefit from thrombolysis or angioplasty. However, more patients with ST elevation do so. The diagnosis of MI has thus been subdivided into ST-elevation MI with a high response rate to thrombolysis or angioplasty, and non-ST-elevation MI, which identifies those who are not very responsive and thus not offered these treatments.

The ability of a diagnostic criterion to predict treatment response is known as its *validity*. The most valid test result for an evolving MI would be the one that identified all those, and only those, who responded to thrombolysis or angioplasty. Note that MI now envelops other diagnostic groups or sets. This is the case for many diagnoses, diabetes mellitus being an important example. One of the diagnoses it envelops is incipient diabetic nephropathy.

If a gold-standard test (i.e., diagnostic criterion) is based on a measurement, another factor that needs determining is the best cutoff point. For example, the upper limit of the normal range for the albumin excretion rate (AER) is 20 µg/min, based on samples taken from healthy laboratory volunteers.

This cutoff point is also used to decide if a diabetic patient has incipient diabetic nephropathy by assuming that all those above this level are at significantly increased risk of nephropathy, e.g., within 2 years. However, if only a small proportion of patients with an initial rate between 20 and 40 µg/min develop nephropathy (as shown in Fig. 2.3), then nephropathy will be incipient for a very few only. If the risk of nephropathy rises rapidly above 40 µg/min, this might be a more suitable cutoff point for incipient diabetic nephropathy.[1]

---

1 Llewelyn DEH, Garcia-Puig J (2004). How different urinary albumin excretion rates can predict progression to nephropathy and the effect of treatment in hypertensive diabetics. *J Renin Angiotensin Aldosterone Syst* 5:141–145.

Thus, empirical evidence should be sought for the validity of a diagnostic criterion, not for just choosing a cutoff point on theoretical grounds, e.g., 2 standard deviations above the logarithmic mean.

The particular evidence regarding a particular patient's diagnosis throughout this Handbook is presented as *Suggested by* and *Confirmed by*. *Suggested by* introduces features that make it probable that the diagnosis will be *confirmed by* another set of tests, which are thus worth doing.

The confirming features usually indicate that some specific advice or treatment should be given. However, in urgent cases, treatment may begin sooner, when the danger of avoiding delay is greater than giving it prematurely and unnecessarily. In other cases, the result of treatment may be the only practical confirmatory test.

So, if the treatment can be stopped when the initial response is not promising, this is referred to as a therapeutic gold-standard test. This is done sometimes in a double-blind crossover manner—the so-called N-of-1 trial. The design is double-blind so that neither the patient nor the doctor knows what treatment is being taken until the trial of therapy is complete, when they both decide if the preliminary response is worth pursuing with continuous treatment.

A perfectly valid diagnostic criterion would identify all those and only those with a presenting complaint who would respond to a particular treatment by their presenting complaint resolving, not returning, and leaving them with perfect health. The perfect treatment given to those with a perfect diagnostic criterion would cause no adverse effects and cause all those with a presenting complaint and diagnostic criterion to get better, who would not otherwise get better without that treatment.

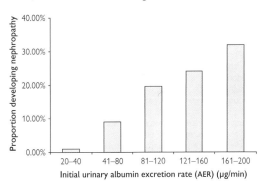

Figure 2.3 Proportion of patients developing diabetic nephropathy 2 years after initial albumin excretion rate (AER) value, as shown.

Working diagnoses and final diagnoses

Many patients have symptoms, physical signs, and tests results that do not satisfy diagnostic criteria. Some diagnostic criteria are not easily accessible; for example, they depend on histology or an appearance at major surgery. We may thus have to begin treatment when there are no recognized criteria.

For example, most antibiotics are prescribed for a chest infection before it is confirmed by culturing bacteria. However, when we decide to treat, we always assume that if a randomized, controlled trial were to be done on such a group of patients, more would benefit from treatment than from placebo (but we would think so with more confidence when there is a diagnostic criterion).

If we are asked to explain why we chose that particular treatment, we could say that we imagine the presence of the disease process for the time being. This is called a "working diagnosis." It is equivalent to a scientific hypothesis during an experiment. If the patient gets better in the expected way and if there was no practical purpose for doing further tests, then we would then assume that we were correct. This would be called a "final diagnosis." It would be the same as a hypothesis becoming a scientific theory because there is no immediate intention to do another experiment to test it.

In both cases, we would be citing an imagined process, knowing that it was theoretical and not proven (i.e., by direct observation of everything being imagined). In the case of a treatment, we would not have been able to prove that the patient would not have gotten better anyway without the treatment. In order to prove this, we would have to do the impossible by turning the clock back and not giving the treatment, to see what happens.

It should also be remembered that even if diagnostic criteria are present, this does not guarantee a response to treatment. Diagnostic criteria are there for consistency between different doctors' diagnoses, and they also allow randomized trials to be done and the knowledge to be shared. Thus, if the diagnostic criteria were chosen carefully to be valid in terms of predicting outcome, then more patients would respond to treatment (and fewer to placebo in a clinical trial) when using the criterion than when not using it. If we stray away from such published clinical-trial criteria when giving treatments, then we have to accept that we are guessing treatment response by extrapolation, and not basing it on formal, documented experience in that clinical trial.

If the patient failed to respond to the treatment that might lead to a final diagnosis, then we would carry out further tests to discover if there is evidence for some other diagnosis or to look for further evidence for the original diagnosis that simply did not respond to the treatment. This further evidence might be a successful response to some other treatment that could work for the original working diagnosis.

The practical purpose of a diagnosis from the patient's point of view is to predict the outcomes of a distressing complaint, with or without treatment. Sophisticated technology is there to improve the validity of diagnostic criteria in terms of their ability to predict what will happen to the patient's symptoms. A diagnosis represents imagination that includes clinical findings and test results, so it can never be proven to be true in its entirety by a single test. The number of detailed imaginary models (e.g., at the molecular level) under the umbrella term of *diagnosis* is limited only by the human imagination.

Science is concerned with imaginative theories or models that can be tested against observed facts, documented, and then shared with others. If no aspect of a theory can be tested by any form of observation, it cannot be the subject of scientific study.

The process of imagining more models of disease (and discarding some of them because they do not fit the facts) results in scientific models becoming more detailed. One effect of this is that diagnoses may become subdivided, e.g., MI has become subdivided into ST-elevation MI responsive to thrombolysis or angioplasty, and non-ST-elevation MI, which is not.

So a working or final diagnosis is simply the title to a model, hypothesis, or theory that explains and connects the combination of pre-treatment facts (e.g., chest pain with ST elevation) to an outcome of treatment with or without a treatment (e.g., lowering of raised ST segments after thrombolysis). In addition to this imaginative view of diagnosis, there is also the public, logical approach, which is the main subject of this book.

Dynamic diagnoses

It is important to understand that clinical diagnosis is not a static classification system based on diagnostic criteria or their probable presence. It is a dynamic process.

Diagnostic algorithms classify patients by following a logical pathway. This works bests when interpreting components of diagnostic criteria. Other systems use findings such as symptoms and physical signs to predict the probable presence of diagnostic criteria.

All of these methods can be regarded as diagnosing a snapshot of what is happening at a particular time. However, the diagnostician will be trying to imagine the presence of a dynamic process that changes with time. This could be over seconds, minutes, hours, days, weeks, months, or years, and the response in terms of investigation and treatment has to be timed appropriately.

There may be several processes taking place at the same time, some progressing over years (e.g., atheromatous changes), some over minutes to hours (e.g., a thrombosis in a coronary artery), some over minutes or seconds (e.g., ventricular tachycardia), and others instantaneously (e.g., a cardiac arrest). This means that a diagnostic process leading to treatment may have to happen repeatedly and for a number of diagnoses at the same time.

It might be more appropriate to think of the process as one of feedback control. In this way, the doctor would be acting as an external control mechanism to assist those of the patient that are failing. After the initial history and examination, the feedback information may come from electronic monitoring, nursing observations, ward rounds, or hospital clinic or primary-care follow-up.

The mechanisms of interest to the diagnostician are of three types. The first type is mechanisms that control the internal milieu by keeping temperature, tissue perfusion, blood gases, and biochemistry constant. The second type is those mechanisms that control the body's structure by effecting repair in response to any damage. The third type consists of those that control the external milieu of day-to-day living.

These three types are all interdependent. If one mechanism fails, it may unmask other weaknesses by causing other failures. It may not be enough to treat the main failure. It is often necessary also to treat the causes and consequences, as they may be unable to recover on their own. For example, a coronary thrombosis may be treated with thrombolysis, but any resulting rhythm abnormalities may need to be treated, as well as the causative risk factors (e.g., smoking) that could result in recurrence. So when we explain our diagnostic thought processes, it helps to think of each diagnosis as a subheading with its own evidence and decision.

The process of taking a history and examining a new patient may take about an hour. If the patient is acutely ill, there may have to be an urgent, life-saving diagnosis and treatment with a reassessment every few minutes until the patient is stable. The presenting complaint and a quick examination may also suggest a minor complaint such as a viral sore throat that is best managed by simple measures and by having the patient return in a few days.

What all these diagnostic approaches have in common is a cycle of evidence gathering, working diagnosis (with or without a diagnostic criterion), and management. The management may involve tests, treatments, and their results, which produce further evidence, a revised diagnosis, and further management.

The probability of any diagnosis being confirmed with diagnostic criteria or becoming the final diagnosis by responding to treatment may not be very high initially. However, you can reassure the patient that the follow-up process will allow further attempts to take place until you get it right.

In many cases the problem will resolve spontaneously before you can arrive at any diagnosis that suggests a treatment. In other cases you may have to observe the patient closely as the mystery disease progresses so that new evidence becomes available. In this way, uncertainty may be overcome by cycles of follow-up and review.

Transparency and replication

Physicians work closely with patients, relatives, other physicians, and members of other disciplines. They frequently hand over care to others who have to understand what is happening, and if they agree, to continue with the plan. There is little place in all of this for mystery and obscurity, which may arouse suspicion about the doctor's motives or competence.

An experienced doctor would know quickly if the evidence did not add up. He or she would check with the patient to see if the presenting complaint is accurate and to check if the evidence given justifies accepting the main diagnosis. It is also easy to see if all the necessary treatments have been given. The same can be done for all the other diagnoses.

If there is doubt about the diagnoses because there is insufficient evidence, then other diagnoses may also have to be considered and added to the list. One reason for such doubt would be if the patient still has symptoms that are slow to resolve. If there is doubt as to whether the answers are sensible, then the history and examination has to be repeated. If the same findings are discovered again, then they can be said to have been corroborated or replicated.

Evidence is of two types. The first type is the *particular* evidence displayed in that particular situation for a particular patient. It has to be given with a time and place and in enough detail to allow a listener to question the witness or to repeat the observations so that they can be replicated along with the reasoning process and decision. (The same principles are used in the legal profession.)

The second part of the evidence is experience from many similar past situations and their outcomes, which demonstrated that a high proportion were successful. This is *general* evidence, in contrast to the particular evidence. For a treatment, it would consist of what happened in a clinical trial to some patients on the treatment and to others on a placebo or something else. The problem is that such general or scientific evidence is not available for much of what we do in medicine, especially when using different diagnostic criteria or gold-standard tests.

General scientific evidence is based on observations made on groups of individuals (who each have their own particular observations). If a listener is going to accept such observations as general scientific evidence, the results and methods have to be described in sufficient detail to be repeated by someone else and thus for the study result to be replicated, if necessary. If the study and its description is of high quality and published in a reputable journal (which reflects the quality), then the reader may not feel obliged to repeat it.

One criterion is that there was a sensible hypothesis and thus a good reason for doing the study (i.e., that it was not just a chance observation). Another important criterion would be that the numbers of observations made were high, so that the statistical probability of replicating the study result was high (e.g., there was a 95% chance of getting a repeat result between two clinically acceptable confidence limits).

Modern medicine involves careful evidence-gathering and the use of imagination to decide on the best action. These actions are then explained to others with diagnoses and evidence for those diagnoses. There is thus a private, imaginative stage and then a public, transparent stage to allow others to decide if they can agree. If it is not possible to provide a clear rationale in a way that can be understood by others who will be affected by an action, then the wisdom of the action should be reconsidered.

One way of providing such a transparent rationale is to set out a diagnostic opinion in writing with clear, particular evidence in support of each diagnosis, for others to discuss (see Box 2.1). This format for supporting a diagnosis with evidence that suggests or confirms the diagnosis is used throughout this book.

Box 2.1 Diagnoses with particular evidence and management

Acute follicular tonsillitis
- *Evidence:* severe sore throat, sweats, and severe malaise for 2 days. Bilaterally swollen tonsils, large and red with small white patches. WBC 18.33°× 10⁹/L, neutrophils 90%
- *Management:* throat swab sent. Start penicillin V 500 mg po qd, acetaminophen 1 g po qd, and review with bacteriology

Probable type II diabetes mellitus
- *Evidence:* glycosuria +, random blood sugar 150 mg/dL
- *Management:* for fasting blood sugar when current, acute illness resolved. Healthy diet meanwhile

Controlled thyrotoxicosis
- *Evidence:* presented 2 months ago with **anxiety, weight loss**, abnormal thyroid function tests in Osler Hospital
- *Management:* continue taking carbimazole, 5 mg po qd

Anxiety about meningitis
- *Evidence:* voiced concerns during history
- *Management:* details of this summary explained to patient

Inadequate home care
- *Evidence:* lives alone with no friends nearby
- *Management:* assist patient to contact family

Differences of opinion about a diagnosis

Differences of opinion can sometimes cause consternation; a common reaction is that someone has to be wrong. Different opinions can all be valid if they are based on documented experience and framed as probability statements with a sensible element of doubt. For example, if a physician makes a number of different predictions with 50% certainty and 50% turn out to be correct overall, this shows good overall judgment.

Different members of the team can thus hold different valid opinions about a diagnosis for a particular patient on the basis of their different personal experiences. A doctor may be wrong about a prediction for a particular patient and yet be correct 75% of the time for such predictions with a 75% probability when they are all taken together in the long run.

However, if a single opinion has to be adopted by a team to decide what should be done for a particular patient, then traditionally the opinion of the most senior member present is adopted (usually after this person has listened carefully to others).

If an opinion is totally certain, then it implies that all other opinions must be wrong. An opinion held with certainty also raises questions about the holder's judgment because, in the long run, it is unlikely that 100% of predictions will be correct. An opinion may become distorted consciously or subconsciously because the holder stands to gain personally from its implementation. It is therefore important to be able to reassure patients and team members if there are differences of opinion.

It is also important not to confuse opinions about outcomes with rules that a team has agreed to abide by. A team member may point out that a rule should be followed; this is not an overconfident opinion but a fact, if it was agreed at a particular time and place. Overconfidence is also different from decisiveness. One can be decisive by choosing an option with a low probability of success because it represents the best of a number of poor options.

Differences of opinion may occur because the particular facts on which they are based are different. The first thing to do when there is a difference of opinion, therefore, is to check the particular facts for the patient and, if necessary, review the methods and conventions used by the team to get agreement. This process may allow facts to be replicated (see Transparency and Replication, p. 30).

The second thing to do is to clarify the personal and published experience on which the opinion and probability are based. This would include the facts that identified the group of patients who were followed and the details of outcomes, such as the diagnostic criteria used or the treatment results.

Clarification of the facts often leads to agreement by revealing oversights and misunderstandings or pooling of experience. Meta-analysis is a technique for combining data from different publications. Bayesian statisticians also combine documented data with personal, undocumented, subjective experience. Decision analysis can be used to ask patients' opinions of how they would feel about different outcomes, so that this can be taken into account when interpreting the meta-analyses and the personal experiences of doctors.

Many opinions are straightforward, and failure to hold some of them might be considered culpable (e.g., that bacterial meningitis should always be treated with antibiotics). There are also particular schools of thought, and these are often represented by local guidelines (e.g., which antibiotic should be used as first-line treatment). If teams agree to abide by such guidelines, then differences of opinion are minimized and teamwork is made easier.

Clinical audit is designed to detect poor performance that might be due to poor choice of guidelines for diagnosis or for treatment. However, there is less formal scientific evidence in the literature to guide us in choosing between diagnostic criteria than between treatments. As in other Oxford Handbooks, the blank spaces in this book are there for you to express your own opinions.

History-taking skills and imagination

History taking with imagination

The aim of the diagnostic process is to build an imaginative picture of what is happening to the patient. *Diagnosis* is derived from the Greek "to see through" (i.e., the history, physical examination, special investigations, and response to treatment).

The diagnosis must not imply that there is only some single hidden process that needs to be discovered. The diagnosis (or diagnostic formulation) may have to include various causes, consequences, interactions, and other independent processes. As well as internal medical processes, it has to include external factors such as circumstances at home and the effects on self-care, employment, and leisure.

Clearly, the most informative part of this broad diagnostic process will be the history. The history also enables patients and supporters to identify the issues that they want addressed in terms of discomfort, loss of function, and difficulties with day-to-day existence. Gold standards for final diagnoses are best based on the outcome of patients' symptoms combined with the result of histology, biochemistry, or some other measurements. So, final diagnoses are often based on initial history-taking skills from which outcomes can be assessed.

Observe normal social conventions. Introduce yourself politely and invite the patient and any accompanying persons to do the same. Check details such as the patient's date of birth, address, etc.

It is then important to establish very clearly why the patient has sought help. This is known as the chief (or presenting) complaint. Ask the patient about its severity and duration and always record this. Be prepared to act immediately to give symptomatic relief (e.g., for pain) if the patient is distressed.

In some cases, the chief complaint may not explain the decision to seek help. The patient may be too ill, shy, guilty, or embarrassed to describe what is happening accurately. In other cases, it may be someone else who is unduly worried (e.g., the wife of a lethargic husband, parents of a child or caregivers of an elderly person who can no longer cope). Be alert and explore the real reason if there is doubt.

Having established the chief complaint(s), establish the factual details of place and time. It is the ability to give a place and time that establishes the complaints as facts. (Medicine shares this convention with pure science and law.)

Listen to what the patient says without prompting first, but, if necessary, ask where they were and what they were doing when the problem was first noticed. This will help the patient to recall what happened and also stimulate your own diagnostic imagination.

Establish the speed of initial onset and subsequent change in severity with time. This helps you to imagine the kind of pathological process that is taking place. An onset within seconds suggests a fit or heart rhythm abnormality; over minutes, a bleed or clotting process; hours to days, an acute infection; days to weeks, a chronic infection; weeks to months, a tumor; and months to years, a degenerative process.

The site may be anatomical, e.g., abdominal pain, or systemic, e.g., a cough. By convention, facts are details that include a time and place that can be checked.

If there are other complaints, note the same details (the time courses of other new symptoms are often the same, however). Ask about other associated, aggravating, and relieving factors, especially as a result of the patient's own actions and those of others. Ask what the patient thinks is going on.

You will have to continue with cycles of evidence, diagnosis, action, more evidence, revised diagnoses, further action, etc. Establish not only what the patient's complaints are and document them, but also the patient's own fears and actions. This will be the starting point for your own explanation and suggestions to the patient later about what is to be done.

Write out your history in a systematic way, for example, as shown in the next section. Go over it with the patient, if possible, to check that it is right.

The case history: an example

Ms. AM, age 31 (DOB: 2/28/77)
23 Smith Street, My Town
Emergency admission: October 16, 2005 at 7 p.m.

Chief complaint (CC): severe sore throat, sweats, and severe malaise for 2 days

History of presenting illness (HPI): The patient was well until last Thursday afternoon, October 14, when she developed a sore throat at work as a secretary at an insurance company. It was relieved that day by warm drinks and acetaminophen, but when she woke the following morning it was very severe. It was no longer relieved by acetaminophen (she found swallowing very painful) and she was too unwell to get up. There had been no previous sore throats. She thought that her neck was getting stiff. Her friend had died of meningococcal meningitis a few years previously and this worried her. She called her PCP and was seen at the clinic that day. The doctor was concerned that she lived alone and looked very unwell and had her admitted to the hospital.

The most striking symptom in this case is the severe sore throat that is getting worse. This is an example of a feature with a short list of causes—a good lead. Most readers will have experienced a sore throat and be aware that it is usually due to a viral pharyngitis, tonsillitis (due to a hemolytic streptococcus), glandular fever, or something else in a relatively small proportion of cases (see p. 100). Very rarely, these causes include the beginning of a meningococcal infection. This loomed large in the patient's mind because of the fate of her friend. The history is compatible with all of these possibilities.

If a better lead with an even shorter differential diagnosis turns up later, you may use that. Use the other findings to try to confirm one cause of the shortest lead (and thus eliminate the others). Consider if the remaining abnormal findings could resolve if the confirmed diagnosis were treated. If not, look for another coexisting diagnosis.

This handbook contains a selection of findings with short differential diagnoses. Single and small combinations of findings of this kind form the foundation of the process of arriving at a working diagnosis (i.e., until the diagnosis is final and no further tests or treatment changes are contemplated). With growing experience, you will learn to recognize more combinations that usually point to a single or a few diagnoses and have to resort less often to working through the possibilities in a conscious way, using the concepts described in this book.

However, you will continue to be faced with new or strange situations throughout your career; this is what makes medical practice such a challenge. The approaches you develop early in your career to deal with new situations will stand you in good stead for the remainder of your career.

The next step is the past medical history (PMH).

The past medical history

> **PMH**: Thyrotoxicosis discovered 6 months ago. (Anxiety, weight loss, abnormal thyroid function tests in Osler Hospital.) Taking carbimazole, 5 mg daily.

The past medical history (PMH) in this case has three components: the diagnosis, the evidence, and the management. Thyrotoxicosis is the *diagnosis*, which summarizes what is imagined to have happened. Anxiety, weight loss, and abnormal thyroid function tests summarize the *evidence* for imaging what had happened. The *management* was taking carbimazole, 5 mg daily.

In many cases, the patient would not be able to provide these details and they would have to be extracted from the hospital or primary care records, in which case it is helpful to name the hospital (the fictitious Osler Hospital, in this case) or primary care center or doctor responsible.

It is important to note, however, that a comprehensive PMH in this format can be written immediately after any consultation—in the hospital or primary care center—with results and dates. It can be included with any communication so that the recipient does not have to hunt for the details. It is very helpful for those that follow the initial consultation (and this may include you). From time to time in the hand-written follow-up notes you may wish to take stock and write down a current PMH that sets out the numbered list of diagnoses, with the evidence and management in parentheses.

In this case, the past history also raises the possibility of recurrence of thyroid disease causing the sore throat, but the only thyroid condition that would do this is acute thyroiditis (viral or autoimmune). This is a rare condition and is not included in lists of common causes of a sore throat.

The message to be taken away from this example is that if the patient has had a condition in the PMH, possible links should be recalled or looked up to see if any of these could explain the presenting problem. In this sense, a history of chronic or recurrent conditions can be used as a lead. So, any type of lead with a short list of possible associations should be considered.

The drug history

The drug history (DH) is often placed at the very end of the history, before the examination findings; it is a matter of personal choice. However, if the patient is on medication, then it indicates that there is an active medical condition, not just a past medical history. Therefore, there is something to be said for documenting the drug history immediately after the past medical history so that past and current conditions can be considered together.

> **Drug history**: Acetaminophen 1 g q6hr (for ? viral pharyngitis: sore throat for 2 days with fever, and general malaise) with carbimazole 5 mg daily for thyrotoxicosis (see **PMH** for evidence)
> • Alcohol 10 units per week
> • Nonsmoker
> • No other recreational drugs

Diagnostic significance of the drug history

Note that the indication for acetaminophen is given in the form of one possible diagnosis (other differentials could have been included) and the evidence for the diagnosis. This is good practice (not often followed). The evidence for thyrotoxicosis has been given already in the past medical history. Recreational drugs have also been covered in this drug history, but they are often included with the social history.

If you look up the side effects of carbimazole, you will see that they include agranulocytosis, which could explain the sore throat. If this was known when the HPI was being written out, it could be included as a possible causal factor in the HPI.

Risk factors for future or current illnesses (such as smoking) can exist in the drug history, past medical history, family history (e.g., of diabetes), or social history.

The family history

FH:

Father	aged 56	Hypertension
Mother	aged 55	Diabetes (onset at 50)
Siblings	male:	Age 34—alive and well
		Age 26—alive and well
	female:	Age 30—alive and well
Children—none		

The family history (FH) rarely contains features that form powerful leads. In general, there will be risk factors in the family history. For example, the fact that the patient's mother had type 2 diabetes means that there is an increased risk of the patient developing type 2 diabetes mellitus. This may have no immediate bearing on the current problems (but she should be checked for diabetes if only to exclude its presence so far). The patient could nonetheless be advised to adopt a healthy diet and lifestyle.

The social history

The social history (SH) is always relevant. The activities of daily living can be considered under the heading of domestic, work, and leisure. Imagine what any person has to do from waking up in the morning to going to sleep at night and consider whether the patient needs support with any of these activities.

Fit, young adults who are expected to recover completely may miss school, college, or work, and the timing of their return will have to be considered. Patients who are more dependent on others such as children and the elderly may need special provisions. Patients with permanent disabilities may need help with most if not all activities of daily living.

SH: Alone in an apartment at present (roommate on vacation for another week)

Parents live 200 miles away

Works as secretary for insurance firm

The review of systems

The review of systems (ROS) may take place at various points in the history. Some clinicians include it after the history of chief complaint or the past medical history or at the very end. In the diagnostic thought process, putting it at the very end allows it to be used to draw together the conclusions reached at the end of the history regarding diagnoses and risk factors.

The social history will be fresh in your mind in terms of the patient's ability to deal with daily living. You can sum up relevant information with a "sieve" to remind you of what is happening in structural and functional terms in the different systems:

- Social and domestic issues
- Locomotor structure and function
- Skin, temperature regulation, and endocrine function
- Cardiovascular structure and circulation
- Respiratory structure and blood gases
- Alimentary tract and metabolism
- Genitourinary and renal function
- Neurological and psychiatric issues

If a direct question turns up a positive response, it has to be treated with caution. It may be a false-positive response to a leading question. A positive response should be treated as an extra chief complaint and added to the original list.

However, if there is a negative response to a direct question, this is more reliable (unless the patient is very forgetful or is purposely withholding information). The absence of *all* symptoms under a heading indicates that there is no symptomatic evidence of an abnormality in that system. If there is a normal physical examination for that system too, then there will be no clinical evidence at all of an abnormality in that system. This does not indicate with certainty that there is no abnormality. A later clinical assessment or test (e.g., a chest X-ray) might discover something.

Locomotor symptoms

- No pain or stiffness in the neck, shoulder, elbow, wrist, hand, or back
- No pain or stiffness in the hip, knee, or foot
- No pain or stiffness in any joints and muscles

Negative responses make locomotor abnormalities unlikely. If any are positive, then a GALS examination screen is performed under the headings of **G**ait, **A**rms, **L**egs, **S**pine. This should be done after the general examination but before the neurological examination so that care can be taken with painfully inflamed or damaged joints.

Skin, lymph node and endocrine symptoms

- No heat or cold intolerance (e.g., wanting to open or close windows when others are comfortable)
- No sweats and shivering
- No drenching night sweats
- No episodes of rigors
- No rashes and itching
- No skin lumps or lumps elsewhere

Negative responses make abnormal thyroid metabolism, and some skin, lymphoid, and immune reactions unlikely.

Cardiovascular (CV) symptoms
- No tiredness and breathlessness on exertion (nonspecific)
- No syncope and dizziness
- No leg pain on walking

Negative responses make cardiac output and peripheral vascular disease unlikely.
- No ankle swelling

A negative response makes a right-sided venous return abnormality unlikely.
- No exertional dyspnea
- No orthopnea
- No paroxysmal nocturnal dyspnea

Negative responses make left heart venous return abnormality unlikely.
- No palpitations
- No central chest pain on exertion or at rest

Negative responses make a cardiac abnormality less likely.

Respiratory symptoms
- No chronic breathlessness
- No acute breathlessness

Negative responses make abnormality of overall respiratory and blood gas abnormality unlikely.
- No hoarseness
- No cough, sputum, hemoptysis
- No wheeze

Negative responses make airway disease unlikely.
- No pleuritic chest pain

A negative response makes acute pleural reactions and chest wall disease unlikely.

Gastrointestinal (GI) symptoms
- No loss of appetite (nonspecific)
- No weight loss (nonspecific)
- No jaundice, dark urine, pale stools

Negative responses make metabolic gut and liver disease unlikely.
- No nausea or vomiting (nonspecific)
- No hematemesis or melena
- No dysphagia
- No indigestion
- No abdominal pain
- No diarrhea or constipation
- No recent change in bowel habit
- No rectal bleeding ± mucus

Negative responses make gastrointestinal disease unlikely.

Genitourinary (GU) symptoms
- Menstrual history—date of menarche, duration of cycle and flow normal
- Volume of flow and associated pain normal
- Any pregnancy outcomes normal
- No dyspareunia and vaginal bleeding
- No vaginal discharge

Negative responses make gynecological disease unlikely.
- No hematuria or other odd color
- No urgency or incontinence
- No dysuria
- No loin pain or lower abdominal pain

Negative responses make urological disease unlikely.
- No impotence or loss of libido
- No urethral discharge

Negative responses make male urological disease unlikely.

Nervous system symptoms
- No loss or disturbance of
  - Vision (loss, blurring, or double vision)
  - Hearing (loss or tinnitus)
  - Smell and taste
- No numbness, pins and needles, or other disturbance of sensation
- No disturbance of speech
- No weakness of limbs
- No imbalance
- No headache
- No sudden headache and loss of consciousness
- No dizziness and blackouts
- No vertigo
- No seizures
- No transient neurological deficit

Negative responses make neurological disease unlikely.

Psychiatric symptoms
- No fatigue, not tired all the time
- No mood change
- No odd voices or odd visual effects
- No anxiety and sleep disturbance
- No loss of self-confidence
- No new strong beliefs
- No phobias, no compulsions or avoidance of actions
- No use of recreational drugs

Patients may, of course, hide or forget many symptoms. There is a school of thought that regards symptom reviews as being of little value, and that only symptoms that are volunteered are worthwhile investigating. Many doctors do not conduct systemic reviews and only ask these questions if other symptoms have been volunteered already in that system. By drawing together all the findings in the history it would appear as follows:

Miss AM   Aged 31 (DOB: 28/2/74)
23 Smith Square, Old Town.
Emergency admission: October 16, 2005 at 7.00 pm

CC: Severe sore throat, sweats, and severe malaise for 2 days.

HPI: The patient was well until last Thursday afternoon, October 14, when she developed a sore throat at work as a secretary at an insurance company. It was relieved that day by warm drinks and acetaminophen but when she woke the following morning it was very severe. It was no longer relieved by acetaminophen (she found swallowing very painful) and she was too unwell to get up. There had been no previous sore throats. She thought that her neck was getting stiff. Her friend had died of meningococcal meningitis a few years previously and this worried her. She called her PCP and was seen at the clinic that day. The doctor was concerned that she lived alone and looked very unwell and had her admitted to the hospital.

PMH: Thyrotoxicosis discovered 6 months ago. (Anxiety, weight loss, abnormal thyroid function tests in Osler Hospital.) Taking carbimazole, 50 mg daily.

DH: Acetaminophen 1 g q6hr (for ? viral pharyngitis: sore throat for 2 days with fever, and severe malaise)
Carbimazole 5 mg for thyrotoxicosis (see **PMH**)
Alcohol 10 units per week
Nonsmoker
No other recreational drugs

FH:

Father	aged 56	Hypertension
Mother	aged 55	Diabetes (onset at 50)
Siblings	male:	Age 34—alive and well
		Age 26—alive and well
	female:	Age 30—alive and well
Children—none		

SH: Alone in an apartment at present (roommate on vacation for another week)
Parents live 200 miles away

NAD

NAD is an abbreviation for "no abnormality detected." However, it is often regarded with suspicion and many readers of the notes will assume cynically that NAD means "not actually done." If direct questions were asked, then all the answers should be documented. If none were asked, then write, "Review of systems not done."

The preliminary diagnosis

Most of the diagnostic information is contained in the history. Much of the physical examination is directed at looking for information to help to confirm or exclude the diagnostic possibilities raised by the history. It is therefore worth pausing at the end of the history to think about the diagnostic possibilities so far.

In some professional examinations, the candidate is asked only to take a history and to give diagnostic conclusions and a management plan of investigations and treatment options.

Following is a reasonable differential for the main diagnosis:

- ? **Viral pharyngitis** ("?" means a reasonable probability, e.g., 20%–80%)
- ? **Glandular fever**
- ? **Acute follicular tonsillitis**
- ? **Agranulocytosis due to carbimazole**
- ?? **Meningococcal meningitis** ("??" means a low probability, e.g., <20%)

Other diagnoses might be

- Inadequate domestic support currently for acute illness
- ?? Undiscovered type 2 diabetes mellitus

The part of the physical examination to concentrate on would be the appearance of the pharynx and tonsils to see if the latter resembled strawberries and cream, suggestive of acute follicular tonsillitis, or simple redness with no pus, suggestive of a pharyngitis possibly of viral origin. Look for enlarged lymph nodes in the neck to support a brisk response to infection, and neck stiffness that would support meningitis.

The special investigations would include an urgent white cell count (WBC) to see if there were absent or low white cells, confirming agranulocytosis; raised neutrophil white cells, suggesting bacterial infection; or raised lymphocytes, suggesting viral infection. Urine should be tested for sugar and a fasting blood sugar test done.

The immediate treatment options would be to continue the acetaminophen for pain relief and offer additional analgesia such as codeine phosphate.

You will hear of many different approaches to history taking. Make up your own mind and write out your approach on the blank pages provided near here or inside the front cover of the book. Write out your own plan like the one in the following section.

Although there are benefits to taking a systematic approach, especially if you are a student or doctor faced with an unfamiliar problem, consultations may have to be very rapid with shortcuts. The circumstances may disrupt any attempt to be systematic, for example, when examining a fractious child, or when faced with several injured or very sick patients.

To be effective, you should think in an orderly way by identifying the most urgent issue first, then running through in your mind the other issues to be considered. For each issue keep thinking: What are the facts (symptoms, signs, and test results)? What do I imagine is going on (the diagnoses)? What should I do (tests, treatments, and advice)? When you write down an account later, do so in response to the same questions. Within each of these questions, consider what is happening in each system. You can do this using sieves.

Medical diagnostic sieves

The diagnostic possibilities discovered thus far were triggered by the findings in the history. It might be helpful to reflect on whether some other possibilities have been temporarily forgotten, or if some other conditions are present that might be caused or complicated by the diagnostic possibilities considered already.

This is when sieves can be useful. Reflect if there is something else that you should have considered in each system from a structural or functional point of view:

• Social system (home, work, or environment) and locomotor function
• Nervous system (psychiatric or neurological)
• Cardiovascular system (physiological or structural)
• Respiratory system (blood gas regulation or structural)
• Gastrointestinal system (metabolic or GI tract)
• Genitourinary system (reproductive or metabolic)
• Skin and reticuloendothelial system
• Endocrine and autonomic system

Surgical diagnostic sieves

If there is a structural abnormality, use the surgical sieve:
• Congenital
• Infective
• Traumatic
• Neoplastic
• Degenerative

There are many variations of these sieves. They are merely self-propelling memory joggers that enhance recall; we stimulate our minds to recognize something that we may be about to forget.

Management sieves

Consider if there is a test or treatment that you may have forgotten to undertake. Think big, first by considering the environmental level, and then work down via the whole patient to small methods by considering electromagnetic radiation.

Tests produce results and treatments have outcomes. Therapeutic tests are useful and legitimate. So the distinction between a test and a treatment can be a fine one, and the same sieve can be applied to both.

Look at each possibility triggered by the diagnostic sieve and consider if there is a test or treatment that you have forgotten by considering the following action sieve.

This may take a few minutes of reflection, but the patient will be grateful. You will learn more if you do this before looking up what you have forgotten in a book.

Have I forgotten to decide about something at any of the following levels?

- Environmental level, e.g., social services assessment and intervention?
- Whole-patient level, e.g., explanation from the doctor, or assessment, treatment, or advice from nurses, occupational therapists, physiotherapists, dietetics, or speech therapy?
- Organ level, e.g., surgical and endoscopic?
- Cellular level, e.g., cytology, hematology, transfusion, transplantation?
- Molecular level, e.g., biochemical tests and drug therapy?
- Electronic level, e.g., electrocardiogram (ECG), electroencephalogram (EEG), electroconvulsive therapy (ECT), or direct-current (DC) cardioversion?
- Radiation level, e.g., radiology and radiotherapy?

Use a plan for writing out the history

Write out your history in the same way each time, and it will act as a checklist to ensure that you have not forgotten something that you will later wish to rely on as evidence for your diagnosis and decisions. The one on the right-hand page is an example; write down your own version inside the front or back cover—best with a pencil so you can change it later.

History taker's name: Date of assessment:
Patient's name: DOB: Age: Occupation:
Patient's address:

Admitted as an emergency/from the waiting list on (date) at (time)

Chief complaints (CC)
First symptom—duration
Second symptom—duration

History of presenting illness (HPI)

1. Nature of complaint (e.g., pain in chest), circumstances and speed of onset, progression (change with time—picture a graph), aggravating and relieving factors, associated symptoms (describe under (2), below)
2. Next associated symptom, etc., described as in (1).

Add response to direct questions from chasing up some diagnostic possibilities that come to mind as the history is taken (some think that this should not be done as the responses may contain too many false positives)

Past medical history (PMH)

First diagnosis and when; evidence; treatment; name of doctor
Second diagnosis, etc.

Drug history (DH)

Name, dose, and frequency; diagnostic indication; evidence; prescriber
Next drug, etc.
Alcohol and tobacco consumption
Drug sensitivities and allergies

Developmental history

(In pediatrics and psychiatry): Pregnancy, infancy, childhood, puberty, adulthood

Family history (FH)

Ages of	Illnesses
(Arrange around family tree if preferred)	Mention especially:
Parents	tuberculosis,
Siblings	asthma, eczema,
Children	diabetes, epilepsy,
Spouse	hypertension

Social history (SH)

Home and domestic activity support—job and financial security—travel and leisure. (Consider the effect of all these on the illness and the effect of the illness on these factors.)

Physical examination skills and leads

Physical examination skills

At the end of the history in the previous chapter the patient was thought
to have
• ? Viral pharyngitis
• ? Infectious mononucleosis
• ? Acute follicular tonsillitis
• ? Agranulocytosis due to carbimazole
• ?? Meningococcal meningitis
• Inadequate domestic support currently for acute illness
• ?? Undiscovered type 2 diabetes mellitus

Recall what you imagined after the history. Give a subjective impression of
how well the patient appears to be on a spectrum from being completely
fit and well, being unwell to some degree, to moribund. Be prepared to
respond appropriately.

An ability to make a subjective diagnosis of degrees of well-being and
imminent outcome depends on experience of observing a large number
of patients and knowing what happened to them. There are early warning
scores that you may be expected to use in some centers based on pulse,
respiratory rate, and other factors.

When you are being assessed by an examiner, do things deliberately so
that you can be clearly seen to be doing the right thing. Students and
many doctors are being assessed continuously during their day-to-day
work, so there is much to be said for doing everything in a deliberate and
transparent way at all times.

The techniques of the physical examination are not covered in detail
in this *Oxford American Handbook of Clinical Diagnosis*. However, the
sequences of examination and documentation are described here. The
skills themselves are best learned by watching experts, copying them, and
practicing as much as possible. Consult books that specialize in describing
practical examination techniques in detail.

Watch others, read other books, and choose your own sequences.
Write out your chosen sequence on the blank pages provided here and
inside the front cover of this book if you wish. Write out your findings in
the patient's record in the same order, to reduce the chance of forgetting
something. However, in some centers you will be provided with a stan-
dardized form, which you will be expected to use.

The general examination

Before examining the patient, look for other clues, e.g., state of dress, nebulizer masks, sputum cups, medication packets, etc. The general examination is directed mainly at assessing the patient's appearance, demeanor, and state of distress; often, the skin and lymph nodes are considered here as well. Abnormal odors are also noted at this time, such as fruity breath in diabetic ketoacidosis, alcohol on the breath, the odors of urine or stool in incontinent patients.

During the history, the order of questioning could be decided entirely by thought processes (for example, probing indirectly for a symptom to chase up a diagnostic possibility that comes to mind), but the physical examination is different. It is more efficient to adopt a routine that is smooth and quick and not to jump about looking for physical signs that might support the diagnostic idea of that moment.

You have already been looking at the patient's face, general appearance, and immediate vicinity (e.g., walking stick, medication packets, etc.) when taking the history, so for the general examination, begin with the hands and work your way up by inspecting (and, when appropriate, palpating) the arms to the shoulders. Examine the patient's scalp, ears, eyes, cheeks, nose, and lips. Take the patient's temperature. Examine inside the patient's mouth, then the neck, breasts, axillae, and then the skin of the abdomen, legs, and feet.

Plan of the general physical examination

General exam
- Appearance
- Level of distress
- Odors

Hands, arms, and shoulders
- Fingernails
- Clubbing
- Finger nodules
- Finger joints deformity
- Rashes
- Pain and stiffness in the elbow, shoulder, neck

Head and neck
- Neck stiffness
- Patchy hair loss
- Eardrum redness
- Perforated eardrum

Eyes, face, and neck
- Facial redness, general appearance
- Red eye
- Iritis
- Conjunctival pallor
- Temperature—high or low
- Mouth lesions
- Lumps in the following areas:
  - Face
  - Submandibular region
  - Anterior neck
  - Anterior triangle of neck
  - Posterior triangle
  - Supraclavicular region

Trunk
- Breast discharge
- Nipple eczema
- Breast lumps
- Gynecomastia in males
- Axillary lymphadenopathy
- Sparse body hair
- Hirsutism
- Scar pigmentation
- Abdominal striae

Legs
- Inguinal and generalized lymphadenopathy
- Sacral, leg, and heel sores

Cardiovascular system

Think first of cardiac output and inspect and feel the hands for warmth or coldness. Feel the radial pulse, take the blood pressure and check the other pulses in the arms and neck. Next think of venous return and look at the jugular venous pressure (JVP). Then examine the heart itself (palpate, percuss, and then listen to it). Finally, consider cardiac output and venous return by feeling skin temperature, palpating pulses, and looking for congestion and edema of the legs, liver, and lungs.

Cardiac output
- Peripheral cyanosis
- Radial pulse
  - Rate
  - Rhythm (compare cardiac apex rate if irregular)
  - Amplitude
  - Vessel wall
- Compare pulses for volume and synchrony
  - Radial, brachial, carotid (femoral, popliteal, posterior and anterior tibials after examining the heart)
- Blood pressure (BP) standing and lying in right arm; repeat on left

Venous return
- Jugular venous pressure (JVP)

The heart itself
- Trachea displaced?
- Apex beat displaced?
- Parasternal heave
- Palpable thrill
- Auscultation
  - Rate, rhythm
  - Extra heart sounds
    —Gallops (S3, S4)
    —Systolic murmurs
    —Diastolic murmurs
    —Friction rubs

Cardiac output and venous return
- Skin temperature
- Posterior and anterior tibials, popliteal, femoral pulses
- Venous skin changes
- Vein abnormalities
- Calf swelling
- Leg edema
- Sacral edema
- Liver enlargement and hepatojugular reflux
- Basilar lung crackles

Respiratory system

Think of general respiratory structure and function. *Inspect* and think of oxygen and carbon dioxide levels, then the ventilation process, which depends on the chest wall and its movement. *Palpate* by feeling for tactile vocal fremitus. *Percuss* and then *auscultate*. Listen for wheezes and rhonchi, thus assessing airways from small (high pitched) to large (low pitched).

General inspection
- Tremor and muscle twitching
- Cyanosis of the tongue and lips
- Clubbing

Chest inspection
- Respiratory rate and depth
- Distorted chest wall
- Poor expansion
- Paradoxical movement

Palpation
- Mediastinum
  - Position of trachea
  - Position of apex beat

Tactile vocal fremitus
- Present or absent (or increased)
- Symmetry

Percussion
- Hyperresonant, resonant, normal, dull, or stony dull

Auscultation
- Diminished breath sounds
- Bronchial breathing
- Crackles
- Rubs
- Wheezes, rhonchi (high or low pitched or polyphonic, during inspiration or expiration or both)

Alimentary and genitourinary systems

Think first of metabolic issues related to general nutrition (obese, average, thin, cachexia) and ensure that the patient is weighed. Check the mucous membranes, e.g., for signs of vitamin deficiency. Look for nongastrointestinal (e.g., skin, eye) signs of hypovolemia and liver disease. Next turn your mind to anatomical aspects of the gastrointestinal (GI) and genitourinary (GU) systems together by inspecting, palpating, and auscultating. Finally, perform examinations (when indicated) that need special equipment.

Inspection
- Obesity
- Cachexia
- Oral lesions
- Jaundice
- Hepatic skin stigmata
- Loss of skin turgor
- Low eye tension

Palpation
- Supraclavicular nodes

Inspection of the abdomen
- Abdominal scars
- Veins
- General distension
- Visible peristalsis
- Poor movement

Palpation
- General tenderness
- Localized tenderness
- Hepatic enlargement
- Splenic enlargement
- Renal enlargement
- Abdominal masses

Percussion
- Dull or resonant
- Shifting dullness

Auscultation
- Silent abdomen
- Tinkling bowel sounds
- Bruits

Inspection and palpation again
- Groin lumps (lymph nodes?)
- Scrotal masses
- Rectal abnormalities
- Prostate exam
- Melena, fresh blood
- Vaginal and pelvic abnormalities

Nervous system

If there are no neurological symptoms or signs detected up to this point, then it is customary to perform an abbreviated examination. Comment on the fact that the patient was conscious and alert, speech was normal, and there were no cranial nerve abnormalities noted when looking at the face during the history and general examination. Also, you should be able to note the patient's gait and movements around the hospital bed or consultation room. According to the GALS system, note and record the *Gait*, appearance, and movement of the *Arms*, *Legs* and *Spine*.

If the patient was not conscious and alert, then the level of consciousness should be addressed with the Glasgow Coma Scale (GCS).

The brief neurological examination consists of checking coordination and reflexes (thus testing sensory and motor function of the nerves and central connections involved). The findings may be recorded as in Box 4.1.

Box 4.1 Short CNS examination

- Conscious and alert
- Speech normal
- Facial appearance and movement normal
- Finger–nose pointing normal
- Hand tapping and rotating normal
- Heel–toe test normal (ran heel from opposite knee to toe and back)
- Foot tapping (examiner's hand) normal

Reflexes	*Right*	*Left*
Biceps normal	+	+
Supinators normal	+	+
Triceps normal	+	+
Knees normal	+	+
Ankles normal	+	+
Plantars normally flexor	↓	↓

The full neurological assessment

The system of examination described here is typical. The blank pages are there for you to write your comments and amendments. The general approach is to assess the conscious level (if the patient is not conscious and alert, then it will not be possible to conduct a full neurological examination, which needs the patient's cooperation).

The cranial nerve sequence follows in their numbered sequence. Motor function can be assessed next, beginning with inspection for wasting and involuntary movements and then palpation, by testing tone and strength. The upper limbs are examined first and then the lower limbs. Sensation is then tested in the upper then lower limbs and, finally, coordination, reflexes, and gait.

The order can be changed by addressing the area of abnormality suggested by the history. For example, if the patient complains of difficulty in walking, then it would be sensible to examine gait, then motor function and sensory function, and cranial nerves last.

General
- Conscious level
- Glasgow Coma Score (GCS)
- Speech
- Gait abnormalities

Cranial nerves
- Absent sense of smell
- Visual field defects
- Decreased acuity
- Absent corneal reflex
- Loss of facial sensation
- Deviation of tongue
- Nystagmus
- Facial weakness
- Deafness
- Loss of taste
- Palatal weakness
- Neck or shoulder weakness

Eye
Opthalmoscopy
- Corneal opacity
- Lens opacity
- Papilledema
- Pale optic disc
- Cupped disc
- Hypertensive retinopathy
- Dot and blot hemorrhages
- New vessel formation
- Pale or black retinal patches

Other eye findings
- Ptosis
- Pupil
  - Constriction
  - Irregularities
  - Dilatation
- Diplopia

Motor function

Upper limbs
- Arm posture
- Hand tremor
- Wasting of hand
- Wasting of arm
- Tone abnormalities

Weakness of
- Shoulder abduction
- Elbow flexion
- Elbow extension
- Wrist extension
- Handgrip
- Finger adduction and abduction
- Thumb abduction and opposition
- Arm incoordination

Lower limbs
- Limitation of movement
- Wasting
- Fasciculation
- Tone abnormalities

Weakness of
- Hip flexion
- Knee extension and flexion
- Foot
  - Plantar flexion
  - Dorsiflexion
  - Eversion
- Bilateral spastic paraparesis
- Spastic hemiparesis

Sensation
Upper limb sensation
- Hypesthesia of
  - Palm
  - Dorsum hand
  - Lateral arm
  - Ulnar border arm
- Dissociated sensory loss
- Progressive sensory loss
- Cortical sensory loss

Lower limb
- Hypesthesia of
  - Inguinal area
  - Anterior thigh
  - Shin
  - Lateral foot
- Progressive downward loss
- Dissociated sensory loss
- Multiple areas of loss

Reflexes
- Brisk or diminished in biceps, supinator, triceps, knee, ankle, and plantars
- Abnormal reflexes: Babinski

Mental status examination

Think of the sequence of perception, affect, drive and arousal, cognitive processes (check memory of different duration, ability to reason with that memory and then the nature of beliefs arrived at with such reasoning), and then actions in response to these:

- *Perception:* attentiveness and any hallucination, visual or auditory
- *Mood:* depression or elation
- *Mental:* rate of speech, level of anxiety
- *Cognition* (6/10 or less correct implies impairment)
- *Orientation:* time to nearest hour, year, address of hospital
- *Short-term memory:* repeat a given name and address, name 2 staff
- *Long-term memory:* own age, date of birth, current president, dates of wars
- *Concentration:* count backwards from 20 to 1
- *Beliefs:* patient's perception and insight of health, self-confidence, any extreme convictions
- *Activity:* physical and social activity, employment, physical signs of drug use

Writing out the examination findings

At the end of the history in the previous chapter, the patient was thought to have

- ? Viral pharyngitis
- ? Infectious mononucleosis
- ? Acute follicular tonsillitis
- ? Agranulocytosis due to carbimazole
- ?? Meningococcal meningitis
- Inadequate domestic support currently for acute illness
- ?? Undiscovered type 2 diabetes mellitus

The physical examination in such a patient would focus on findings that may occur in any of the possible diagnoses brought to mind by the history. If they are absent, this absence is specified, together with all positive findings. The positive and negative findings may be written out as follows.

Looks unwell, flushed
Wt not recorded
Temperature 38.5°C, Pulse 100, BP 105/60

Head, eyes, ears, nose, throat (HEENT)/NECK

Bilaterally swollen tonsils, large red with small white patches
Bilateral tender multiple lymph node enlargement in neck. No lymph node swelling in axillae or groins

Cardiovascular system (CVS)

Pulse 110/min regular low volume
BP 100/60
Heart sounds normal
No murmurs

Respiratory system (RS)

Chest shape and movement normal
Breath sounds normal

GI system

Not jaundiced
Liver 1 finger breadth below costal margin
Spleen not palpable

Central nervous system (CNS)

Conscious and alert
No neck stiffness
Hand and leg coordination normal
Reflexes all normal and symmetrical

The problem list and positive-finding summary

It is customary to summarize the history and examination by listing the positive findings or presenting them in a brief summary. This is how clinical problems are posed in journals and examinations. If negative findings are added, then they give an indication of what the writer was thinking. There is a place for this in a case presentation, but the problem list or positive finding summary is a preliminary device.

Note that a few laboratory findings are also included in the list below for completeness. Although these were not discussed above under history or physical exam, they are included in problem lists.

Problem list
- Severe sore throat for 2 days
- Sweats for 2 days
- Severe malaise for 2 days
- Hyperthyroid 2 months ago (now taking carbimazole)
- Lives alone in a flat
- Unwell, flushed
- Temperature 38.5°C
- *Bilaterally swollen tonsils, large and red with small white patches*
- Bilateral tender, multiple–lymph node enlargement in neck
- *Urine testing: + glycosuria*
- *WBC 18.3 × 10³/mm³, neutrophils 90%*

A clear differential diagnosis may well have occurred to the writer by now (some were already being considered at the end of the history). If this is not the case, then the next step is to look at this problem list and consider which feature(s) will be associated with the shortest list of possible causes—the best leads. These are shown in bold italics.

Looking up the lead

A glance at the following extract from Chapter 5 will suggest immediately that the patient probably has acute follicular tonsillitis, but this may be associated with agranulocytosis. The neutrophil cell count is an important deciding factor. It is high, which by definition excludes agranulocytosis and makes a viral infection and infectious mononucleosis unlikely (where there is usually a lymphocytosis). However, in some cases, no streptococcus is found on the swab culture, leaving a question over the definitive diagnosis.

Red pharynx and tonsils

Some differential diagnoses and typical outline evidence

Viral tonsillitis	*Suggested by:* enlarged red mass(es) lateral to back of tongue without white patches
	Confirmed by: clinical appearance, fever, and normal or slightly ↓ WBC and relative lymphocytosis
Acute follicular tonsillitis complicated by peritonsillar abcess (quinsy), scarlet fever, retropharyngeal abscess	*Suggested by:* enlarged red mass(es) lateral to back of tongue with small white patches ("strawberries and cream")
	Confirmed by: clinical appearance and fever (usually high). ↑↑ WBC. Bacterial culture of streptococcus
Infectious mononucleosis due to Epstein–Barr virus	*Suggested by:* very severe throat pain with enlarged tonsils covered with creamy or gray membrane. Petechiae on palate. Profound malaise. Generalized lymphadenopathy, splenomegaly. Lymphocytosis
	Confirmed by: heterophile antibody test positive. Viral titers
Agranulo-cytosis (e.g., caused by carbimazole)	*Suggested by:* sore throat, background history of taking a drug or contact with noxious substance
	Confirmed by: low or absent neutrophil count
Meningococcal meningitis	*Suggested by:* sore throat, red pharynx without purulent patches, neck stiffness and positive Kernig's sign. High blood neutrophil count
	Confirmed by: lumbar puncture showing pus or neutrophil count and organisms on microscopy or culture

The working diagnoses

The finding of white patches on red tonsils occurs commonly in acute follicular tonsillitis but less commonly in infectious mononucleosis or anything else, including viral pharyngitis, thus making other conditions improbable. Despite all of this, it is still possible that there could be agranulocytosis due to carbimazole sensitivity. However, the raised leukocyte count with 90% neutrophils excludes this diagnosis because a low or absent WBC is obviously a necessary condition for the diagnosis of agranulocytosis. There is no need, therefore, to stop the carbimazole immediately.

The glycosuria and random blood sugar of 151 mg/dL makes the diagnosis of diabetes mellitus (DM) probable. If the patient has no symptoms of diabetes and an active intercurrent illness (as in this case), two fasting sugars >126 mg/dL would be needed to satisfy the World Health Organization (WHO) criteria so that the diagnosis would be acceptable to other doctors.

Look at the other positive findings and consider if they would all resolve if the acute follicular tonsillitis resolved. Use common sense, experience, and imagination from your knowledge of physiology. The only remaining problems would be the glycosuria, prior thyrotoxicosis, and the patient living alone when very ill.

The main *working diagnosis* therefore is
• Acute follicular tonsillitis

The other diagnoses are
• Probable type II diabetes mellitus
• Controlled thyrotoxicosis
• Inadequate home care

The plan is
• Start
  • Penicillin V 500 mg four times a day (qid)
  • Acetaminophen 650 mg qid
• Continue
  • Carbimazole 5 mg once a day (qd)
• Help patient to contact family

General examination physical signs

General principles

The findings discussed here are presented in a sequence of the general examination. While taking the patient's history you will be looking at the patient's face. If you are asked to look at the hands, look at the patient's face and note any recognizable features of significance as you introduce yourself and greet the patient. Then begin with the fingernails and joints, backs and fronts of the hands, arms, and elbows, moving up to the neck and scalp, then down to the face, mouth, throat, breasts, axillae, trunk, and groin. Note any skin abnormalities.

Fingernail abnormality

Classify fingernail changes by naming them first. Some have very few causes.

Classification

Clubbing due to many causes (see pp. 76–77)	*Suggested by*: angle lost between nail and finger (no gap when nails of same finger on both hand apposed, bogginess of nail bed, increased nail curvature both longitudinally and transversely, and drumstick finger appearance). *Confirmed by*: see p. 76
Terry's lines due to many causes (see p. 78)	*Suggested by*: nail tips having dark pink or brown bands *Confirmed by*: see next page (p. 78)
Nail fold infarcts due to vasculitis due to many causes (see next page, 79)	*Suggested by*: dark blue-black areas in nail fold *Confirmed by*: see next page (p. 79)
Koilonychia due to iron deficiency anemia (occasionally ischemic heart disease [IHD] or syphilis)	*Suggested by*: spoon-shaped nails *Confirmed by*: ↓*Hb*, ↓*ferritin* from iron deficiency (basal or exercise ECG for IHD; *serology* for syphilis)
Onycholysis due to psoriasis, hyperthyroidism	*Suggested by*: nail thickened, dystrophic, and separated from the nail bed *Confirmed by*: clinical appearance and evidence of cause, e.g., skin changes of psoriasis or ↑FT4 (free T4), ± ↑FT3 (free T4) and ↓TSH (thyroid-stimulating hormone)
Beau's lines due to any period of severe illness	*Suggested by*: transverse furrows *Confirmed by*: history of associated condition
Longitudinal lines due to lichen planus, alopecia areata, Darier's disease	*Suggested by*: transverse furrows (ending in triangular nicks and nail dystrophy in Darier's disease)

Onychomedesis due to any period of severe illness	*Suggested by:* shedding of nail *Confirmed by:* history of associated condition
Muehrcke's lines due to hypo-albuminemia	*Suggested by:* paired white, parallel, transverse bands *Confirmed by:* serum albumin <2.0 g/dL
Nail pitting due to psoriasis and alopecia areata	*Suggested by:* small holes in nail *Confirmed by:* rash on extensor surfaces with silvery scales (psoriasis) or circumscribed areas of hair loss (alopecia areata)
Splinter hemorrhages due to infective endocarditis (sometimes due to manual labor)	*Suggested by:* fine, longitudinal hemorrhagic streaks under the nail *Confirmed by:* history of manual labor (or fever, changing heart murmurs, and bacterial growth on several ***blood cultures***)
Chronic paronychia due to chronic infection of nail bed	*Suggested by:* red, swollen, and thickened skin in nail fold *Confirmed by:* response to antibiotics (erythromycin for bacterial infection or nystatin for fungal infection)
Mees' lines due to arsenic poisoning or renal failure, Hodgkin's disease, heart failure	*Suggested by:* single, white, transverse bands *Confirmed by:* presence of associated conditions
Yellow nails due to lymphedema, bronchiectasis, hypoalbuminemia	*Suggested by:* color *Confirmed by:* presence of associated condition

Clubbing

Clubbing is present when the angle is lost between the nail and finger; alternatively, there is no gap when the nails of the same finger on both hands are apposed.

Some differential diagnoses and typical outline evidence

Subacute bacterial endocarditis	*Suggested by:* general malaise, weight loss, fever, PMH of heart valve disease or congenital heart disease, heart murmurs
	Confirmed by: growth on **blood cultures** of organism, e.g., *Streptococcus viridans*, etc. Endocardial vegetations (but not always) on **echocardiography**
Cyanotic congenital heart disease	*Suggested by:* long past history, central cyanosis
	Confirmed by: **echocardiography**
Lung carcinoma	*Suggested by:* malaise, increased cough, weight loss, hemoptysis. Smoking history. Opacity (suggestive of mass, ± pneumonia ± effusion) on **chest X-ray (CXR)** and **computerized tomography (CT) scan**
	Confirmed by: **Bronchoscopy** appearances and histology
Bronchiectasis	*Suggested by:* chronic cough, productive of copious purulent, often rusty-colored sputum
	Confirmed by: **CXR** and **CT scan** appearances (thickened tram line [dilated] bronchi). **Bronchoscopy** appearances
Lung abscess	*Suggested by:* cough, very ill, spiking fever, PMH of lung disease
	Confirmed by: **CXR**: mass containing fluid level (air above pus)
Empyema	*Suggested by:* cough, very ill, fever, stony dull over one lung
	Confirmed by: high neutrophil WBC. **CXR**: long opacity on one view. Aspiration of pus, culture and sensitivity

Pulmonary fibrosis	*Suggested by:* cough, fine crackles, especially bases
	Confirmed by: **CXR**: bilateral diffuse nodular shadows or honeycombing (late finding)
Cirrhosis	*Suggested by:* long history of alcohol intake, ascites, prominent abdominal veins. In males: spider nevi, Gynecomastia
	Confirmed by: ↓*serum albumin*, abnormal *liver function tests (LFTs)* and ↑ bilirubin (sometimes). *Liver biopsy* findings
Crohn's disease	*Suggested by:* history of chronic diarrhea and abdominal pain, low weight
	Confirmed by: **colonoscopy** and biopsy, **barium** enema and **barium meal** and follow-through
Ulcerative colitis	*Suggested by:* history of intermittent diarrhea with blood and mucus, low weight
	Confirmed by: **colonoscopy** and biopsy

Terry's lines: dark pink or brown bands on nails

Some differential diagnoses and typical outline evidence

Cirrhosis	*Suggested by:* long history of alcohol intake, ascites, prominent abdominal veins. In males: spider nevi, gynecomastia
	Confirmed by: ↓*serum albumin,* abnormal *liver function tests* and ↑ bilirubin (sometimes). *Liver biopsy* findings
Congestive cardiac failure	*Suggested by:* dyspnea, orthopnea, paroxysmal nocturnal dyspnea (PND), ↑JVP, gallop rhythm, basal inspiratory crackles, ankle edema
	Confirmed by: **CXR** and echocardiography
Diabetes mellitus	*Suggested by:* thirst, polydipsia, polyuria, fatigue, FH
	Confirmed by: **fasting blood glucose** ≥120 mg/dL on two occasions OR fasting, random or glucose tolerance test (GTT) glucose ≥200 mg/dL once only with symptoms
Cancer somewhere	*Suggested by:* weight loss and anorexia with symptoms developing over months, bone pain
	Confirmed by: careful history, examination, CXR, complete blood count (CBC), erythrocyte sedimentation rate (ESR), and follow-up
Old age	*Suggested by:* age >75 years
	Confirmed by: normal follow-up

Vasculitic nodules on fingers

These nodules and dark lines in nail folds are focal areas of infarction, which suggest local vasculitis.

Some differential diagnoses and typical outline evidence

Systemic lupus erythematosus	*Suggested by:* swelling of distal interphalangeal (DIP) joints, any other large joints, malar rash, pleural effusion, especially in Afro-Caribbean females. Multisystem dysfunction
	Confirmed by: CBC: ↓Hb (hemoglobin), ↓WBC. ESR: ↑ or ↑CRP (C-reactive protein) *Anti-nuclear antibody* positive, especially if directed at *double-stranded DNA*
Subacute bacterial endocarditis (Osler nodes)	*Suggested by:* general malaise, pallor, low-grade fever, changing heart murmurs
	Confirmed by: CBC: ↓Hb, ↑WBC. ESR: ↑↑, ↑↑CRP. Growth of streptococci, e.g., *S. viridans* after *serial blood cultures*

Hand arthropathy

Look at the finger joints (the interphalangeal [IP] joints), the knuckles (metacarpophalangeal [MCP] joints), and compare them. Finally, look at the wrist.

Some differential diagnoses and typical outline evidence

Primary (post-menopausal) osteoarthritis	*Suggested by:* Heberden's nodes (paired bony nodes on terminal IP joints)
	Confirmed by: **X-ray** appearances of affected joints
Rheumatoid arthritis	*Suggested by:* swelling and deformity of phalangeal joints (with ulnar deviation) and wrist, rheumatoid nodules
	Confirmed by: positive **rheumatoid factor**. **X-ray** appearances of affected joints
Psoriatic arthropathy	*Suggested by:* swelling and deformity of distal (or all) IP joints
	Confirmed by: dry rash with silvery scales (especially near elbow extensor surface). **X-ray** appearances of affected joints
Systemic lupus erythematosus	*Suggested by:* swelling and deformity of all (or distal) IP joints, butterfly facial rash, signs of pleural or pericardial effusion, renal impairment
	Confirmed by: positive **anti-nuclear factor, double-stranded DNA antibodies**

Hand and upper limb rashes

Look at the back of the hands and forearm, the palms and forearm elbow flexures, the extensor surface of the elbows, and then the upper arm.

Some differential diagnoses and typical outline evidence

Atopic eczema	*Suggested by:* vesicles, erythema, scaling, lichenification, fissures on flexor surfaces, wrists, palms. FH
	Confirmed by: no evidence of contact precipitant
Contact dermatitis and irritant	*Suggested by:* vesicles, erythema, scaling, lichenification, fissures related to contact with chemical or object, e.g., oil, nickel alloy
	Confirmed by: response by improvement on removal of precipitant (and recurrence with re-exposure)
Psoriasis	*Suggested by:* dry rash with silvery scales (especially near elbow extensor surface)
	Confirmed by: clinical appearance if obvious, otherwise, **histology**

Lumps around the elbow

Inspect and, with care not to hurt, palpate around the elbow.

Some differential diagnoses and typical outline evidence

Osteoarthritis	*Suggested by:* joint deformity, intermittent pain and swelling, paired Heberden's nodes over distal IP joints in primary osteoarthritis
	Confirmed by: clinical appearance usually. If there are doubts, negative **rheumatoid factor, X-ray** shows loss of joint space (due to atrophy of cartilage)
Rheumatoid nodules	*Suggested by:* mobile subcutaneous nodule
	Confirmed by: history or joint changes of rheumatoid arthritis and positive **rheumatoid factor**
Xanthomatosis	*Suggested by:* pale subcutaneous plaques attached to underlying tendon
	Confirmed by: **hyperlipidemia** on blood testing
Gouty tophi	*Suggested by:* irregular hard nodules, risk factors or PMH of gout
	Confirmed by: ↑**plasma urate. Biopsy:** urate crystals present

Neck stiffness

Distinguish between limited range of neck movement and neck stiffness throughout range of movement.
• Limited neck range of movement

Some differential diagnoses and typical outline evidence

Chronic cervical spondylitis with osteophytes	*Suggested by:* no fever or associated symptoms *Confirmed by:* limitation in range of neck movement but no stiffness within free range of movement. Normal WBC, no fever, no neurological signs, X-ray appearance of neck

• Neck stiffness throughout range of movement

Bacterial meningitis	*Suggested by:* gradual headache over days, photophobia, vomiting. Fever, high neutrophil count. Petechial rash in meningococcal meningitis *Confirmed by:* **lumbar puncture**: turbid cerebrospinal fluid (CSF). ↑CSF neutrophil count with ↓ glucose. Bacteria on microscopy. Growth of bacteria on culture of CSF
Viral meningitis	*Suggested by:* gradual headache over days. Fever, high lymphocyte count, normal neutrophil count *Confirmed by:* **lumbar puncture**: clear CSF. ↑CSF lymphocyte count with normal glucose. No bacteria on microscopy. No growth of bacteria on CSF culture
Meningismus due to viral infection	*Suggested by:* gradual headache over days. Fever, high lymphocyte count, normal neutrophil count *Confirmed by:* **lumbar puncture**: clear CSF. Normal CSF white cell count. No bacteria on microscopy. No growth of bacteria on CSF culture
Subarachnoid hemorrhage	*Suggested by:* sudden onset of headache over seconds. Variable degree of consciousness. No fever. Normal white cell count *Confirmed by:* CT or magnetic resonance imaging (MRI) **brain scan. Lumbar puncture**: blood-stained CSF that does not clear in successive bottle collection, or presence of xanthochromia in CSF (12 hours to 2 weeks after hemorrhage)

Acute cervical spondylitis	*Suggested by:* gradual neck pain (occasionally a headache) over hours or days. Immobile neck. Usually past history of similar episodes. No fever
	Confirmed by: above history
Posterior fossa tumor	*Suggested by:* headache, papilledema
	Confirmed by: **CT** or **MRI scan** appearances
Anxiety with semi-voluntary resistance	*Suggested by:* improvement with reassurance or temporary distraction
	Confirmed by: resolution after rest and observation

Hair loss in a specific area

Examine overall and then gently part hair to examine the scalp. Use a magnifying glass if hair is abnormal.

Some differential diagnoses and typical outline evidence

Alopecia areata	*Suggested by:* well-circumscribed loss with exclamation-mark hairs
	Confirmed by: above clinical appearance
Alopecia totalis	*Suggested by:* total hair loss on head and body
	Confirmed by: above clinical appearance
Polycystic ovary syndrome	*Suggested by:* bitemporal recession and occipital thinning. Hirsutism on trunk. Onset near puberty. Obesity
	Confirmed by: ↑ testosterone and ↓SHBG (sex hormone-binding globulin). ↑LH (luteinizing hormone), ovarian ultrasound
Testosterone-secreting ovarian tumor	*Suggested by:* bitemporal recession and occipital thinning. Rapid onset over months
	Confirmed by: ↑↑ testosterone and ↓LH, ovarian ultrasound scan and laparoscopy

Diffuse hair loss

Examine trunk, pubic, and limb hair too.

Some differential diagnoses and typical outline evidence

Cytotoxic drugs	*Suggested by:* mainly head hair loss. History of recent cytotoxic drugs
	Confirmed by: improvement after stopping cytotoxic drug
Iron deficiency	*Suggested by:* mainly head hair loss. Koilonychia, pallor of conjunctive
	Confirmed by: ↓Hb, ↓MCV (mean corpuscular volume), ↓MCHC (mean corpuscular hemoglobin concentration), ↓ ferritin
Severe illness	*Suggested by:* mainly head hair loss. History of recent severe illness
	Confirmed by: improvement with restoration of health
Hypogonadism	*Suggested by:* loss of hair from axilla, pubic area
	Confirmed by: testosterone ↓ or estrogen ↓ with FSH ↑ and ↑LH in primary gonadal failure; ↓LH or normal, ↓FSH or normal in secondary hypogonadism
Recent pregnancy	*Suggested by:* mainly head hair loss. Recent pregnancy
	Confirmed by: improvement after delivery

External ear abnormalities

Inspect the pinna for scars and other abnormalities. Examine the auditory meatus by first pulling the pinna up and back to straighten the cartilaginous bend. (In infants, the pinna is pulled back and down.) Swab any discharge, and remove any wax.

Some differential diagnoses and typical outline evidence

Congenital anomalies	*Suggested by:* accessory tags, auricles and preauricular pit, sinus, or fistula and atresia
	Confirmed by: above clinical appearances
Infected preauricular sinus	*Suggested by:* looking like infected sebaceous cyst
	Confirmed by: deep tract that lies close to the facial nerve
Chondrodermatitis nodularis chronica helicis	*Suggested by:* painful nodular lesions on the upper margin of the pinna in men
	Confirmed by: excision of skin and underlying cartilage
Pinna hematoma resulting in a "cauliflower" ear	*Suggested by:* history of blunt trauma
	Confirmed by: appearance of bleeding in the subperichondrial plane that elevates the perichondrium to form a hematoma
Exostosis (localized bony hypertrophy) may cause build-up of wax or debris or conductive deafness	*Confirmed by:* smooth, often multiple (bilateral) swellings of the bony ear canals
Wax (cerumen) may cause conductive deafness if it impacts	*Suggested by:* dark brown, shiny, soft mass
	Confirmed by: improvement in hearing after removal
Foreign bodies in the ear	*Suggested by:* visible foreign body and inflammation (in child or learning-disabled patient)
	Confirmed by: retrieval of foreign body

Painful ear

Consider referred pain from the neck (C3, C4, and C5), throat, and teeth and examine these as well. Insert the largest comfortable aural speculum gently.

Some differential diagnoses and typical outline evidence

Otitis externa (swimmer's ear) due to eczema, psoriasis, trauma, Pseudomonas, fungal infection	*Suggested by:* pain, discharge, and tragal tenderness *Confirmed by:* acute inflammation of the skin of the meatus, ***culture*** of swab
Malignant necrotizing otitis externa	*Suggested by:* pain, discharge, and tragal tenderness in a diabetic, elderly, or immunosuppressed person, facial palsy *Confirmed by:* ***X-ray*** showing local bone erosion, nuclear bone scan, and tagged white cell scan
Furunculosis (staphylococcal abscess in hair follicle) often diabetic	*Suggested by:* acutely painful throbbing ear *Confirmed by:* appearance of a boil in the meatus
Bullous myringitis (associated with influenza infection or Mycoplasma pneumoniae)	*Suggested by:* extremely painful hemorrhagic blisters on the drum and deep meatal skin, and fluid behind the drum *Confirmed by:* above clinical appearance
Barotrauma (aerotitis)	*Suggested by:* history of ear pain during descent in an aircraft or in diving *Confirmed by:* relief by decompression (e.g., holding nose and swallowing)
Temporomandibular joint dysfunction	*Suggested by:* earache, facial pain, and joint clicking or popping related to malocclusion, teeth-grinding or joint derangement, and stress *Confirmed by:* tenderness exacerbated by lateral movement of the open jaw, or trigger points in the pterygoids

Ear discharge

Examine the eardrum quadrants in turn. Note color, translucency, and any bulging or retraction of the membrane. Note size, position, and site (marginal or central) of any perforations. Drum movement during a Valsalva maneuver also depends on a patient's Eustachian tube.

Some differential diagnoses and typical outline evidence

Acute otitis media (due to pneumococcus, hemophilus, streptococcus, and staphylococcus, occasionally complicated by mastoiditis)	*Suggested by:* rapid onset over hours of pain and fever, irritability, anorexia, or vomiting after viral upper respiratory tract infection *Confirmed by:* bulging red drum or profuse purulent discharge for 48 hours after drum perforates
Otitis media with effusion (serous, secretory, or glue ear) usually in young children	*Suggested by:* gradual onset over weeks or months of deafness and intermittent ear pain *Confirmed by:* loss of drum's light reflex or retraction relieved by grommets
Chronic suppurative otitis media (may be associated with cholesteatoma, petrositis, labyrinthitis; facial palsy; meningitis; intracranial abscess)	*Suggested by:* purulent discharge, hearing loss, but no pain *Confirmed by:* central drum perforation
Cholesteatoma (locally destructive stratified squamous epithelium)	*Suggested by:* foul discharge, deafness, headache, ear pain, facial paralysis, and vertigo *Confirmed by:* continuing mucopurulent discharge, pearly white soft matter (keratin) in attic or posterior marginal perforation

Chronic otitis externa	*Suggested by:* watery discharge, itching
	Confirmed by: erythema and weeping of meatus
Auditory canal trauma	*Suggested by:* bloody discharge
	Confirmed by: history of trauma, laceration, and erythema
CSF otorrhea	*Suggested by:* history of head or facial trauma or surgery
	Confirmed by: halo sign on filter paper

Striking facial appearance

This is best recognized when meeting the patient for the first time, but there is a wide normal variation.

Some differential diagnoses and typical outline evidence

Parkinson's disease	*Suggested by:* mask-like (akinetic) face ± hand or head tremor
	Confirmed by: response to dopaminergic drugs
Chorea (Huntington's chorea or drug effect)	*Suggested by:* choreiform—jerky, purposeless facial movement or athetosis (writhing facial movement)
	Confirmed by: Family history, or response to withdrawal of drug or dose reduction (if due to drug effect)
Bilateral upper motor neuron lesion (due to amyotrophic lateral sclerosis, cerebrovascular disease, myasthenia gravis)	*Suggested by:* paucity of movement of face
	Confirmed by: other features of cause and *MRI* or *CT scan*
Thyrotoxicosis	*Suggested by:* anxious looking with lid retraction and lag
	Confirmed by: ↓TSH and ↑T3 or ↑T4 or both
Hypothyroidism	*Suggested by:* puffy face, obesity, cold intolerance, tiredness, constipation, bradycardia
	Confirmed by: ↑TSH, ↓FT4
Acromegaly	*Suggested by:* large, wide face, embossed forehead, jutting jaw (prognathism), widely spaced teeth and large tongue
	Confirmed by: insulin-like growth factor (IGF) ↑. Failure to suppress growth hormone (GH) to <2 mU/L with *oral GTT*. *Skull X-ray* confirms bony abnormalities. *Hand X-ray* shows typical tufts on terminal phalanges. *MRI* or *CT scan* showing enlarged pituitary fossa

Cushing's syndrome pituitary-driven Cushing's disease, or autonomous adrenal Cushing's, or glucocorticoid therapy	*Suggested by:* round, florid face (and trunk with purple striae) with thin arms, legs, and hirsutism. Inability to rise from squatting position (due to proximal myopathy) *Confirmed by:* midnight cortisol ↑ and/or failure to suppress on dexamethasone, or drug history of glucocorticoids

Proptosis of eye(s) or exophthalmos

A prominent eye is suggested by sclera showing between the cornea and upper lid margin; this may also result from lid retraction due to sympathetic overactivity or lung disease. If in doubt, look down on eyes from above. (In myopia there is a large eyeball but the sclera is not visible.)

Some differential diagnoses and typical outline evidence

Ophthalmic Graves' disease (± thyrotoxicosis)	*Suggested by:* bilateral (usually) exophthalmos, goiter, pretibial myxedem,a and lid retraction
	Confirmed by: titer of thyroid antibodies ↑↑ (with ↓TSH or normal, and T3 or T4 ↑ or normal). CT scan appearance
Orbital cellulitis (medical emergency)	*Suggested by:* pain, fever, unilateral lid swelling, decreased vision and double vision. Neurological signs in advanced disease
	Confirmed by: **CT** or **MRI scan** appearance and response to antibiotics
Corticocavernous fistula	*Suggested by:* unilateral engorgement of eye surface vessels, lid and conjunctiva, pulsatile with bruit over eye.
	Confirmed by: **CT** or **MRI scan** appearance
Orbital tumors— rarely primary, often secondary, especially isthiocytosis	*Suggested by:* unilateral proptosis and displacement of the eyeball. Lymph node, liver, or spleen enlargement
	Confirmed by: **CT** or **MRI scan** appearance

Red eye

Gritty pain suggests an external cause. Aching pain suggests an internal cause. Light sensitivity always accompanies inflammation in the eye. Fluoresceine (Fl) yellow dye glows green with a blue examination light and stains all epithelial breaks.

Some differential diagnoses and typical outline evidence

Spontaneous subconjunctival hemorrhage	*Suggested by:* painless, bright red area on conjunctiva (oxygenated blood) and no light sensitivity
	Confirmed by: clinical appearance and resolution over days. No Fl staining of cornea (not done often)
Conjunctivitis due to bacterial infection	*Suggested by:* red eyes, dilated blood vessels on the eyeball and tarsal (lid) conjunctiva with a purulent discharge ± bilateral ± gritty pain
	Confirmed by: above clinical appearance. Not light sensitive and no Fl stain of cornea
Conjunctivitis due to viral infection	*Suggested by:* red eyes with dilated vessels on the eyeball only, sometimes in one quadrant around the cornea with a watery "tap-running" discharge. Gritty pain ± impaired vision
	Confirmed by: Fl stain showing dendritic (branching) pattern and resolution with topical antiviral
Conjunctivitis due to allergy	*Suggested by:* red eyes with pink, swollen conjunctiva and white, stringy mucoid discharge
	Confirmed by: no Fl stain and no visual loss and resolution with chromoglycate (over 6 weeks) or steroid eye drops
Corneal ulcer (ulcerative keratitis) due to abrasion or herpes simplex, Pseudomonas, Candida, Aspergillus, protozoa	*Suggested by:* painful, light-sensitive, deeply red eye with yellowish abscess in the cornea. Purulent discharge
	Confirmed by: slit-lamp examination after **fluoresceine instillation** showing hypopyon (pus in the eye)

Episcleritis	*Suggested by:* localized red eye with superficial vessel dilatation. Mild pain. No visual loss or light sensitivity
	Confirmed by: Instillation of one drop of phenylephrine 2.5% causing a blanching of the lesion
Scleritis	*Suggested by:* localized area of dark red, dilated, superficial and deep vessel on the sclera with aching pain and tenderness
	Confirmed by: failure to blanch with one drop of 2.5% phenylephrine
Acute closed-angle glaucoma (emergency)	*Suggested by:* severely painful red eyeball with marked visual loss, accompanied by nausea and vomiting ± history of haloes around lights and severe headache with blurred vision
	Confirmed by: dull gray cornea, nonreacting and irregular pupil with raised ocular pressures
Iritis or uveitis (see p. 96)	*Suggested by:* redness around cornea and haze in front of iris and severe light sensitivity (photophobia)
	Confirmed by: small, nonreacting and irregular pupil. Slit-lamp examination showing flare, cells, and hypopyon (pus in eye)

Iritis (anterior uveitis)

Redness in the cornea next to the iris (circumcorneal injection) occurs, with a muddy appearance of fluid in front of the iris.

Some differential diagnoses and typical outline evidence

Trauma (usually surgical)	*Suggested by:* impact accident, recent surgery
	Confirmed by: slit-lamp examination showing blood in the front of the eye and D-shaped distortion of the pupil if torn from its base or perforation if the pupil is pointing
Infection: herpes simplex, zoster, TB, syphilis, leprosy, protozoa, fungi	*Suggested by:* general malaise, fever, leukocytosis
	Confirmed by: **bacteriological culture** of eye swab or **viral immunology**
Autoimmune diseases: ankylosing spondylitis, Reiter's disease, juvenile chronic arthritis, immune ocular disease	*Suggested by:* arthritis, anemia, no obvious fever, raised ESR
	Confirmed by: **immunology** (seronegative for rheumatoid factor). **Protein electrophoresis**
Sarcoidosis	*Suggested by:* history of dry cough, breathlessness, malaise, fatigue, weight loss, enlarged lacrimal glands, erythema nodosum. Raised serum angiotensin converting enzyme (ACE)
	Confirmed by: **CXR** appearances (e.g., bilateral lymphadenopathy), **tissue biopsy** showing non-caseating granuloma. Slit lamp shows large keratic precipitates
Ulcerative colitis	*Suggested by:* history of diarrhea with mucus and blood
	Confirmed by: **colonoscopy** and **histology of biopsy**
Crohn's disease	*Suggested by:* history of abdominal pain, diarrhea, weight loss
	Confirmed by: **colonoscopy, barium enema** and **meal** and follow-through

Clinical anemia

This is often noticed as subconjunctival pallor (± face, nail, and palmar pallor).

Some differential diagnoses and typical outline evidence

Microcytic due to iron deficiency, thalassemia, etc. (see p. 433)	*Suggested by:* history of blood loss or FH of hemoglobinopathy (especially in patients of Mediterranean origin) and sideroblastic anemia
	Confirmed by: CBC: ↓Hb and ↓MCV, in thalassemia ↓↓MCV
Macrocytic (see p. 434)	*Suggested by:* FH of pernicious anemia, antifolate, and cytotoxic drugs or alcohol
	Confirmed by: CBC: ↓Hb and ↑MCV. *Film:* hypersegmented polymorphs in B_{12} deficiency
Normocytic (see p. 435)	*Suggested by:* history of chronic intercurrent illness, e.g., chronic renal failure, anemia of chronic disease, etc.
	Confirmed by: CBC: ↓Hb and MCV normal
Hypoplastic or aplastic	*Suggested by:* gradual onset without blood loss and potentially causal medication
	Confirmed by: CBC: ↓Hb and MCV normal and **bone marrow** atrophic
Leukemia	*Suggested by:* gradual onset and large spleen or lymph node (LN) (can fall ill suddenly with rapid deterioration in acute leukemia)
	Confirmed by: ↓Hb and MCV normal, ↑↑WBC, and bone marrow replaced by leukemic cells

Fever

Temperature is >37°C (99°F). Fever is not a good lead. The causes suggested here are broad.

Some differential diagnoses and typical outline evidence

Infection	*Suggested by:* low-grade or high fever with raised white cell count and usually symptoms and signs pointing to a focus
	Confirmed by: **serology ± cultures** of blood and other body fluids
Thrombus, tissue necrosis, neoplasm, autoimmune diseases, drugs	*Suggested by:* low-grade fever, history of severe illness or trauma
	Confirmed by: specific tests, e.g., **CXR, Doppler ultrasound scan of leg veins**

Possible hypothermia

Temperature is <35°C (95°F)—but confirm with low-reading thermometer—it could be lower. Also confirm with rectal temperature.

Some differential diagnoses and typical outline evidence

True hypothermia due to prolonged exposure to cold or hypothyroidism	*Suggested by:* history of immersion or cold-weather exposure. Temperature <35°C (95°F) with low-reading rectal thermometer
	Confirmed by: temperature chart using low-reading rectal thermometer

Mouth lesions

Examine lips, buccal mucosa, teeth, tongue, tonsils, and pharynx.

Some differential diagnoses and typical outline evidence

Local aphthous ulcers	*Suggested by:* red, painful ulcer with associated lymph node enlargement
	Confirmed by: spontaneous resolution within days
Local infection and gingivitis	*Suggested by:* vesicles in herpes simplex, creamy white plaques in oral candidiasis
	Confirmed by: spontaneous resolution or after antibiotic or antifungal treatment within days
Carious teeth	*Suggested by:* intermittent toothache, broken and/or severely discolored teeth
	Confirmed by: formal dental examination
Traumatic ulceration	*Suggested by:* jagged ulcers or lacerations
	Confirmed by: history of trauma, injury, ill-fitting dentures, shallow, painful ulcers
Vitamin deficiency e.g., B_{12}, riboflavine, nicotinic acid	*Suggested by:* atrophic glossitis, fissured tongue; "raw beef" tongue in B_{12} deficiency, magenta in riboflavin deficiency
	Confirmed by: response to vitamin supplements
Hereditary hemorrhagic telangiectasias	*Suggested by:* telangiectasias on the face, around the mouth, on the lips and tongue, epistaxis, anemia
	Confirmed by: family history and examination of relatives
Peutz–Jegher's syndrome (associated with intestinal polyps)	*Suggested by:* peri-oral pigmentation (not the tongue)
	Confirmed by: finding polyps on **colonoscopy**

Red pharynx and tonsils

Some differential diagnoses and typical outline evidence

Viral pharyngitis	*Suggested by:* sore throat, pain on swallowing, fever, cervical lymphadenopathy and injected fauces. ↑ lymphocytes, leukocytes normal in WBC
	Confirmed by: negative **throat swab** for bacterial culture, self-limiting: resolution within days
Acute follicular tonsillitis (streptococcal)	*Suggested by:* severe sore throat, pain on swallowing, fever, enlarged tonsils with white patches (like strawberries and cream). Cervical lymphadenopathy especially in angle of jaw. Fever, ↑ leukocytes in WBC
	Confirmed by: **throat swab** for culture and sensitivities of organisms
Infectious mononucleosis due to Epstein–Barr virus	*Suggested by:* very severe throat pain with enlarged tonsils covered with creamy membrane. Petechiae on palate. Profound malaise. Generalized lymphadenopathy, splenomegaly
	Confirmed by: ↑ atypical lymphocytes in WBC. **Heterophile antibody** test positive. **Viral titers**
Candidiasis of buccal or esophageal mucosa	*Suggested by:* painful dysphagia, white plaque, history of immunosuppression, diabetes, or recent antibiotics
	Confirmed by: **esophagoscopy** showing erythema and plaques, **brush cytology ± biopsy** shows spores and hyphae
Agranulocytosis	*Suggested by:* sore throat, background history of taking a drug or contact with noxious substance
	Confirmed by: low or absent neutrophil count
Meningococcal meningitis	*Suggested by:* headache, photophobia, vomiting, sore throat, red pharynx without purulent patches, neck stiffness. High blood neutrophil count
	Confirmed by: lumbar puncture showing pus or neutrophil count and organisms on microscopy or culture

Parotid swelling

Swelling from anterior border of masseter muscle (teeth clenched) to lower half of ear, and from the zygomatic arch to angle of the jaw.

Some differential diagnoses and typical outline evidence

Parotid duct obstruction (usually due to stone)	*Suggested by:* intermittent infection or no discharge from duct *Confirmed by:* **plain X-ray** showing radio-opaque stone or **sialography** to show filling defect
Parotid tumor	*Suggested by:* no obvious features of alterative nonmalignant or infective condition *Confirmed by:* urgent surgical referral for **biopsy** or exploration
Mumps parotitis	*Suggested by:* acute painful swelling of whole gland(s), contact with others cases *Confirmed by:* bilateral swelling or associated pancreatitis or orchitis (rising mumps **viral titer** if doubt)
Suppurative parotid infection	*Suggested by:* hot, tender, fluctuant swelling with high fever. No discharge from duct orifice *Confirmed by:* ↑WBC, response to **drainage** ± antibiotics
Nonsuppurative parotitis from ascending infection along parotid duct	*Suggested by:* unilateral swelling, oral sepsis, or poor general condition *Confirmed by:* fever, ↑WBC discharge from duct orifice. Resolution with antibiotics
Parotid Sjögren's syndrome	*Suggested by:* dry mouth and eyes with no tears *Confirmed by:* rheumatoid factor positive ± anti- Ro(SSA) and anti-La(SSB) positive
Parotid sarcoidosis	*Suggested by:* history of dry cough, enlarged lacrimal glands, erythema nodosum, raised serum ACE. *Confirmed by:* CXR appearances (e.g., bilateral lymphadenopathy) and tissue biopsy showing noncaseating granuloma

Lump in the face (non-parotid lesion)

Swelling is anterior to border of the masseter muscle (teeth clenched).

Some differential diagnoses and typical outline evidence

Preauricular lymph node inflammation	*Suggested by:* tender nodular swelling in front of ear
	Confirmed by: above clinical features
Preauricular lymphoma	*Suggested by:* non-tender nodular swelling in front of ear
	Confirmed by: **biopsy** with or without or excision
Basal cell carcinoma	*Suggested by:* painless ulcer with rolled edge
	Confirmed by: **biopsy**
Sebaceous cyst	*Suggested by:* fluctuant swelling with central punctum
	Confirmed by: **incision**
Subcutaneous abscess	*Suggested by:* tender, fluctuant swelling
	Confirmed by: **incision** when pointing
Dental abscess	*Suggested by:* tenderness of underlying tooth (tap gently)
	Confirmed by: **dental exploration**
Skin melanoma	*Suggested by:* painless swelling with pigment and red edge
	Confirmed by: **wide excision biopsy**

Submandibular lump—not moving with tongue or on swallowing

This occurs below the mandible and above the digastric muscle.

Some differential diagnoses and typical outline evidence

Parotitis	*Suggested by:* acute, painful swelling of whole gland(s), contact with others cases
	Confirmed by: bilateral swelling or associated pancreatitis or orchitis (rising **mumps titer** if doubt)
Nonsuppurative sialitis from ascending infection along duct	*Suggested by:* unilateral swelling, oral sepsis, or poor general condition
	Confirmed by: discharge from duct orifice. Resolution with antibiotics
Suppurative salivary infection	*Suggested by:* hot, tender, fluctuant swelling with high fever. No discharge from duct orifice
	Confirmed by: **ultrasound scan**, response to drainage ± antibiotics
Salivary duct obstruction (usually due to stone)	*Suggested by:* intermittent infection or no discharge from duct
	Confirmed by: **ultrasound scan** response to stomaplasty
Salivary Sjögren's syndrome	*Suggested by:* dry mouth and eyes with no tears
	Confirmed by: rheumatoid factor positive, anti-Ro(SSA) and anti-La(SSB) positive
Salivary sarcoidosis	*Suggested by:* dry cough, enlarged lacrimal glands, and erythema nodosum
	Confirmed by: **CXR** appearances (e.g., bilateral lymphadenopathy) and tissue biopsy showing noncaseating granuloma
Salivary tumor due to adeno-carcinoma, squamous cell tumor, etc.	*Suggested by:* no obvious features of alternative nonmalignant or infective condition
	Confirmed by: urgent surgical referral for **biopsy** or **exploration**

Submandibular lymph node inflammation	*Suggested by:* tender, solid, nodular swelling between the mandibular branches, especially at age <20 years
	Confirmed by: above clinical features or **ultrasound scan**
Submandibular lymph node malignancy	*Suggested by:* non-tender solid nodular swelling between the mandibular branches, especially at age >20 years
	Confirmed by: **ultrasound scan, biopsy** ± excision
Ranula	*Suggested by:* transilluminable cyst lateral to midline, with domed, bluish discoloration in floor of mouth lateral to frenulum
	Confirmed by: clinical appearance, **ultrasound scan**, and **histology** after excision
Submental dermoid	*Suggested by:* midline cyst and age <20 years
	Confirmed by: **histology** after excision

Anterior neck lump—moving with tongue and swallowing

This suggests extrathyroid tissue.

Some differential diagnoses and typical outline evidence

Thyroglossal cyst	*Suggested by:* fluctuant cystic lump in midline or just to the left
	Confirmed by: **ultrasound scan**, **radioisotope scan** (cyst is cold), CT scan, **histology** of excised tissue
Ectopic thyroid tissue	*Suggested by:* solid lump in midline or just laterally
	Confirmed by: **ultrasound scan**, **radioisotope scan** (nodule may take up iodine), CT scan, **histology** of excised tissue

Neck lump—moving with swallowing but not with tongue

This suggests a goiter (or attached to thyroid gland). The following are preliminary diagnoses (see also pp. 107, 108).

Some differential diagnoses and typical outline evidence

Thyrotoxic goiter	*Suggested by:* sweating, fine tremor, tachycardia, weight loss, lid lag
	Confirmed by: ↑FT4, ± ↑FT3 and ↓↓TSH. Ultrasound scan, isotope scan
Hypothyroid goiter	*Suggested by:* cold intolerance, tiredness, constipation, bradycardia
	Confirmed by: ↑TSH, ↓FT4. Ultrasound scan ± thyroid antibodies positive
Euthyroid goiter	*Suggested by:* no sweating, no fine tremor, no weight change, no cold intolerance, no tiredness, no lid lag, normal bowel habit, normal pulse rate
	Confirmed by: normal FT4, and normal TSH

Bilateral neck mass—moving with swallowing but not with tongue

This is a central mass crossing the midline.

Some differential diagnoses and typical outline evidence

Graves' disease	*Suggested by:* clinical thyrotoxicosis, exophthalmos, pretibial myxedema. No nodules
	Confirmed by: ↑FT4 or ↑FT3 and ↓↓TSH and TSH receptor antibody positive. Diffuse increased uptake on *thyroid isotope scan*
Hashimoto's thyroiditis	*Suggested by:* clinically euthyroid or hypothyroid (or rarely transient thyrotoxicosis). Multiple nodules in large gland
	Confirmed by: FT4↑ transiently then ↓FT4 and ↑TSH, thyroid antibodies titer ↑↑. Diffuse poor uptake on *thyroid isotope scan*
"Simple" goiter	*Suggested by:* clinically euthyroid. Not nodular
	Confirmed by: normal FT4 or FT3 and normal TSH and negative *thyroid antibodies*
Toxic multinodular goiter	*Suggested by:* multiple nodules and clinically thyrotoxic
	Confirmed by: ↑FT4 or ↑FT3, and ↓TSH and nodules on *ultrasound scan* or *thyroid isotope scan*
Nontoxic multinodular goiter	*Suggested by:* multiple nodules and clinically euthyroid
	Confirmed by: normal FT4 or FT3 and normal TSH. Nodules on *ultrasound scan* or *thyroid isotope scan*
Thyroid enzyme deficiency (rare)	*Suggested by:* presentation in childhood, clinically hypothyroid or euthyroid. Not nodular
	Confirmed by: ↓FT4 or ↓FT3 and ↑TSH but with abnormal (high or low) *radio-iodine uptake*

Solitary thyroid nodule

Some differential diagnoses and typical outline evidence

Autonomous toxic thyroid nodule	*Suggested by:* single nodule and clinically thyrotoxic (weight loss, frequent bowel movement, ↑ pulse rate, sweats, tremor)
	Confirmed by: ↑FT4 or FT3, ↓TSH and single hot nodule thyroid isotope (iodine or technetium) scan.
Thyroid carcinoma: papillary 60% follicular 25% medullary 5% lymphoma 5% anaplastic <1%	*Suggested by:* single nodule and clinically euthyroid.
	Confirmed by: normal FT4 or FT3, normal TSH and single cold nodule thyroid isotope (iodine or technetium) scan. Solid on ultrasound scan. Malignant cells on needle aspiration or removal.
Thyroid adenoma	*Suggested by:* single nodule and clinically euthyroid
	Confirmed by: normal FT4 or FT3, normal TSH and single cold nodule thyroid isotope (iodine or technetium) scan. Solid on ultrasound scan. No malignant cells on needle aspiration or removal
Thyroid cyst	*Suggested by:* single nodule and clinically euthyroid
	Confirmed by: normal FT4 or FT3, normal TSH and single cold nodule thyroid isotope (iodine or technetium) scan. Cystic on ultrasound scan. Disappears on needle aspiration and no malignant cells then or if removed

Lump in anterior triangle of neck

This is below the digastric and in front of the sternocleidomastoid muscles.

Some differential diagnoses and typical outline evidence

Lymph node inflammation	*Suggested by:* tender, solid nodular swelling, especially at <20 years of age
	Confirmed by: above clinical features, CT scan
Acute abscess	*Suggested by:* hot, tender, fluctuant swelling with high fever
	Confirmed by: clinical features and discharge of pus after incision, ultrasound scan, CT scan
Tuberculous ("cold") abscess	*Suggested by:* fluctuant swelling with low-grade or no fever
	Confirmed by: acid-fast bacillus (AFB), culture and sensitivity of aspirate
Branchial cyst	*Suggested by:* fluctuant swelling at anterior border of sternocleidomastoid muscle, patient <20 years of age
	Confirmed by: ultrasound scan, CT scan, surgical anatomy, appearance and **histology** on excision
Cystic hygroma	*Suggested by:* fluctuant swelling that transilluminates well, patient <20 years of age
	Confirmed by: ultrasound scan, CT scan, surgical anatomy, appearance and histology on excision or regression with sclerosing agent
Pharyngeal pouch	*Suggested by:* intermittent, fluctuant swelling (usually on left) and dysphagia
	Confirmed by: **barium swallow** fills pouch
Carotid body tumor (chemodectoma)	*Suggested by:* mobile arising from carotid bifurcation soft (upper third of sternocleidomastoid) and gently pulsatile
	Confirmed by: ultrasound scan, CT scan, surgical anatomy, appearance and **histology** on excision
Hodgkin's or non-Hodgkin's lymphoma	*Suggested by:* non-tender solid nodular swelling between the mandibular branches, especially at >20 years of age, fever, weight loss. Chest pain with alcohol in Hodgkin's lymphoma
	Confirmed by: ultrasound scan, CT scan, **biopsy** with or without or excision

Lump in posterior triangle of neck

This is behind the sternocleidomastoid and in front of trapezius muscles.

Some differential diagnoses and typical outline evidence

Acute abscess	*Suggested by:* hot, tender, fluctuant swelling with high fever
	Confirmed by: clinical features and discharge of pus after incision, ultrasound scan, CT scan
Cystic hygroma	*Suggested by:* fluctuant swelling that transilluminates well, patient <20 years of age
	Confirmed by: ultrasound scan, CT scan, surgical anatomy, appearance and **histology** on excision or regression with sclerosing agent
Lymph node inflammation	*Suggested by:* tender, solid nodular swelling, especially at <20 years of age
	Confirmed by: clinical features, ultrasound scan, CT scan
Hodgkin's or non-Hodgkin's lymphoma	*Suggested by:* non-tender, solid nodular swelling. Chest pain with alcohol in Hodgkin's
	Confirmed by: ultrasound scan, CT scan, **biopsy** with or without or excision
Metastasis in lymph node	*Suggested by:* non-tender, solid nodular swelling
	Confirmed by: ultrasound scan, CT scan, **biopsy** ± excision
Tuberculous ("cold") abscess	*Suggested by:* non-tender, cystic swelling, especially at >50 years of age
	Confirmed by: ultrasound scan, CT scan, **aspiration biopsy** or excision, culture of AFB

Supraclavicular lump(s)

Some differential diagnoses and typical outline evidence

Lymph node inflammation	*Suggested by:* tender, solid nodular swelling, especially at <20 years of age
	Confirmed by: clinical features
Lymphoma	*Suggested by:* rubbery, matted nodes
	Confirmed by: lymph node **biopsy**
Lymph node secondary to gastric or lung carcinoma	*Suggested by:* rock-hard, fixed nodes, Virchow's node in left supraclavicular fossa (Troisier's sign)
	Confirmed by: lymph node **biopsy, gastroscopy, bronchoscopy**
Aneurysm of subclavian artery	*Suggested by:* pulsatile cyst
	Confirmed by: **ultrasound scan** and **MRI scan** or **angiography**

Galactorrhea

This characterized by spontaneous or expressible milky fluid.

Some differential diagnoses and typical outline evidence

Primary hyper-prolactinemia	*Suggested by:* infertility, oligomenorrhea, or amenorrhea
	Confirmed by: ↑*prolactin* and normal TSH and T4. *Pituitary CT* or *MRI scan:* normal or microadenoma
Prolactinoma	*Suggested by:* infertility, oligomenorrhea, or amenorrhea. In large tumors, field defects and loss of secondary sexual characteristics
	Confirmed by: ↑ *prolactin* and normal TSH and T4. Micro- or macroadenoma on *CT* or *MRI* scan pituitary
Pregnancy	*Suggested by:* amenorrhea, frequency of urine, etc., in woman of childbearing age
	Confirmed by: pregnancy test positive
Primary hypothyroidism	*Suggested by:* cold intolerance, tiredness, constipation, bradycardia
	Confirmed by: ↑TSH, ↓FT4
Drugs	*Suggested by:* taking metoclopramide, chlorpromazine, and other major tranquilizers
	Confirmed by: ↑*prolactin* and ↑TSH and ↓T4, resolution and lowering of *prolactin* after stopping suspected drug
Idiopathic galactorrhea	*Suggested by:* galactorrhea alone, no other findings
	Confirmed by: normal *prolactin* and TSH and T4

Nipple abnormality

Some differential diagnoses and typical outline evidence

Paget's disease of nipple with underlying carcinoma	*Suggested by:* breast nipple eczema
	Confirmed by: in situ malignant change on **histological examination** of skin scrapings
Duct ectasia and chronic infection	*Suggested by:* green or brown nipple discharge
	Confirmed by: chronic inflammation on **histology** of excised ducts
Duct papilloma	*Suggested by:* bleeding from nipple
	Confirmed by: excision of affected ducts. Benign **histology** of excised ducts
Mamillary fistula	*Suggested by:* discharge from para-areolar region, patient age 30–40 years
	Confirmed by: excision of affected ducts. Benign **histology** of excised ducts

Breast lump(s)

Some differential diagnoses and typical outline evidence

Benign fibrous mammary dysplasia	*Suggested by:* generally painful breast lumpiness, greatest near axilla. Cyclically related to periods
	Confirmed by: relief on **aspiration** of cysts, diuretics or estrogen suppression
Fibroadenoma	*Suggested by:* smooth and mobile lump ("breast mouse") usually in patients 15–30 years of age
	Confirmed by: appearance on mammogram *Confirmed by* benign **histology** after excision
Cyst(s)	*Suggested by:* spherical, fluctuant lump, single or multiple, painful before periods
	Confirmed by: cysts on **mammography,** benign tissue after excision
Acute or chronic abscess	*Suggested by:* fluctuant lump, hot and tender, acute presentation often in puerperium. Chronic after antibiotics
	Confirmed by: response to drainage, chronic abscess excision and **histology** to exclude carcinoma
Fat necrosis or sclerosing adenosis	*Suggested by:* firm, solitary, localized lump
	Confirmed by: appearance on mammogram *Confirmed by* benign **histology** after excision
Carcinoma (infiltrating ductal cancer or invasive lobar cancers)	*Suggested by:* some of the following: fixed, irregular, hard, painless lump, nipple retraction, fixed to skin (peau d'orange) or muscle and local, hard or firm, fixed nodes in axilla. Metastases to lymph nodes, or via blood to bones, brain, liver, lung, and abdominal cavity
	Confirmed by: ill-defined speculate borders, faint linear or irregular calcification, and abnormal adjacent structures on mammography. Malignant **histology after aspiration** or excision

Gynecomastia

These findings should have been discovered during the general examination. Breast swelling occurs in males, with a disc of firm tissue. If there is no disc, it is fatty tissue only.

Some differential diagnoses and typical outline evidence

Immature testis	*Suggested by:* adolescence and no testicular lump
	Confirmed by: normal testosterone, estrogen, and LH levels; normal ultrasound scan of testis
Digoxin, spironolactone	*Suggested by:* taking of drug and no testicular lump
	Confirmed by: improvement when drug stopped
High alcohol intake	*Suggested by:* high alcohol intake and no testicular lump
	Confirmed by: improvement when alcohol stopped
Hepatic cirrhosis	*Suggested by:* long history of high alcohol intake (usually), spider nevi, abnormal liver size (large or small) and consistency (fatty or hard)
	Confirmed by: very abnormal biochemical liver function tests, ↓LH, ↑**estrogens**, ↓**testosterone**
Testicular tumors	*Suggested by:* scrotal mass ± pain, tenderness if hemorrhage occurs (sometimes arising in undescended testis)
	Confirmed by: testicular ultrasound, inguinal exploration, ↑α-*fetoprotein*, ↑β-*hCG*
Hypogonadism (primary to testicular disease, or secondary to low LH from pituitary defect or tumor)	*Suggested by:* sparse pubic hair, no drug or alcohol history, poor libido
	Confirmed by: **testosterone**↓, LH↑ (in primary testicular disease), LH↓ or normal (when secondary to pituitary diseases)
Lung carcinoma	*Suggested by:* smoking history, hemoptysis, weight loss, clubbing
	Confirmed by: **CXR, bronchoscopy** with biopsy
Klinefelter's syndrome	*Suggested by:* poor sexual development, infertility, eunuchoid
	Confirmed by: 47, XXY **karyotype**
Obesity	*Suggested by:* no breast tissue, only mammary fat
	Confirmed by: improvement with weight loss

Axillary lymphadenopathy

Axillary lymphadenopathy ± tenderness.

Some differential diagnoses and typical outline evidence

Reaction to infection, e.g., viral prodrome, HIV infection, etc.	*Suggested by:* tender, solid nodular swelling(s), especially at <20 years of age *Confirmed by:* clinical features
Infiltration by secondary tumor, e.g., breast	*Suggested by:* non-tender, solid nodular swelling(s) *Confirmed by:* **excision biopsy**
Histiocytosis or primary tumor	*Suggested by:* non-tender, solid nodular swelling(s) *Confirmed by:* **excision biopsy**
Drug effect	*Suggested by:* drug history, e.g., phenytoin, retroviral drug *Confirmed by:* improvement when drug withdrawn

Hirsuitism in females

Upward extension of pubic hair in females. Hirsute upper lip and chin and sideburns can also occur.

Some differential diagnoses and typical outline evidence

Racial skin sensitivity	*Suggested by:* family history, normal menstrual periods (and fertility if applicable)
	Confirmed by: LH normal, **testosterone** normal
Polycystic ovary syndrome	*Suggested by:* gradual increase in hirsutism since puberty, thin head hair, irregular periods, infertility
	Confirmed by: **testosterone** ↑, SHBG↓, LH↑ (tests done in follicular phase of menstrual cycle). Ultrasound scan showing cystic ovaries
Ovarian or adrenal carcinoma	*Suggested by:* change in hair pattern over months, deeper voice, breast atrophy, no periods, clitoromegaly
	Confirmed by: ↓LH and ↑↑**testosterone**. Ultrasound scan and laparoscopy findings
Cushing's syndrome pituitary-driven Cushing's disease, or autonomous adrenal Cushing's, or glucocorticoid therapy	*Suggested by:* round, florid face (and trunk with purple striae) with thin arms and legs, hirsutism. Inability to rise from squatting position (due to proximal myopathy)
	Confirmed by: ↑24-hour urinary free cortisol, midnight cortisol ↑, and/or failure to suppress cortisol after 48 hours on dexamethasone 0.5 mg 6 hourly or drug history of glucocorticoids

Abdominal striae

White striae are healed pink or purple striae.

- Pink striae

Some differential diagnoses and typical outline evidence

Pregnancy	*Suggested by:* no periods and obvious pregnant uterus
	Confirmed by: **pregnancy test** positive and ultrasound scan of abdomen or pelvis
Simple obesity	*Suggested by:* large abdomen and usually rapid weight increase
	Confirmed by: above clinical findings

- Purple striae

Some differential diagnoses and typical outline evidence

Glucocorticoid steroid therapy	*Suggested by:* truncal obesity, purple striae, bruising, moon face and buffalo hump
	Confirmed by: drug history: taking high dose of glucocorticoid
Cushing's disease (ACTH driven)	*Suggested by:* truncal obesity, purple striae, bruising, moon face and buffalo hump. Pigmented creases indicate high ACTH, especially in ectopic ACTH (from a carcinoma or carcinoid tumor)
	Confirmed by: ↑24-hour urinary free cortisol, midnight cortisols ↑, and/or failure to suppress cortisol after dexamethasone, ↑ACTH and bilaterally large adrenals on *CT* or *MRI scan*
Cushing's syndrome due to adrenal adenoma	*Suggested by:* truncal obesity, purple striae, and bruising. No pigmentation in skin creases
	Confirmed by: ↑24-hour urinary free cortisol, midnight cortisol ↑, and/or failure to suppress cortisol after dexamethasone, ↓ACTH and unilateral large adrenal on *CT* or *MRI scan*

Obesity

The definition of obesity is body mass index (BMI) >30.

Some differential diagnoses and typical outline evidence

Simple obesity	*Suggested by:* limb and truncal obesity
	Confirmed by: TSH and FT4 normal. 24-hour urinary cortisol normal
Hypothyroidism	*Suggested by:* cold intolerance, tiredness, constipation, bradycardia
	Confirmed by: ↑TSH, ↓FT4
Cushing's syndrome	*Suggested by:* moon face, truncal obesity, hirsutism, buffalo hump, abdominal striae, proximal weakness
	Confirmed by: ↑24-hour urinary free cortisol, midnight cortisol ↑, and/or failure to suppress cortisol after dexamethasone

Pigmented creases and flexures (and buccal mucosa)

This condition suggests excess adrenocorticotropic hormone (ACTH) secretion.

Some differential diagnoses and typical outline evidence

Addison's disease = primary adrenal failure due to autoimmune destruction or tuberculosis	*Suggested by:* fatigue, low BP, and postural drop *Confirmed by:* low 9 AM cortisol with poor response to ACTH stimulation test and ACTH↑
(Pituitary) Cushing's disease	*Suggested by:* facial and truncal obesity with striae, limb wasting, and proximal myopathy *Confirmed by:* ↑24-hour urinary free cortisol and/or failure to suppress cortisol after dexamethasone. Midnight cortisol ↑ and ACTH ↑
Ectopic ACTH secretion	*Suggested by:* general weakness, proximal myopathy, usually evidence of lung cancer or other malignancy *Confirmed by:* ↓ serum potassium and ↑↑ midnight cortisol and ↑ACTH

Spider nevi (nevus araneus)

These are red, pin-head-sized spots with radiating blood vessels that empty when the center is pressed by a pin-head-sized object.

Some differential diagnoses and typical outline evidence

Normal	*Suggested by:* small numbers on chest (≤3), usually in a young woman on the chest and upper back
	Confirmed by: no increase with time
Taking estrogens	*Suggested by:* small numbers on chest in a young woman on estrogen-containing contraceptive pill
	Confirmed by: decrease when pill stopped in due course (no urgency)
Pregnancy	*Suggested by:* moderate numbers in a pregnant woman
	Confirmed by: decrease when pregnancy over
Liver failure	*Suggested by:* large numbers on chest, also on neck and face, jaundice, features of liver failure
	Confirmed by: ↓*albumin*, ↑*prothrombin time (PT)*

Thin, wasted, cachectic

Some differential diagnoses and typical outline evidence

Low-calorie intake (e.g., anorexia nervosa alcoholism, drug abuse, any prolonged systemic illness e.g., severe COPD)	*Suggested by:* dietary history *Confirmed by:* dietician's assessment, as inpatient if necessary
Thyrotoxicosis	*Suggested by:* normal appetite and adequate intake, frequent loose bowel movement, lid retraction and lag, sweats, tachycardia *Confirmed by:* ↓↓TSH, ↑FT4
AIDS	*Suggested by:* signs of opportunistic infection, e.g., oral candidiasis, oral hairy leukoplakia, Kaposi's sarcoma, lymphadenopathy *Confirmed by:* detection of HIV *antibodies* in serum, HIV RNA *in plasma*
Malignancy	*Suggested by:* progressive weight loss and malaise, poor appetite *Confirmed by:* metastases in liver on *ultrasound scan*, bone metastases on *plain X-rays*, *endoscopy* for gut tumors, *bronchoscopy*, etc.
Tuberculosis	*Suggested by:* cough, night sweats, hemoptysis, CXR: abnormal shadowing *Confirmed by:* AFB in sputum on microscopy, mycobacteria on culture, response to antibiotics

Purpura

This covers a spectrum from small, pin-point petechiae to large areas of "bruising" in skin that do not blanch when compressed.

Some differential diagnoses and typical outline evidence

Thrombocytopenia due to autoimmune process or idiopathic (ITP), SLE	*Suggested by:* petechiae and history of associated condition *Confirmed by:* ↓**platelet count** but RBC and WBC normal
Pancytopenia due to aplastic anemia, hypersplenism, myelodysplasia, disseminated vascular anticoagulation	*Suggested by:* petechiae and history of associated condition *Confirmed by:* ↓**platelet count**, ↓WBC, and ↑Hb
Platelet dysfunction due to aspirin, NSAIDs, renal failure	*Suggested by:* bruising and drug history *Confirmed by:* less bruising when aspirin stopped or other cause removed
Congenital vasculopathy due to Osler–Weber–Rendu syndrome, etc.	*Suggested by:* bruising from punctiform malformations on mucous membranes. Nose bleeds, GI bleeding *Confirmed by:* clinical findings and normal **platelet count** and clotting
Acquired vasculopathy due to senile changes, autoimmune vasculitis (Henoch–Schönlein), steroids, scurvy	*Suggested by:* bruising into associated thin skin with atrophied subcutaneous tissue *Confirmed by:* normal **platelet count** and **clotting**
Acquired coagulopathy due to liver disease, vitamin K deficiency, DIC	*Suggested by:* bruising and history of associated condition *Confirmed by:* prolonged **prothrombin time**
Congenital coagulopathy e.g., Von Willebrand's disease	*Suggested by:* lifelong bruising and bleeding (after tooth extraction, heavy periods) *Confirmed by:* abnormal platelet function (count normal) and long activated partial thromboplastin time (PTT)
Drug effect	*Suggested by:* drug history, e.g., warfarin, steroids *Confirmed by:* improvement or drug withdrawal

Generalized lymphadenopathy

Some differential diagnoses and typical outline evidence

Infectious mononucleosis due to Epstein–Barr virus	*Suggested by:* very severe throat pain with enlarged tonsils covered with creamy membrane. Petechiae on palate. Profound malaise. Generalized lymphadenopathy, splenomegaly
	Confirmed by: **Heterophile antibody** test positive. **Viral titers**
Hodgkin's lymphoma	*Suggested by:* anemia, splenomegaly, multiple lymph node enlargement
	Confirmed by: characteristic histology showing Reed–Sternberg cells
Non-Hodgkin's lymphoma	*Suggested by:* anemia, multiple lymph node enlargement
	Confirmed by: characteristic histology with no Reed–Sternberg cells, tumor markers, flow cytometry
Chronic myeloid leukemia (CML)	*Suggested by:* splenomegaly, variable hepatomegaly, bruising, anemia
	Confirmed by: presence of Philadelphia chromosome, ↑↑WBC, e.g., >100 cells/μL
Chronic lymphocytic leukemia (CLL)	*Suggested by:* anorexia, weight loss, enlarged, rubbery, non-tender lymph nodes. Hepatomegaly, late splenomegaly. Bruising, anemia
	Confirmed by: marked lymphocytosis. Bone marrow infiltration
Acute myeloid leukemia (AML)	*Suggested by:* variable hepatomegaly, bruising, anemia
	Confirmed by: Blast cells in bone marrow biopsy
Acute lymphoblastic leukemia (ALL)	*Suggested by:* variable hepatomegaly, bruising, anemia
	Confirmed by: presence of immunological marker of common (CD10), T-cell, β-cell, null-cell
Sarcoidosis	*Suggested by:* dry cough, breathlessness, malaise, fatigue, weight loss, enlarged lacrimal glands, erythema nodosum
	Confirmed by: **CXR** appearances (e.g., bilateral lymphadenopathy) and **tissue biopsy** showing noncaseating granuloma
Drug effect	*Suggested by:* drug history, e.g., phenytoin, retroviral drug
	Confirmed by: improvement when drug withdrawn

Localized groin lymphadenopathy

This is a nonspecific finding.

Some differential diagnoses and typical outline evidence

Infection somewhere in lower limb or pelvis (usually in past and node remained large)	*Suggested by:* enlarged nodes confined to groin *Confirmed by:* local infection in foot or leg, or no symptoms or signs of generalized condition

Pressure sores

These are blisters or ulcers on the heel or sacrum.

Some differential diagnoses and typical outline evidence

Prolonged contact	*Suggested by:* history of sensory loss, e.g., spinal cord injury, cerebrovascular accident (CVA)
	Confirmed by: response to frequent turning and dressings and wound care
Poor nutrition	*Suggested by:* ↓Hb. Low total serum protein and low potassium
	Confirmed by: formal dietary assessment, response to improved nutrition, nurses turning patient frequently, and dressings and wound care

Cardiovascular symptoms

Chest pain—alarming and increasing over minutes to hours

This refers to chest pain that is not sharp and is not an easily recognized pattern by the patient (e.g., as predictable, familiar angina). Ideally, the detailed history is taken where resuscitation facilities are available. Early, nonspecific ECG changes will suggest an acute coronary syndrome, a blanket term that includes angina or infarction (MI), but serial ECG or enzyme changes may be needed to distinguish between them.

- Normal troponin 12 hours after pain: probability of MI <0.3%
- ↑Troponin indicates episode of muscle necrosis up to 2 weeks before
- ST-segment elevation indicates current ischemia (or rarely ventricular aneurysm).

Some differential diagnoses and typical outline evidence

Angina (new or unstable)	*Suggested by:* central pain ± radiating to jaw and either arm (left usually). Intermittent, brought on by exertion, relieved by rest or nitrates, and lasting <30 minutes. May be associated with transient ST depression or T inversions or, rarely, ST elevation.
	Confirmed by: no ↑*troponin* after 12 hours (excludes MI). Stress test showing inducible ischemia
ST-elevation myocardial infarction (STEMI)	*Suggested by:* central chest pain ± radiating to jaw and either arm (left usually). Continuous, usually over 30 minutes, not relieved by rest or nitrates
	Confirmed by: ST elevation 1 mm in limb leads or 2 mm in chest leads on *serial ECGs* (this is regarded as sufficient evidence to treat with thrombolysis). ↑*troponin* indicates episode of muscle necrosis up to 2 weeks before. ↑*troponin* **may not be present in the first 4 hours after the onset of chest pain.**
Non-ST-elevation myocardial infarction (NSTEMI)	*Suggested by:* central chest pain ± radiating to jaw and either arm (left usually). Continuous, usually over 30 minutes, not relieved by rest or nitrates
	Confirmed by: elevated *troponin* after 12 hours. T-wave and ST-segment changes but no ST elevation on *serial ECGs*
Esophagitis and esophageal spasm	*Suggested by:* past episodes of pain when supine, after food. Relieved by antacids
	Confirmed by: no ↑ in troponin after 12 hours and no ST-segment changes on ECG. Improvement with antacids. Esophagitis on *endoscopy*

Pulmonary embolus arising from leg DVT, silent pelvic vein thrombosis, right atrial thrombus	*Suggested by:* central chest pain, also abrupt shortness of breath, cyanosis, tachycardia, loud second sound in pulmonary area, associated deep vein thrombosis (DVT) or risk factors such as cancer, recent surgery, immobility *Confirmed by:* **V/Q scan** with mismatched ventilation and perfusion, **spiral (helical) CT (CT-pulmonary angiogram)** showing clot in pulmonary artery
Pneumothorax	*Suggested by:* abrupt pain in center or side of chest with abrupt breathlessness. Resonance to percussion over site *Confirmed by:* **expiration CXR** showing dark field with loss of lung markings outside sharp line containing lung tissue
Dissecting thoracic aortic aneurysm	*Suggested by:* 'tearing pain often radiating to back and not responsive to analgesia, abnormal or absent peripheral pulses, early diastolic murmur, low BP, and wide mediastinum on CXR *Confirmed by:* loss of single clear lumen on **CT scan** or **MRI**
Chest wall pain e.g., costochondritis and Tietze's syndrome, strained muscle or rib injury	*Suggested by:* chest pain and localized tenderness of chest wall or chest pain on twisting of neck or thoracic cage *Confirmed by:* no ↑ in troponin after 12 hours, and no ST-segment changes or T-wave changes serially on ECG. Response to rest and analgesics

Chest pain—sharp and aggravated by breathing or movement

This is a common symptom experienced in mild or transient forms by many in the population; it usually resolves with no cause being discovered. It frightens a patient into seeking advice when it is severe or accompanied by other symptoms, such as breathlessness, when a specific cause is more likely to be found.

Some differential diagnoses and typical outline evidence

Pleurisy due to pneumonia	*Suggested by:* being worse on inspiration, shallow breaths, pleural rub, evidence of infection (fever, cough, consolidation, etc.)
	Confirmed by: opacification in lung periphery on CXR and sputum/blood culture
Pulmonary infarct due to embolus arising from DVT in leg, silent pelvic vein thrombosis, silent right atrial thrombosis	*Suggested by:* sudden shortness of breath, pleural rub, cyanosis, tachycardia, loud P2, associated DVT, or risk factors such as recent surgery, cancer, immobility
	Confirmed by: **V/Q scan** mismatch, **spiral CT** showing clot in pulmonary artery
Pneumothorax	*Suggested by:* pain in center or side of chest with abrupt breathlessness. Diminished breath sounds, resonance to percussion over site
	Confirmed by: **expiratory CXR** showing loss of lung markings outside sharp pleural line
Pericarditis caused by MI, infection, especially viral, malignancy, uremia, connective tissue diseases	*Suggested by:* sharp pain worse lying flat or with trunk movement, relieved by leaning forward. Pericardial rub
	Confirmed by: **ECG:** diffuse concave ST elevations and PR depressions. **CXR:** globular heart shadow and relief with pericardial drainage (if hypotensive)
Musculoskeletal injury or inflammation (often Borholm's disease, Cocksackie B infection)	*Suggested by:* associated focal tenderness. Often history of trauma
	Confirmed by: excluding other explanations. Normal troponin

Chest wall pain e.g., chostochondritis or Tietze's syndrome, strained muscle or rib injury	*Suggested by:* chest pain and localized tenderness of chest wall or chest pain on twisting of neck or thoracic cage
	Confirmed by: no ↑**troponin** after 12 hours, and no ST-segment or T-wave changes serially on ECG. Response to rest and analgesics
Referred cervical root pain	*Suggested by:* previous minor episodes, exacerbation by neck movement (producing closure of nerve root foramina related to area of pain)
	Confirmed by: clinical features and MRI scan
Shingles	*Suggested by:* pain (often burning in nature) in a dermatomal distribution, previous exposure to chicken pox or shingles attacks. More common in immunocompromised patients
	Confirmed by: vesicles appearing within days

Severe lower chest or upper abdominal pain

Upper abdominal pain may also be difficult for the patient to separate from lower chest pain, so the causes of chest pain have to be borne in mind as well.

Some differential diagnoses and typical outline evidence

Gastroesophageal reflux/gastritis	*Suggested by:* central or epigastric burning pain, onset over hours, dyspepsia, worse lying flat, worsened by food, alcohol, nonsteroidal anti-inflammatory drugs (NSAIDs)
	Confirmed by: esophagogastroduodenoscopy (EGD) showing inflamed mucosa
Biliary colic	*Suggested by:* postprandial pain, severe and "gripping" or colicky, usually in right upper quadrant (RUQ) and that can radiate to right scapula. Onset over hours
	Confirmed by: ultrasound showing gallstones and biliary dilatation or characteristic findings on endoscopic retrograde cholangiopancreatography (ERCP)
Pancreatitis (often due to gallstone impacted in common bile duct)	*Suggested by:* mid-epigastric pain radiating to back, associated with nausea and vomiting, gallstones. Onset over hours.
	Confirmed by: ↑*serum amylase* to 5 times normal, ↑*serum lipase*
Myocardial infarction (often inferior)	*Suggested by:* continuous pain, usually over 30 minutes, not relieved by rest or (antianginal) medication. Onset over minutes to hours
	Confirmed by: T wave inversion ± ST elevation of 1 mm in limb leads or 2 mm in chest leads on *serial ECGs* or ↑*troponin*

Orthopnea and paroxysmal nocturnal dyspnea (PND)

Orthopnea is shortness of breath when lying flat. (Try to confirm by observing what happens when patient lies flat.) It is most often associated with congestive heart failure (CHF) when pulmonary venous pressure and alveolar edema, especially in the upper lung fields, are increased in the recumbent position.

Less frequently it occurs with pulmonary disease such as chronic obstructive pulmonary disease (COPD) associated with abdominal obesity when abdominal contents press up on the diaphragm in the recumbent position. PND can occur when the patient slides down in bed at night or by bronchospasm due to nighttime asthma.

Some differential diagnoses and typical outline evidence

Pulmonary edema	*Suggested by:* **dyspnea,** displaced apex beat, third heart sound, bilateral basal fine crackles
due to congestive (chronic) left ventricular failure (due to ischemic heart disease, valvular disease)	*Confirmed by:* **CXR** appearances. Impaired left ventricular (LV) function on **echocardiogram**. Abnormal **ECG** reflecting underlying heart disease
COPD	*Suggested by:* smoking history, cough and sputum. Pursed lip breathing, use of accessory muscles, reduced breath sounds, wheezes. Chest hyperinflation. Reduced peak flow rate
	Confirmed by: **CXR:** radiolucent lungs. **Spirometry:** reduced FEV_1, reduced FEV_1/FVC ratio, <12% reversibility, hypoxia $\pm$ $\uparrow$ arterial PCO_2 (rarely, reduced α_1-**antitrypsin** levels)
Asthma	*Suggested by:* wheeze or dry cough. Other specific triggers to breathlessness. Other allergies. Past history of similar attacks unless first presentation
	Confirmed by: reversibility of spirometric abnormalities with bronchodilator treatment, and symptomatic response to treatment

Palpitations

These are very subjective and nonspecific unless forceful, fast, and associated with dizziness or loss of consciousness.

Some differential diagnoses and typical outline evidence

Runs of supraventricular tachycardia (SVT)	*Suggested by:* abrupt onset, sweats and sustained dizziness.
	Confirmed by: baseline ECG or **24-hour ECG** showing tachycardia with normal QRS complexes with absent or abnormal P waves >140/min. **Exercise** ECG to see if precipitated by exercise (and due to IHD)
Episodic heart block Second-degree or third-degree atrioventricular (AV) block	*Suggested by:* onset over minutes or hours, slow and forceful beats. Loss of consciousness, pallor if significant loss of cardiac output
	Confirmed by: nonconducted P waves associated with conducted P waves with fixed or progressive prolonged PR interval, P–R dissociation, and slow QRS rate on 12-lead or **24-hour ECG**
Sinus tachycardia (anxiety, pain, fever, caffeine, hypovolemia, pulmonary embolism, hyperventilation, etc.)	*Suggested by:* gradual onset over minutes of regular palpitations and pulse. History of precipitating cause (usually)
	Confirmed by: 12 lead ECG or monitor strip and resolution by stopping precipitating factors or resolution of potential cause
Atrial fibrillation	*Suggested by:* onset over seconds, irregularly irregular radial and apex pulse, apical–radial pulse deficit, and variable BP
	Confirmed by: ECG showing no P waves and irregularly irregular QRS complexes
Ventricular ectopy unifocal (benign) or multifocal (may have underlying pathology)	*Suggested by:* palpitations felt as early or skipped beats occurring one at a time or in short bursts, noted over hours or days, sometimes associated with anxiety
	Confirmed by: premature wide QRS complexes without preceding P waves on **12 lead ECG** or **24-hour ECG**

Menopause	*Suggested by:* sweats, mood changes, irregular or no more periods, getting worse over weeks or months
	Confirmed by: ↓*serum estrogen*, ↑FSH/LH, and response to hormone replacement therapy
Thyrotoxicosis	*Suggested by:* anxiety, irritability, weight loss, sweating, loose frequent stools, lid retraction and lag, proptosis, brisk reflexes, other signs and symptoms of hyperthyroidism. Onset over weeks or months. 12 lead ECG may show sinus tachycardia, atrial fibrillation, or ventricular arrhythmias
	Confirmed by: ↑FT4, and/or ↑FT3 and ↓TSH
Pheochromocytoma (rare)	*Suggested by:* abrupt episodes of anxiety, fear, chest tightness, sweating, headaches, and marked rises in BP
	Confirmed by: catecholamines (VMA, HMMA) or *free metanephrine* ↑ in urine and blood soon after episode

Cough and pink frothy sputum

This is due to a combination of frothy sputum of pulmonary edema tinged with blood.

Some differential diagnoses and typical outline evidence

Acute pulmonary edema	*Suggested by:* onset over minutes or hours of shortness of breath, orthopnea, displaced apex, loud third heart sound, fine crackles at lung base
	Confirmed by: CXR appearance (see Fig. 19.13, though 19.14 is more typical), poor LV function on echocardiogram
Mitral stenosis causing pulmonary edema	*Suggested by:* months or years of orthopnea, tapping, displaced apex, loud first heart sound, diastolic murmur, fine crackles at lung bases. Enlarged left atrial shadow (behind heart) and splayed carina on CXR
	Confirmed by: large left atrium and mitral stenosis on echocardiogram

Syncope

This is sudden loss of consciousness over seconds. Think of abnormal cardiac or CNS "electrical" activity or a temporary drop in cardiac output and BP that improves as soon as the patient is in a prone position. Seizures can occur from a profound fall in BP, so they are not specific for epilepsy.

Some differential diagnoses and typical outline evidence

Vasovagal attack—simple faint	*Suggested by:* seconds or minutes of preceding emotion, pain, fear, urination, or prolonged standing—with nausea, sweating and darkening of vision. Recovery within minutes. Incontinence is rare.
	Confirmed by: history, positive upright tilt test
Postural hypotension often due to antihypertensive drugs, dehydration, anemia, or blood loss	*Suggested by:* dizziness or sudden loss of consciousness within minutes after getting up from sitting or lying position
	Confirmed by: fall in BP and rise in heart rate (HR) from reclining to standing, confirmation of a causal diagnosis
Stokes–Adams attack due to a variety of cardiogenic causes, e.g., syncope caused by AV conduction block	*Suggested by:* **recurrent episodes** of sudden loss of consciousness with no warning. Pallor, then recovery within seconds or minutes.
	Confirmed by: **24-hour ECG** showing episodes of asystole or heart block, SVT, or ventricular tachycardia (VT)
Aortic stenosis	*Suggested by:* syncope on exercise. Cool extremities, slowly rising carotid arterial pulse, low BP and pulse pressure and heaving apex. Mid-systolic murmur radiating to carotids. ECG showing left ventricular hypertrophy (LVH)
	Confirmed by: **Echocardiogram** and **cardiac catheterization**: stenosed aortic valve
Hypertrophic cardiomyopathy	*Suggested by:* syncope on exercise. FH of sudden death or hypertrophic cardiomyopathy. Angina, breathless, jerky pulse, high JVP with "a" wave, double apex beat, thrill and murmur best at left sternal edge
	Confirmed by: characteristic **echocardiogram** showing increased left ventricular wall thickness, small, well-contracting left ventricle

Micturition syncope	*Suggested by:* sudden loss of consciousness after urination, usually in a man at night. Often history of prostatism
	Confirmed by: history and examination not indicative of other causes of syncope
Cough syncope	*Suggested by:* sudden loss of consciousness after severe bout of coughing
	Confirmed by: history and examination not indicative of other causes of syncope
Carotid sinus syncope	*Suggested by:* sudden loss of consciousness after turning head, e.g., while shaving. More likely with tight collars
	Confirmed by: history and onset of symptoms on careful repeat of movement. Excessive sinus bradycardia with carotid sinus massage
Hypoglycemia	*Suggested by:* preceded by seconds or minutes by hunger, sweating, and darkening of vision. Usually in diabetic on insulin.
	Confirmed by: **blood sugar** <50 mg/dL and exclusion of associated cardiac condition
Epilepsy (may be due to profound fall in BP)	*Suggested by:* preceding aura for a few minutes then tonic phase with cyanosis, clonic jerks of limbs, incontinence of urine and/or feces
	Confirmed by: history from witness. EEG changes, e.g., spike and wave
Pulmonary embolus (PE) or infarct due to embolus arising from DVT in leg, silent pelvic vein thrombosis, silent right atrial thrombus	*Suggested by:* sudden shortness of breath, pleural rub, cyanosis, tachycardia, loud P2, associated DVT, or risk factors such as recent surgery, childbirth, immobility, etc.
	Confirmed by: V/Q scan mismatch, spiral CT showing clot in pulmonary artery

Leg pain on walking—intermittent claudication

This is analogous to the more familiar angina but pain comes on in the legs instead of the chest on exercise. Quantify the effect on daily activity (especially distance walked) and ability to cope at home, work, recreation, and rest.

Some differential diagnoses and typical outline evidence

Arterial disease in legs	*Suggested by:* predictable leg, calf, thigh, or buttock pain (worse on hills, better downhill) that is better with rest (if also present at rest, this implies incipient gangrene). Patient sleeps with leg hanging down, e.g., over edge of bed or in chair. Abnormal pulses, poor perfusion of skin and toes
	Confirmed by: **Doppler ultrasound** or **arteriogram** or **magnetic resonance angiogram (MRA)** showing stenosis and poor flow
Aortoiliac occlusive arterial disease associated with erectile dysfunction = Leriche's syndrome	*Suggested by:* predictable buttock, hip, or thigh pain on exertion and male erectile dysfunction (impotence)
	Confirmed by: arteriogram or MRA showing stenosis and poor flow in the distal aortic or iliac arteries
Neurogenic claudication	*Suggested by:* weakness and pain in leg, calf, thigh, or buttock and pain improving slowly with rest but variable. Worse downhill. No cold toes, normal pulses
	Confirmed by: MRI showing neurospinal canal stenosis or disc compression of cord or cauda equina

Leg pain on standing—relieved by lying down

Think of something relieved by reducing pressure on lying down. Two possibilities are relief of the pressure transmitted down to leg tissues by incompetent venous valves, or relief of pressure by the spinal column on a damaged disc, aggravating its protrusion and pressure on adjacent nerve roots.

Some differential diagnoses and typical outline evidence

Peripheral venous disease and varicose veins	*Suggested by:* generalized ache, associated itching, varicose veins, and venous eczema ± ulcers. Cough impulse felt and Trendelenberg test shows filling down along extent of communicating valve leaks.
	Confirmed by: clinical findings or **Doppler ultrasound** probe to confirm whether or not incompetence is present in the saphenofemoral junction or the short saphenous vein
Disc protrusion (slipped disc)	*Suggested by:* severe referred ache or shooting pains, affected by position. Neurological deficit in root distribution
	Confirmed by: MRI of sacral and dorsal spine showing disc impinging on nerve roots (but may be less obvious as patient lies down in scanner)

Bilateral ankle swelling

Think of increased pressure within the veins or lymphatic vessels or low albumin in the vascular space, bilateral damage to veins, lymphatics, or capillaries due to local inflammation.

Some differential diagnoses and typical outline evidence

Right ventricular failure due to pulmonary vascular disease or CHF	*Suggested by:* jugular venous distension, edema, liver enlargement and pulsation, right ventricular (RV) heave. Onset over months, usually
	Confirmed by: elevation of central venous pressure (CVP) using a central venous catheter or elevation of right arterial (RA) and RV pressures during right heart catheterization, dilated RV on *echocardiogram*
Poor venous return due to abdominal or pelvic masses, post-phlebitic or thrombotic venous damage	*Suggested by:* onset over months. Worse on prolonged standing or sitting, varicosities, venous eczema, pigmentation or ulceration. Non-pitting edema if chronic
	Confirmed by: clinically with Trendelenberg test showing filling along extent of communicating valve leaks or on venous *Doppler ultrasound*
Low albumin states caused by liver failure, nephrotic syndrome, malnutrition, etc.	*Suggested by:* generalized edema often including face after lying down. Onset usually over months
	Confirmed by: low *serum albumin*
Bilateral cellulitis often associated with diabetes mellitus	*Suggested by:* warm, red, and tender legs, thrombophlebitis and tracking, ulcers, etc. Onset over days
	Confirmed by: positive *blood cultures* (usually streptococcal or staphylococcal) (*blood sugar* ↑ in diabetes)
Inferior vena cava (IVC) obstruction due to prolonged immobility, carcinoma, and oral combined contraceptive use)	*Suggested by:* bilateral leg-swelling onset over hours, associated risk factors (obesity, smoker, FH). Symptoms of PE.
	Confirmed by: *CT abdomen*, low flow on *Doppler ultrasound scan,* or filling defect on *venogram*.

Bilateral thromboses	*Suggested by:* onset over hours, risk factor of obesity, history of immobility, carcinoma, oral contraceptive use. Associated with PE. Leg(s) firm, warm, tender
	Confirmed by: no flow on **Doppler ultrasound scan**
Impaired lymphatic drainage	*Suggested by:* firm, non-tender, non-pitting edema of gradual onset over months to years
	Confirmed by: obstruction to flow on **lymphangiogram** (rarely done)

Cardiovascular signs

Thoughts on interpreting cardiovascular signs

The findings are discussed in a sequence of the CV examination, thinking of cardiac output, beginning with hand warmth, checking the radial pulse, and measuring the BP. Continuing to think of cardiac output, examine the carotids. Next think of venous return by inspecting the JVP. Finally, inspect, palpate, percuss, and auscultate the heart. Examine the legs, and again think of cardiac output (e.g., temperature of skin, peripheral pulses) and venous return (e.g., pitting edema, leg veins, and liver enlargement).

Peripheral cyanosis

This includes cyanosis of the hands but not the lips or tongue.

Main differential diagnoses and typical outline evidence

Raynaud's phenomenon due to exposure of hands to cold or vibration	*Suggested by:* normal pulse and BP, history of blue hands after exposure to cold, vibrating tools, etc.; history of scleroderma
	Confirmed by: hands and feet assume normal color in warm room
Arterial obstruction due to atheroma or small vessel disease in diabetics	*Suggested by:* absent or poor or asymmetric radial or dorsalis pedis pulses. Absent hair and skin atrophy in chronic cases
	Confirmed by: **Doppler ultrasound** measure of low blood flow and **angiography**
Hemorrhage due to external or internal bleeding	*Suggested by:* pallor, sweating, low BP, high pulse rate, observable external bleeding or melena or massive trauma expected to cause internal bleeding
	Confirmed by: low **Hb** (although Hb is often normal early after a bleed) and **response to blood transfusion** or volume expansion and control of bleeding
Low cardiac output e.g., due to large MI or severe valvular disease	*Suggested by:* pallor, cold extremities, sweating, low BP
	Confirmed by: poor LV function on **echocardiogram**, low cardiac output measured by a Swan-Ganz catheter

Central cyanosis

This includes cyanosis of the lips, tongue, and hands.

Main differential diagnoses and typical outline evidence

Right-to-left cardiac shunt due to congenital heart disease, e.g., tetralogy of Fallot, Eisenmenger's syndrome, tricuspid atresia, Ebstein's anomaly, pulmonary AV fistula, transposition of the great vessels	*Suggested by:* breathlessness, clubbing, systolic or continuous murmur, right ventricular heave *Confirmed by:* **echocardiogram** and **cardiac catheterization**
Right-to-left pulmonary shunt due to decreased perfusion of lung tissue from extensive collapse or consolidation or alveolar filling	*Suggested by:* breathlessness, poor chest movement, dullness to percussion and absent breath sounds over a large area of the chest *Confirmed by:* **chest X-ray** and **bronchoscopy**
Hemoglobin abnormalities due to congenital NADH diaphorase, Hb M disease, or acquired methemoglobinemia or sulfhemoglobinemia	*Suggested by:* no clubbing, no murmurs, normal chest movement, no chest signs. History from childhood or exposure to toxic drugs, e.g., aniline dyes *Confirmed by:* **Hb electrophoresis**

Tachycardia (pulse rate >100bpm)

Main differential diagnoses and typical outline evidence

Fever	*Suggested by:* warm skin, erythema, sweats, temperature >38°C
	Confirmed by: elevated temperature, fever pattern
Hemorrhage	*Suggested by:* signs of blood loss, pallor, sweats, low BP, poor peripheral perfusion
	Confirmed by: low *Hb* (can be normal in initial stages), low central venous pressure
Hypoxia	*Suggested by:* cyanosis, respiratory distress
	Confirmed by: pulse oximetry or ↓PaO$_2$
Thyrotoxicosis	*Suggested by:* sweating, fine tremor, weight loss, lid lag, frequent bowel movements, sweats, weight loss
	Confirmed by: ↑FT4, ± ↑FT3 and ↓TSH
Severe anemia	*Suggested by:* subconjunctival and nail-bed pallor, tiredness, poor exercise tolerance
	Confirmed by: ↓*Hb* (and indices)
Heart failure (LVF, RHF, CHF) associated with ischemic heart disease, myocarditis, etc.	*Suggested by:* third heart sound, fine crackles at bases, raised JVP
	Confirmed by: CXR showing large heart, pulmonary congestion; poor LV function on **echocardiogram**, low cardiac output measured by a Swan-Ganz catheter
Pulmonary embolus (PE)	*Suggested by:* history of sudden breathlessness, cyanosis, raised JVP, loud P2. ECG: right axis deviation
	Confirmed by: **V/Q scan** showing mismatched defects, **pulmonary angiography** of spinal CT showing filling defect in pulmonary artery
Drugs e.g., amphetamines, β-agonists, anticholinergic agents, cocaine	*Suggested by:* drug history
	Confirmed by: normal pulse rate if drug stopped

Bradycardia (<60 bpm)

Main differential diagnoses and typical outline evidence

Athletic heart (nonpathologic)	*Suggested by:* young and fit, asymptomatic
	Confirmed by: above clinical findings. Normal chronotropic response to exercise. Normal echocardiogram
Drugs	*Suggested by:* history e.g., beta blockers
	Confirmed by: improvement when drug withdrawn
Sinoatrial disease	*Suggested by:* elderly, ischemic heart disease
	Confirmed by: ECG: Slow atrial rate with sinus P waves or abnormal P waves
Ventricular or supraventricular ectopy or bigeminy	*Suggested by:* known ischemic heart disease
	Confirmed by: comparison of pulse rate to ECG: premature ectopic beats may not generate a pulse if early enough to not allow sufficient ventricular filling
Myocardial infarction (MI)	*Suggested by:* central, crushing chest pain (can be atypical pain)
	Confirmed by: ECG: Q waves, raised ST segments, and inverted T waves. ↑CPK-MB or *troponin*. Bradycardia is most frequently seen with inferior MI
Hypothyroidism	*Suggested by:* constipation, weight gain, dry skin, dry hair, slow-relaxing reflexes, other symptoms and signs of hypothyroidism
	Confirmed by: ↑TSH, ↓T4
Hypothermia	*Suggested by:* history of exposure to cold temperature and immobility
	Confirmed by: Core temperature <35°C

Pulse irregular

Main differential diagnoses and typical outline evidence

Atrial fibrillation caused by ischemic heart disease, thyrotoxicosis, etc.	*Suggested by:* irregularly irregular pulse
	Confirmed by: ECG showing no P waves, and irregularly irregular normal QRS complexes
Atrial flutter with variable heart block caused by ischemic heart disease, etc.	*Suggested by:* irregularly irregular pulse
	Confirmed by: ECG showing "saw tooth" F waves, and irregularly irregular normal QRS complexes
Atrial or ventricular ectopics caused by ischemic heart disease, etc.	*Suggested by:* pulse with early or dropped beats, compensatory pause with ventricular ectopy
	Confirmed by: ECG showing underlying sinus rhythm with early QRS complexes. Atrial ectopic beats have a narrow or wide QRS and are preceded by an early P wave. Ventricular ectopic beats have a wide QRS, are not preceded by an early P wave, and usually are followed by a compensatory pause.
Wenkebach heart block caused by ischemic heart disease, etc.	*Suggested by:* regular rate with periodic slightly longer pauses
	Confirmed by: ECG showing AV conduction with progressive prolongation of P-R interval with normal QRS complex followed by a P wave not followed by a QRS complex. The next P-R interval is abruptly shorter.

Pulse amplitude high (bounding pulse)

This is an indication of the width of the pulse pressure. It can be confirmed by a large difference between the systolic (SBP) and diastolic (DBP) blood pressure.

Main differential diagnoses and typical outline evidence

Aortic insufficiency	*Suggested by:* striking "water hammer" quality. Systolic BP high (e.g., >160 mmHg) and diastolic BP very low (e.g., <50 mmHg) early diastolic murmur, forceful, displaced apex impulse
	Confirmed by: **echocardiogram** and **cardiac catheterization** showing diastolic leaking of the aortic valve
Atherosclerosis	*Suggested by:* older age. Systolic BP high (e.g., >160 mmHg) and diastolic BP not low (e.g., >80 mmHg)
	Confirmed by: **echocardiogram** to exclude aortic incompetence
Severe anemia	*Suggested by:* pallor. Systolic BP high (e.g., >160 mmHg) and diastolic BP normal (e.g., <85 mmHg)
	Confirmed by: **Hb↓** (e.g., <10 grm/dL)
Bradycardia of any cause with normal myocardium	*Suggested by:* slow heart rate (e.g., <50 bpm)
	Confirmed by: ECG showing slow rate and type of rhythm
Hyperkinetic circulation e.g., due to hypercapnia, thyrotoxicosis, fever, Paget's disease, AV fistula	*Suggested by:* warm peripheries and features of cause, e.g., cyanosis, tremor, lid lag, fever, skull deformity, etc.
	Confirmed by: high pCO_2 (if hypercapnia) or ↑FT4, ± ↑FT3 and ↓TSH (if thyrotoxic) or fever or ↑ hydroxyproline (if Paget's disease)

Pulse amplitude low (thready pulse)

This is an indication of the width of the pulse pressure. It can be confirmed by a small difference between the systolic and diastolic blood pressure.

Main differential diagnoses and typical outline evidence

Poor cardiac contractility due to ischemic heart disease, cardiomyopathy, cardiac tamponade, constrictive pericarditis	*Suggested by:* quiet heart sounds, ↑JVP, peripheral edema, basal lung crackles *Confirmed by:* poor LV function on **echocardiogram**
Hypovolemia due to blood loss, dehydration	*Suggested by:* cold peripheries, thirst, dry skin and mucous membranes, low urine output *Confirmed by:* **blood urea nitrogen (BUN)**↑, **Hb**↓ (in blood loss) or ↑ (if hemo-concentrated)
Poor vascular tone, hypotension e.g., due to septic shock	*Suggested by:* warm peripheries, thirst, dry skin, ↓urine output *Confirmed by:* hypotension, other evidence of sepsis (positive blood cultures, azotemia)
Aortic stenosis	*Suggested by:* slowly rising carotid pulse, characteristic systolic murmur *Confirmed by:* **echocardiogram** and **cardiac catheterization**

Blood pressure high (hypertension)

High blood pressure is defined as systolic BP >140 mmHg and diastolic BP >90 mmHg. The level treated depends on presence of risk factors. Generally, any sustained systolic BP over 140 is treated, but in diabetics, >130 systolic or >85 diastolic is treated.

Main differential diagnoses and typical outline evidence

Temporary hypertension with no risk factors	*Suggested by:* normal blood pressure <140 mmHg systolic and <90 mmHg diastolic when repeated *Confirmed boy:* **24-hour ambulatory blood pressure monitoring**
Essential hypertension 95% of cases	*Suggested by:* sustained hypertension *Confirmed by:* **24-hour ambulatory blood pressure monitoring.** No symptoms or signs of specific cause, normal BUN and electrolytes, and prompt control on treatment
Hypertension of pregnancy (pre-eclampsia sometimes progressing to eclampsia)	*Suggested by:* only occurring during pregnancy. Very high BP and seizures in eclampsia *Confirmed by:* resolution or improvement when pregnancy over or terminated
Renovascular hypertension due to renal artery stenosis or primary renal disease	*Suggested by:* established renal impairment too soon to be caused by hypertension *Confirmed by:* **BUN** and **creatinine** raised, **Hb↓** (in established renal failure), hyper-reninemia. **Ultrasound** or **isotope scan** of kidneys and ureters. Arteriogram or MR angiogram of the renal arteries
Endocrine hypertension due to primary hyperaldostero-nism (Conn's syndrome if tumor too), Cushing's syndrome, pheo-chromocytoma	*Suggested by:* proximal muscle weakness in Cushing's syndrome or severe aldosteronism. Paroxysms of vascular symptoms in pheochromocytoma *Confirmed by:* ↑ **aldosterone** and ↓ **renin**, ↑ 24-hour urinary free cortisol, etc., in Cushing's syndrome. ↑**VMA** and **metanephrines** ↑ in pheochromocytoma

Vascular hypertension due to coarctation of the aorta, subclavian artery stenosis	*Suggested by:* upper extremity hypertension (right arm), normal in legs (and left arm in subclavian artery stenosis). Delayed arterial pulse between upper and lower extremities suggests coarctation of the aorta. *Confirmed by:* **MRA/angiography**
Drug induced due to NSAIDs, estrogen, steroids, erythropoietin	*Suggested by:* drug history *Confirmed by:* resolution or improvement when drug stopped

Blood pressure very low (hypotension)

Main differential diagnoses and typical outline evidence

Cardiogenic— low output due to poor myocardial contraction, valvular stenosis or regurgitation, etc.	*Suggested by:* very low BP, fast or slow heart rate, peripheral and central cyanosis, quiet heart sound ± abnormal murmur, cool extremities. High or normal JVP, abnormal heart rhythms, enlarged heart, echocardiogram findings of systolic or diastolic dysfunction, valve stenosis, or regurgitation
	Confirmed by: echocardiogram with findings indicating low cardiac output, right heart catheterization showing low cardiac output
Low circulating blood volume due to hemorrhage (GI etc.) dehydration, etc.	*Suggested by:* very low BP, fast heart rate, peripheral cyanosis, JVP low, cool extremities. Background evidence of cause
	Confirmed by: low CVP, ECG, normal heart on CXR. Improvement with blood, plasma expander, intravenous (IV) fluids with CVP monitoring
Loss of vascular tone ("distributive" shock) due to septicemia, adrenal failure, etc.	*Suggested by:* very low BP, fast heart rate, peripheral cyanosis, JVP low or normal, warm extremities. Background evidence of cause
	Confirmed by: low CVP, normal heart on CXR. Improvement in BP and CVP with blood transfusion, volume expansion (IV fluids), glucocorticoids, and antibiotics

Postural fall in blood pressure (orthostatic hypotension)

To be significant, the blood pressure must fall >30 mmHg, remain low for at least 1 minute, and be accompanied by dizziness.

Main differential diagnoses and typical outline evidence

Drug induced due to excessive dose of hypotensive agent (opiates, benzodiazepines, other sedatives, antidepressants)	*Suggested by:* drug history *Confirmed by:* by resolution or improvement after stopping or reducing drug
Autonomic neuropathy due to diabetes mellitus or tabes dorsalis (rarely)	*Suggested by:* history of long-standing diabetes (common) or tabes dorsalis (rare). Also, diarrhea, abdominal distension, and vomiting (gastroparesis), impotence, urine frequency *Confirmed by:* **ECG monitor of beat-to-beat variation:** <10 beats per minute (bpm) change in heart rate on deep breathing at 6 breaths/minute or getting up from lying
Idiopathic orthostatic hypotension	*Suggested by:* no other features except elderly *Confirmed by:* isolated phenomenon
Volume depletion due to mild or early dehydration or hemorrhage	*Suggested by:* history of vomiting or diarrhea or poor po intake or melena or hematochezia; poor skin turgor, dry axillae; labs showing azotemia with BUN rise disproportionate to creatinine rise *Confirmed by:* low urine Na or FENa; anemia; evidence of hemorrhage; response to fluids or blood transfusion

BP/pulse difference between arms

This refers to asymmetric pulses or BP differential >15 mmHg.

Main differential diagnoses and typical outline evidence

Old or acute thrombosis in atheromatous artery or aneurysm or dissection of ascending aorta	*Suggested by:* associated peripheral vascular disease *Confirmed by:* **MRA/angiography**
Supravalvular aortic stenosis (congenital)	*Suggested by:* "elfin-like" facies, ejection systolic murmur, angina, and syncope *Confirmed by:* **angiography**
Subclavian steal syndrome	*Suggested by:* associated neurological symptoms. Exercising right arm induces cerebral ischemia. *Confirmed by:* **angiography** showing abnormal subclavian artery
Thoracic inlet syndrome	*Suggested by:* bracing shoulder aggravating BP difference *Confirmed by:* **MRA/angiography** showing abnormal subclavian artery
Aortic arch syndrome, Takayasu's syndrome	*Suggested by:* in young Asian female with cerebral and peripheral ischemic symptoms *Confirmed by:* **angiography** showing abnormal subclavian artery

BP/pulse difference between arms and legs

A BP difference >15 mmHg. A wide cuff must be used for the thigh. The patient's arms and leg must be level when measuring BP.

Main differential diagnoses and typical outline evidence

Old or acute thrombosis in atheromatous artery or aneurysm or dissection of descending thoracic or abdominal aorta or iliac arteries, especially in diabetics	*Suggested by:* associated peripheral vascular disease. Atrophic skin and hair loss on lower legs *Confirmed by:* Doppler ultrasound of legs to try to find remediable flow reduction. **Angiography** to try to identify surgically remediable arterial stenosis
Coarctation of aorta	*Suggested by:* ejection systolic murmur presenting in childhood or early adult life, rib notching on CXR *Confirmed by:* stenosis on angiography

Prominent leg veins ± unilateral leg swelling

Main differential diagnoses and typical outline evidence

Varicose veins ± incompetent communicating valves	*Suggested by:* veins distended and tortuous made worse when standing. Cough impulse felt and Trendelenberg test shows filling down along extent of communicating valve leaks
	Confirmed by: clinical findings usually, but if doubt, use *Doppler ultrasound* probe to confirm whether or not incompetence is present in the saphenofemoral junction or short saphenous vein behind the knee
Thrombophlebitis	*Suggested by:* tender, hot veins with redness of surrounding skin
	Confirmed by: resolution on antibiotics
Deep vein thrombosis (DVT)	*Suggested by:* immobility, prominent dilated veins; warm, tender, swollen calf; other risk factors for DVT
	Confirmed by: reduced flow on compression *Doppler ultrasound*, blockage seen on *venography*

Unilateral leg and ankle swelling

Main differential diagnoses and typical outline evidence

Deep vein thrombosis	*Suggested by:* immobility, prominent dilated veins, warm, tender, swollen calf and positive Homan's sign
	Confirmed by: reduced flow on compression *Doppler*, blockage seen on *venography*
Ruptured Baker's cyst	*Suggested by:* sudden onset while straightening knee, warm, tender, swollen calf
	Confirmed by: **D-dimer** titers not raised, normal flow on compression *Doppler*, no blockage seen on *venography*. Leaking from joint capsule on arthrography
Cellulitis from infection secondary or primarily due to insect bites	*Suggested by:* tender, hot, red leg and fever
	Confirmed by: resolution on antibiotics
Unilateral varicose veins	*Suggested by:* distended and tortuous veins made worse when standing
	Confirmed by: **Doppler ultrasound probe** to confirm where incompetence is present
Chronic venous insufficiency from old deep vein thromboses	*Suggested by:* past history, veins distended and made worse on standing
	Confirmed by: **Doppler ultrasound** probe to where incompetence is present
Venous insufficiency from obstruction by tumor or lymph node	*Suggested by:* onset over weeks, veins distended
	Confirmed by: **Doppler ultrasound** and **venography** to explore where obstruction is present
Lymphedema from lymphatic obstruction due to primary lymphatic hypoplasia	*Suggested by:* unilateral swelling that is worse premenstrually, in warm weather, and with immobility. No venous dilatation
	Confirmed by: **Doppler ultrasound** to show normal venous flow. MRI or CT or **lymphangiogram** (rarely) to show hypoplastic lymphatics

Subacute lymphatic obstruction secondary to neoplastic obstruction	*Suggested by:* unilateral swelling developing over months. No venous dilatation
	Confirmed by: **Doppler ultrasound** to show normal venous flow. MRI or CT or **lymphangiogram** (rarely) to show site of obstruction
Acute lymphatic obstruction due to streptococcal lymphangitis	*Suggested by:* sudden unilateral swelling developing over hours. No venous dilatation but lymphangitic streaks
	Confirmed by: clinical features and response to penicillin. **Doppler ultrasound** to show normal venous flow

Bilateral leg and ankle swelling

Main differential diagnoses and typical outline evidence

Bilateral varicose veins or old deep vein thromboses	*Suggested by:* veins distended and tortuous made worse when standing
	Confirmed by: **Doppler ultrasound** probe to confirm where incompetence is present
Low albumin due to poor nutrition, malabsorption, liver failure, nephrotic syndrome, protein-losing enteropathy	*Suggested by:* history of facial puffiness in morning and evidence of possible cause of low albumin
	Confirmed by: low **serum albumin** (<3.0 g/dL to be significant)
Congestive cardiac failure (i.e., right heart failure due to left heart failure) caused by ischemic heart disease, mitral stenosis, cardiomyopathy, etc.	*Suggested by:* raised JVP, large liver, fine rales at lung bases or higher, third heart sound. Echocardiogram showing systolic or diastolic dysfunction or valve dysfunction
	Confirmed by: **CXR:** large heart, distension of veins in upper lobes of lung, and fluffy lung infiltrates. **Echocardiogram:** ventricular dysfunction
Cor pulmonale (right heart failure) from pulmonary hypertension due to long-standing lung disease, old pulmonary emboli, etc.)	*Suggested by:* raised JVP, large liver, third heart sound, loud pulmonary second sound, and RV heave
	Confirmed by: **CXR** showing pulmonary disease, ECG showing right axis deviation. **Echocardiogram:** right ventricular dysfunction
Lymphedema due to primary lymphatic hypoplasia	*Suggested by:* bilateral swelling that is worse premenstrually, in warm weather, and with immobility. No venous dilatation.
	Confirmed by: **Doppler ultrasound** to show normal venous flow. Occasional **lymphangiography** to show hypoplastic lymphatics

Raised jugular venous pressure

This is measured with the patient lying at 45°. It is undetectably low if the external jugular empties when the compressing finger is released. An elevated JVP with *a* and *v* waves that is accurately assessed means that right atrial pressure is abnormally high.

Main differential diagnoses and typical outline evidence

Fluid overload due to excessive IV or oral fluids	*Suggested by:* elevated double pulsations JVP with *a* and *v* waves. History of high input of IV or oral fluids. Renal insufficiency or failure. Echocardiogram showing normal or hyperdynamic systolic function
	Confirmed by: response to reduced fluid intake and spontaneous diuresis (or diuretics) or fluid removal
Congestive cardiac failure (i.e., right-sided failure due to left-sided failure)	*Suggested by:* elevated JVP with *a* and *v* waves. Dyspnea, rales on pulmonary exam. CXR consistent with pulmonary edema. Echocardiogram showing LV systolic or diastolic dysfunction or valve dysfunction
	Confirmed by: **echocardiogram** showing ventricular dysfunction, **right heart catheterization** showing elevated RA and pulmonary capillary wedge pressure, decreased cardiac output
Cor pulmonale Right heart failure due to pulmonary vascular disease	*Suggested by:* elevated JVP; large *a* waves may be present. Pulmonary exam with hyperresonance and low diaphragms. Sometimes wheezing or rhonchi, but not rales. ECG showing tall P wave in lead 2
	Confirmed by: echocardiogram showing dilated RV with reduced systolic function, flattened intraventricular septum indicating elevation of RV pressure, no LV systolic or diastolic dysfunction or valve dysfunction. Right heart catheterization showing elevation of RA, RV, and PA systolic pressure, elevation of pulmonary vascular resistance, but normal pulmonary capillary wedge pressure
Right-sided congestive heart failure with atrial fibrillation	*Suggested by:* elevated JVP with a single pulsation, *a* waves absent, irregularly irregular pulse
	Confirmed by: ECG showing no P waves and normal QRS complexes. Other findings of congestive heart failure mentioned above
Complete heart block	*Suggested by:* intermittent elevations of JVP when the atria contract when AV valves are closed. Bradycardia
	Confirmed by: ECG showing no association between P waves and QRS complexes

Tricuspid regurgitation	*Suggested by:* elevated JVP with single pulsation, large *v* waves in mid-systole. Holosystolic murmur present in the low sternal area
	Confirmed by: **echocardiogram** showing large right atrium and tricuspid incompetence
Pericardial effusion sufficient to compromise heart function	*Suggested by:* pulsatile JVP with *a* wave and rapid descent. Very breathless. Quiet heart sounds. Globular heart shadow on CXR. Low-voltage QRS complexes on ECG
	Confirmed by: Echocardiogram showing moderate or large pericardial effusion, excessive respiratory variation of the inflow velocity of mitral and tricuspid valves, diastolic collapse of the RA or RV
Constrictive pericarditis	*Suggested by:* JVP rising with inspiration (Kussmaul sign), *a* waves have rapid descent. Quiet heart sounds. Large liver and ascites.
	Confirmed by: small heart shadow on CXR. **Echocardiogram** shows small cavity and little contraction
Jugular vein obstruction	*Suggested by:* no JVP pulsation, external jugular vein also distended
	Confirmed by: **ultrasound** scan to explore site of obstruction

Abnormal apical impulse

Look for displacement from normal site in mid-clavicular line, heave, and character of impulse (tapping, double).

Main differential diagnoses and typical outline evidence

Obesity, emphysema, pleural effusion, pericardial effusion or dextrocardia	*Suggested by:* impalpable apical impulse
	Confirmed by: evidence of intervening factors or apical impulse palpable on right (dextrocardia)
Large left ventricle due to mitral incompetence, aortic incompetence, right-to-left VSD shunt	*Suggested by:* apical impulse displaced to the left and heaving
	Confirmed by: large left ventricle on **echocardiogram** with corresponding valve lesion
Hypertrophied left ventricle due to hypertension or aortic stenosis	*Suggested by:* apex not displaced but heaving. ECG meeting voltage criteria for LVH
	Confirmed by: hypertrophied left ventricular wall on **echocardiogram**
Hypertrophic cardiomyopathy	*Suggested by:* double apex beat, angina, breathlessness, syncope on exercise, jerky pulse, high JVP with *a* wave, thrill and murmur best at left sternal edge. Rapid and notched carotid upstroke
	Confirmed by: **echocardiogram** showing hypertrophied septum and left ventricular walls with small left ventricular cavity
Ventricular aneurysm	*Suggested by:* double apical impulse. Persistently raised ST segments on ECG
	Confirmed by: thinning and paradoxical movement of ventricular wall on **echocardiogram**

Mitral stenosis	*Suggested by:* tapping left ventricular impulse (palpable first heart sound) and rumbling diastolic murmur radiating to the axilla. ECG showing left atrial enlargement without LVH *Confirmed by:* **echocardiogram** and ***cardiac catheterization***
Right ventricular hypertrophy due to pulmonic stenosis or pulmonary hypertension	*Suggested by:* upper sternal heave *Confirmed by:* ECG findings and **echocardiogram**.
Major valve stenosis or regurgitation or muscular outflow tract obstruction	*Suggested by:* palpable thrill or loud murmur *Confirmed by:* ECG findings and **echocardiogram** and ***cardiac catheterization***

Extra heart sounds

The third and fourth heart sounds (S3 and S4), respectively, are early and late diastolic ventricular filling sounds. S3 can be heard in healthy children, but S4 is abnormal even in children.

Main differential diagnoses and typical outline evidence

LVH due to hypertension, aortic stenosis, or hypertrophic cardiomyopathy	*Suggested by:* fourth heart sound. Increased LV voltage on ECG
	Confirmed by: LV hypertrophy on *echocardiogram*
Decompensated heart failure in cardiomyopathy, constrictive pericarditis	*Suggested by:* third heart sound
	Confirmed by: Elevated JVP, pulmonary rales, CXR findings of CHF
Severe heart failure	*Suggested by:* third and fourth heart sound giving gallop
	Confirmed by: raised JVP, crackles at lung bases, pulmonary edema on CXR and systolic or diastolic dysfunction or valve dysfunction on *echocardiogram*

Diastolic murmur

Find where it is heard best (e.g., at the apex or left sternal edge).

Main differential diagnoses and typical outline evidence

Mitral stenosis	*Suggested by:* mitral facies, tapping apex beat, loud first heart sound, rumbling diasystolic murmur best at apex with patient lying on left side
	Confirmed by: **echocardiogram** and cardiac catheter displaying valve lesion
Mitral stenosis with pliable valve	*Suggested by:* opening snap
Aortic insufficency	*Suggested by:* high BP, wide pulse pressure, laterally displaced apex beat, early diastolic murmur best at left or right sternal edge
	Confirmed by: **echocardiogram** and **cardiac catheterization** displaying valve lesion

Systolic murmur

Main differential diagnoses and typical outline evidence

Aortic stenosis	*Suggested by:* crescendo–decrescendo systolic murmur at upper right sternal border radiating to the carotid arteries. Cool extremities, slowly rising carotid pulse, low BP and pulse pressure, heaving apex and soft or absent aortic component of the second heart sound (A_2). ECG with criteria for LVH
	Confirmed by: **echocardiogram** and **cardiac catheterization showing** stenosed aortic valve
Hypertrophic cardiomyopathy	*Suggested by:* angina, breathlessness, syncope on exercise, double peaked carotid pulse, high JVP with *a* wave, double apex beat, normal aortic component of second heart sound (A_2), and systolic murmur best at left sternal edge
	Confirmed by: **echocardiogram** showing hypertrophied septum and left ventricular walls with small ventricular cavity showing evidence of subvalvular outflow obstruction
Aortic sclerosis	*Suggested by:* normal pulse and BP ± no heaving apex. Normal ECG
	Confirmed by: **echocardiogram** showing thickening of aortic valve leaflets but not stenosis
Pulmonary high flow	*Suggested by:* normal pulse and BP, normal JVP, and no left parasternal heave. Normal ECG
	Confirmed by: Normal **echocardiogram**
Atrial septal defect (rare) causing high pulmonary flow	*Suggested by:* normal pulse and BP, normal JVP and left parasternal heave present. ECG: peaked P waves, right axis deviation in secundum defect, left-axis deviation in primum defect.
	Confirmed by: **echocardiogram** and **cardiac catheterization** findings
Pulmonary stenosis	*Suggested by:* low pulse, high JVP, and left parasternal heave. Right bundle branch block (RBBB) and right-axis deviation on ECG
	Confirmed by: **echocardiogram** and **cardiac catheterization**

Mitral incompetence due to rheumatic heart disease, valve dysfunction after myocardial infarction	*Suggested by:* holosystolic murmur at apex with radiation to axilla. No large JVP *v* waves. Displaced heaving apex beat *Confirmed by:* CXR: large, round opacity "behind heart" (big left atrium). ECG: M-shaped P wave. **Echocardiogram** and **cardiac catheterization**
Tricuspid incompetence (rare alone) sometimes alone in severe cor pulmonale or after pulmonary embolus	*Suggested by:* holosystolic murmur at left sternal edge (louder on inspiration), no radiation to axilla. Large JVP with mid-systolic *v* waves. Left parasternal heave. ECG: tall-peaked P waves, right-axis deviation and RBBB *Confirmed by:* **Echocardiogram** and **cardiac catheterization** showing tricuspid valve incompetence
Mitral and tricuspid incompetence due to rheumatic heart disease or dilated ventricles in severe heart failure	*Suggested by:* holosystolic murmur with radiation to axilla. Large JVP *v* waves. Displaced heaving apex beat *Confirmed by:* normal ECG and **echocardiogram** showing mitral and tricuspid valve incompetence
Ventricular septal defect (VSD) usually congenital, sometimes rupture of septum after infarction	*Suggested by:* holosystolic murmur loud and rough. Raised JVP. Central cyanosis if right-to-left shunt. Displaced heaving apex beat. RBBB and right-axis deviation on ECG *Confirmed by:* **echocardiogram** and **cardiac catheterization** showing defect

Murmurs not entirely in systole or diastole

Main differential diagnoses and typical outline evidence

Patent ductus arteriosus	*Suggested by:* newborn infant, high pulse volume, diastolic and systolic murmurs to give continuous, "mechanical" murmur: "shee-shoo, shee-shoo"
	Confirmed by: **echocardiogram** and **cardiac catheterization**
Pericarditis with pericardial friction rub (not true murmur)	*Suggested by:* "scratching murmur" heard in systole ± diastole. Chest pain worse when lying back and relieved by lying forward. Raised ST segments or T-wave inversion on ECG
	Confirmed by: **echocardiographic** findings of pericardial effusion

Respiratory symptoms

Sudden breathlessness

This situation may be life threatening; the severity of the underlying condition often creates helpful diagnostic information.

Some differential diagnoses and typical outline evidence

Pulmonary embolus (PE) arising from DVT in leg, pelvic vein, or right atrium	*Suggested by:* central chest pain also with abrupt shortness of breath, cyanosis, tachycardia, loud second sound in pulmonary area, associated DVT or risk factors of silent DVT. PO_2 low, PCO_2 normal or low
	Confirmed by: **Spiral CT** showing filling defect (best) or **V/Q scan** showing ventilation/perfusion mismatch. When **spiral CT** is not available (rare today) and confirmatory test required, **pulmonary angiogram** may be done (shows filling defect)
Pneumothorax	*Suggested by:* pain in center or side of chest with abrupt breathlessness. Resonance to percussion over same side, especially lung apex
	Confirmed by: **expiratory CXR** showing loss of lung markings outside sharp line (see Fig. 19.20)
Anaphylaxis	*Suggested by:* dramatic onset over minutes, history of prior allergen exposure, tachycardia and hypotension, acute bronchospasm with wheeze and dyspnea, flushing and/or sweating, feeling of dread, facial edema, urticaria, warm but clammy extremities
	Confirmed by: clinical presentation and by controlled allergen exposure and examination. Response to intramuscular (IM) adrenaline
Inhalation of foreign body	*Suggested by:* history of putting an object in mouth, e.g., peanut. Sudden stridor, severe cough, low-pitched, monophonic wheeze
	Confirmed by: relief in extremis by performing Heimlich maneuver, etc., or if not in extremis, foreign body seen on **CXR/CT** or **bronchoscopy**

Orthopnea and paroxysmal nocturnal dyspnea (PND)

Orthopnea is shortness of breath when lying flat. (Try to confirm by observing patient lying flat.) This can be explained by increased venous return or less efficient lung movement when the abdominal contents press against the diaphragm. PND is shortness of breath that awakens a patient from sleep; PND usually has similar pathophysiology to orthopnea, but may also occur with nocturnal bronchospasm (e.g., in asthma).

Some differential diagnoses and typical outline evidence

Pulmonary edema from congestive (chronic) LV failure (due to ischemic heart disease, mitral stenosis)	*Suggested by:* displaced apex beat, third heart sound, bilateral basal fine crackles *Confirmed by:* **CXR** appearances (see Fig. 19.13). Impaired LV function on **echocardiogram**. Abnormal ECG reflecting underlying heart disease
COPD	*Suggested by:* dry cough and white sputum, wheeze. Smoking history of ≥10 pack-years. Chest hyperinflation, pursed lips. Reduced breath sounds, accessory muscles of respiration used. Reduced peak flow rate *Confirmed by:* **CXR:** oyperexpanded, radiolucent lungs; bullae. **Spirometry:** <12% reversibility, reduced ratio of forced expiratory volume in 1 second to forced vital capacity (FEV_1/FVC ratio), reduced carbon dioxide diffusing capacity (DL_{CO}). Hypoxia ± hypercapnia. Rarely (young patients, family history): reduced α_1-*antitrypsin* levels
Asthma	*Suggested by:* wheeze or dry cough. Other specific triggers to breathlessness. Other allergies. Past history of similar attacks unless first presentation *Confirmed by:* reduced **peak flows**, FEV_1 that improves >12% with treatment and symptomatic response to treatment

Acute breathlessness, wheeze ± cough

This symptom suggests airway narrowing due to a foreign body, bronchospasm, inflammation or hydrostatic edema.

Some differential diagnoses and typical outline evidence

Asthma	*Suggested by:* wheeze with exacerbations over hours (silent chest if very severe). Anxiety, tachypnea, tachycardia, prolonged expiration, use of accessory muscles. Usually known asthmatic
	Confirmed by: reduced peak flows, FEV_1 that improve by >12% with treatment
COPD	*Suggested by:* wheeze with exacerbations over hours to days often with pursed lips. Long history of cough, breathlessness and wheeze
	Confirmed by: response to bronchodilators, spirometry showing low FEV_1/FVC and little reversibility of FEV_1 (improves by <12%)
Acute viral or bacterial bronchitis	*Suggested by:* onset of wheeze over days. No dramatic progression. Fever, mucopurulent sputum, dyspnea
	Confirmed by: **sputum culture** and sensitivities, response to antibiotics (if bacterial)
Acute left ventricular failure	*Suggested by:* onset over minutes or hours of breathlessness and wheeze, displaced tapping apex beat, third heart sound, bilateral basal late, fine inspiratory crackles and wheeze
	Confirmed by: **CXR:** fluffy opacification greatest around the hilum, fine horizontal linear opacities (Kerley lines), peripherally, large heart. Impaired LV function on **echocardiogram** (see Fig. 19.13)
Anaphylaxis	*Suggested by:* dramatic onset over minutes, acute bronchospasm with wheeze and dyspnea, flushing, sweating and a feeling of dread, facial edema, urticaria and warm but clammy extremities. Tachycardia and hypotension
	Confirmed by: clinical presentation and later by controlled allergen exposure and examination. Response to adrenaline IM

Frank hemoptysis (blood-streaked sputum)

This may have a sinister cause that requires urgent diagnosis and treatment.

Some differential diagnoses and typical outline evidence

Acute viral or bacterial bronchitis	*Suggested by:* days of fever, mucopurulent sputum, dyspnea
	Confirmed by: **sputum culture** and sensitivities, response to appropriate antibiotics
Pulmonary infarction due to embolus from DVT in leg, pelvis, or right atrium	*Suggested by:* sudden shortness of breath, pleural rub, cyanosis, tachycardia, loud P2, associated DVT or risk factors such as recent surgery, childbirth, immobility, etc.
	Confirmed by: **V/Q scan** mismatch, **spiral CT scan** showing clot in artery, **pulmonary angiogram** showing filling defect
Carcinoma of lung	*Suggested by:* weeks or months of weight loss, smoking history, new or worsening cough
	Confirmed by: opacity on CXR and/or CT scan (see Fig. 19.6). Tumor cells on **sputum cytology** or bronchoscopic biopsy
Pulmonary tuberculosis	*Suggested by:* weeks or months of fever, malaise, weight loss, and a contact history. CXR: opacification, especially in apical segments.
	Confirmed by: AFB on **smear sputum, culture** and/or response to treatment (when cultures negative and no other explanation for symptoms)
Upper respiratory infection (URI) abnormalities and bleeding e.g. nasal polyps, laryngeal carcinoma, pharyngeal tumors	*Suggested by:* days of purulent rhinorrhea (blood from URI swallowed or inhaled and coughed back up).
	Confirmed by: **fiber-optic rhinoscopy, CT/MRI,** surgery and biopsy

Lung abscess	*Suggested by:* days or weeks of copious and foul-smelling sputum, fever, chest pain
	Confirmed by: **CXR:** circular opacity with fluid level, **sputum culture**
Bronchiectasis	*Suggested by:* months of copious (often cupfuls) of purulent sputum daily. Coarse, late inspiratory crackles, digital clubbing
	Confirmed by: **CXR:** cystic shadowing; **high-resolution CT chest:** honeycombing and thickened, dilated bronchi (see Fig. 19.18)
Wegener's granulomatosis	*Suggested by:* months of cough, breathlessness, hematuria. Classic triad of URT, LRT, and renal abnormalities. Multisystem vasculitis, e.g., arthritis, myalgia, skin rashes, and nasal bridge collapse
	Confirmed by: ↑titers of **cytoplasmic anti-neutrophil cytoplasmic antibody (cANCA)** antibody and microscopic arteritis on biopsy (see Fig. 19.8)
Goodpastures' syndrome (very rare)	*Suggested by:* profuse hemoptysis, months or years of ill health, renal failure, ↑BP, chest pain
	Confirmed by: anti-glomerular basement antibody (anti-GBM) in serum and/or on **renal biopsy**
Pulmonary arteriovenous malformation	*Suggested by:* hemoptysis alone. No other symptoms. CXR normal
	Confirmed by: vascular red-blue lesion on **bronchoscopy**, enhancing lesion on **CT chest** with contrast, **pulmonary angiography** showing feeding blood vessels

Cough with sputum

The majority of patients presenting with a productive cough will have a short history of days or weeks, but many will have a background of a chronic cough.

Some differential diagnoses and typical outline evidence

Chronic bronchitis (with emphysema, part of the entity COPD)	*Suggested by:* gray sputum, slow progression over years, and a smoker (nearly always)
	Confirmed by: gray sputum >3 months over 2 consecutive years
Acute viral bronchitis	*Suggested by:* onset over hours or days. Fever, white or yellow sputum
	Confirmed by: no consolidation on CXR, quick spontaneous resolution
Acute bacterial bronchitis	*Suggested by:* onset over hours or days. Fever, mucopurulent sputum, dyspnea
	Confirmed by: **sputum culture** and sensitivities, response to appropriate antibiotics
Pneumonia	*Suggested by:* onset over hours or days. Rusty brown sputum (i.e., purulent sputum tinged with blood). Sharp chest pain worse on inspiration, pleural rub, fever, cough, consolidation, etc.
	Confirmed by: patchy shadowing on CXR (see Figs. 19.1a, 19.1b, 19.15), sputum and blood cultures
Bronchiectasis	*Suggested by:* progression over months or years. Finger clubbing, copious (often cupfuls of) purulent sputum daily. Coarse, late inspiratory crackles
	Confirmed by: CXR: cystic shadowing; high-resolution **CT chest**: honeycombing and thickened, dilated bronchi (see Fig. 19.18)
Lung abscess	*Suggested by:* copious, foul-smelling purulent or brown sputum, hemoptysis, high fever, chest pain over weeks. Usually preceded by a prior significant respiratory infection (e.g., pneumonia)
	Confirmed by: fluid level in cavity on **CXR, CT chest**, response to physiotherapy, antibiotics, and aspiration

Persistent dry cough (no sputum)

The duration of symptoms, severity, and progression will affect the causes of a dry cough.

Some differential diagnoses and typical outline evidence

Viral infection with slow recovery	*Suggested by:* original onset over days, fever, sore throat, generalized aches *Confirmed by:* natural history of spontaneous improvement
Chronic asthma	*Suggested by:* progression or static over months or years. Worse at night and early morning. Associated wheeze, exacerbations with exercise or atopic exposure *Confirmed by:* spirometry (reduced FEV_1), peak expiratory flow rate (PEFR) chart—classical diurnal dipping and variability, >12% improvement in **spirometry** with treatment
COPD	*Suggested by:* chronic breathlessness, little variation, a history of smoking. Signs of hyperinflation, reduced breath sounds, hyperresonant percussion, wheezing *Confirmed by:* **CXR** showing generalized loss of lung markings and flat diaphragms. **Spirometry:** reduced FEV_1/FVC, FEV_1 or FVC <12% improvement with β-agonists. Decreased $α_1$-antitrypsin levels in young patents with genetic component
Bronchogenic carcinoma	*Suggested by:* weight loss, chest pain, hemoptysis. Smoker. Opacity with irregular outline on **CXR** or **CT chest** (see Fig. 19.6) *Confirmed by:* tumor cells in sputum or bronchoscopic biopsy
Tuberculosis	*Suggested by:* fever, malaise, weight loss, contact history, characteristic CXR (see Figs. 19.7, 19.10) *Confirmed by:* AFB on smear, **culture of sputum** or biopsy, or response to trial of therapy

Hoarseness

Hoarseness of some weeks' or months' duration may have some sinister causes that need urgent attention.

Some differential diagnoses and typical outline evidence

Laryngeal carcinoma	*Suggested by:* progressive hoarseness over weeks to months. Smoker, including cannabis. Dysphagia, hemoptysis, ear pain
	Confirmed by: **laryngoscopy** and biopsy of glottic, supraglottic or subglottic tumor and staging
Chronic laryngitis	*Suggested by:* onset over months or years. History of recurrent acute laryngitis
	Confirmed by: inflamed cords at **laryngoscopy** and no other pathology
Singer's nodes	*Suggested by:* onset over months. Long history, often occupational in teachers or singers from voice strain, singing, alcohol, fumes, etc.
	Confirmed by: nodules on cord at **laryngoscopy**. Resolution with speech therapy or after **surgical removal**
Functional hoarseness	*Suggested by:* recurrence at times of stress. Able to cough normally
	Confirmed by: no other pathology at **laryngoscopy**
Vocal cord paresis due to vagal nerve trauma, cancer (thyroid, esophagus, pharynx, bronchus) or TB, MS, polio, syringomyelia, (idiopathic in 15%)	*Suggested by:* onset after surgery or otherwise over weeks and months. Bovine cough. Symptoms of cause
	Confirmed by: paresis or abnormal movement of cords on **laryngoscopy** and CXR, **barium swallow,** MRI

Myxedema	*Suggested by:* onset over months or years. Fatigue, puffy face, obesity, cold intolerance, bradycardia, slowly relaxing reflexes
	Confirmed by: swollen vocal cords at **laryngoscopy**. ↑TSH, ↓FT4
Acromegaly	*Suggested by:* swollen vocal cords at **laryngoscopy**. Large, wide face, embossed forehead, jutting jaw (prognathism), widely spaced teeth and large tongue
	Confirmed by: IGF↑, failure to suppress GH to <2 mU/L with **oral** GTT. **Skull X-ray** confirms bony abnormalities. **Hand X-ray** showing typical tufts on terminal phalanges. **MRI** or **CT scan** showing enlarged pituitary fossa
Sicca syndrome	*Suggested by:* onset over months to years. Dry mouth and eyes
	Confirmed by: clinical presentation and inflamed cords at **laryngoscopy** and no other pathology
Granulomas due to syphilis, TB, sarcoidosis, Wegener's	*Suggested by:* onset over months with symptoms and signs in other systems
	Confirmed by: granulomata on cords at **laryngoscopy**. Biopsy of cord or other affected tissues

Unilateral calf or leg swelling

This symptom is included here because of its frequent association with deep venous thrombosis (DVT) and pulmonary embolus (PE). Swelling is usually due to accumulation of extravascular fluid, possibly from increased pressure within the veins or lymphatic vessels.

It can also be due to unilateral damage to the local small veins and capillaries from local inflammation. Unilateral swelling thus implies local inflammation, damage, or obstruction to a vein or lymphatic vessel. The speed of onset allows one to imagine what process might be taking place—traumatic, thrombotic, or infectious.

Some differential diagnoses and typical outline evidence

Deep venous thrombosis	*Suggested by:* onset over hours, presence of risk factors, e.g., obesity, immobility, carcinoma, contraceptive. Associated pulmonary embolism.
	Confirmed by: poor flow on **Doppler ultrasound scan**, filling defect on **venogram (now rarely done)**
Ruptured Baker's cyst (leaking synovial fluid, sometimes no cyst)	*Suggested by:* onset sudden over seconds, e.g., when walking up a step. Usually known to have an arthritic knee
	Confirmed by: normal flow on **Doppler ultrasound scan**, no filling defect on **venogram**. Leakage of contrast from joint capsule if **arthrogram** done soon after the event
Cellulitis	*Suggested by:* firm, warm, tender erythema, tracking (red lines), fever, very tender over vein, ↑WBC, with onset over days
	Confirmed by: skin swabs if discharge from skin, blood cultures, response to antibiotics
Abnormal lymphatic drainage caused by lymphoma or malignant infiltration. Rarely, a hereditary condition affecting young women	*Suggested by:* onset over years, firm, non-tender, non-pitting edema of gradual onset over years
	Confirmed by: **CT scan** or **lymphoscintigraphy** (radionuclide imaging) or (rarely) **lymphangiogram**
Congenital edema (Milroy's syndrome)	*Suggested by:* presence since childhood
	Confirmed by: history and **CT scan** or **lymphoscintigraphy** (radionuclide imaging) or (rarely) **lymphangiogram**

Respiratory signs

Examination of the respiratory system

The findings discussed here are presented in a sequence of those found on inspection, palpation, percussion, and then auscultation. While inspecting the patient, think of the arterial blood gas, and when palpating, think of the mechanisms of ventilation. When percussing, think of the pleural surfaces, contents of the pleural cavity, and lung tissue. When auscultating, think of the state of the lung tissue and the airways.

Appearance suggestive of blood gas disturbance

Look for dyspnea, tachypnea, and slow respiratory rate. Examine the patient's fingers for peripheral cyanosis and the skin for warmth. Look at the tongue and lips for central cyanosis.

Some differential diagnoses and typical outline evidence

Hypoxia	*Suggested by:* cyanosis of fingers and/or lips, restlessness, confusion, drowsiness
	Confirmed by: ↓**PaO$_2$** on **blood gas analysis** (or **pulse oximetry** of <90% (mild) or <80% (severe)
Carbon dioxide retention	*Suggested by:* slow respiratory rate, warm hands, bounding pulse, dilated veins on hands and face, twitching of facial muscles, changed mental status
	Confirmed by: ↑PaCO$_2$ on **blood gas analysis**
Hypocapnia	*Suggested by:* tachypnea, hyperventilation, dizziness, paresthesias of lips
	Confirmed by: ↓PaCO$_2$ on **blood gas analysis**

Respiratory rate low (<10/minute)

Count the number of respirations in a minute.

Some differential diagnoses and typical outline evidence

Carbon dioxide narcosis (very high blood carbon dioxide)	*Suggested by:* warm hands, bounding pulse, dilated veins on hands and face, twitching of facial muscles, drowsy
	Confirmed by: ↑$PaCO_2$ on **blood gas analysis**
Drugs, e.g., opiates, alcohol, benzodiazepines	*Suggested by:* Pin-point pupils (in opiates—track marks). History of ingestion, empty medication bottle
	Confirmed by: **response to drug withdrawal** or antidotes, e.g., naloxone, flumazenil. Drug levels on **toxicology screen**
Raised intracranial pressure	*Suggested by:* papilledema, focal neurology, severe headaches, and vomiting
	Confirmed by: **CT brain** (loss of normal sulci, edema)

Chest wall abnormalities

Inspect the chest shape and then its change on movement for asymmetry, looking up over the abdomen.

Some differential diagnoses and typical outline evidence

Pectus carinatum developmental or associated with emphysema	*Suggested by*: prominent sternum, often associated with in-drawing of the ribs, causing Harrison's sulci above the costal margins *Confirmed by*: CXR
Pectus excavatum developmental defect	*Suggested by*: depression of the lower end or whole sternum *Confirmed by*: CXR
Kyphosis congenital or due to anterior collapse of spinal vertebrae, e.g., spinal TB	*Suggested by*: spine curved forward and laterally *Confirmed by*: **CXR, spinal X-ray**
Scoliosis congenital, neuromuscular disease, previous surgery, TB	*Suggested by*: spine curved laterally *Confirmed by*: **CXR, spinal X-ray**
Absence of part of chest wall bone structure congenital (Poland's syndrome) or post-surgery	*Suggested by*: absence of ribs, pectoralis muscle, clavicle, etc. *Confirmed by*: **CXR, spinal X-ray**

Bilateral poor chest expansion

Some differential diagnoses and typical outline evidence

Obesity	*Suggested by:* insidious onset of breathlessness.
	Confirmed by: examination, BMI >30 kg/m^2
Emphysema (also can come under the term COPD)	*Suggested by:* hyperinflation, poor air entry, hyperresonance, pursed-lip breathing. Hyperinflation and paucity of lung markings on CXR
	Confirmed by: **CT thorax,** obstructive deficit with reduced carbon monoxide diffusing capacity (DL_{CO}) and no reversibility on *pulmonary function testing (PFT)* (see Figs. 19.19a, 19.19b, 19.21)
Pulmonary fibrosis	*Suggested by:* clubbed (60%–70%), fine, late inspiratory bibasilar crackles. Loss of lung volume on CXR (not corresponding to a single lobe)
	Confirmed by: **High-resolution (HR)-CT thorax.** Restrictive deficit with reduced DL_{CO} *on pulmonary function testing* (see Fig. 19.17)
Muscular dystrophy (other rarer myopathies)	*Suggested by:* early age onset, FH, pseudohypertrophy of calf muscles, lower motor neuron (LMN) signs, restrictive deficit on *pulmonary function testing* (especially when lying flat) with preservation of corrected DL_{CO}
	Confirmed by: **muscle biopsy**
Amyotrophic lateral sclerosis (ALS)	*Suggested by:* late-onset mixed upper motor neuron (UMN)/LMN signs, tongue fasciculation, bulbar palsy. Restrictive deficit on *pulmonary function testing* (especially when lying flat) with preservation of corrected DL_{CO}
	Confirmed by: electromyography (EMG)
Guillain–Barré syndrome	*Suggested by:* ascending weakness, autonomic disturbances, recent infection. Restrictive deficit on *pulmonary function testing* (especially when lying flat) with preservation of corrected DL_{CO}. Rapid deterioration of forced vital capacity (FVC) or forced expiratory volume in 1 second (FEV_1)
	Confirmed by: history, characteristic **nerve conduction velocity testing** and CSF findings (increased protein), **response to steroids and plasmapheresis or immunoglobulin (Ig) infusions**

Unilateral poor chest expansion

Some differential diagnoses and typical outline evidence

Pleural effusion	*Suggested by:* reduced breath sounds, reduced tactile vocal fremitus, stony dull percussion note
	Confirmed by: **CXR, CT**, or **ultrasound** of **chest** showing effusion (see Fig. 19.4)
Pneumothorax	*Suggested by:* reduced breath sounds, reduced tactile vocal fremitus, resonant percussion note, tracheal deviation
	Confirmed by: **CXR** showing no lung markings next to chest wall, and line of demarcation with lung tissue. Best seen at lung apex (see Fig. 19.20)
Extensive consolidation	*Suggested by:* reduced breath sounds, bronchial breathing, increased tactile vocal fremitus, reduced percussion note
	Confirmed by: CXR (see Figs. 19.1a, 19.1b, 19.15)
Fractured ribs	*Suggested by:* antecedent trauma, focal tenderness
	Confirmed by: CXR
Flail segment following trauma	*Suggested by:* paradoxical movement of part of chest wall
	Confirmed by: **CXR, spinal X-ray**
Musculoskeletal, e.g., previous thoracoplasty	*Suggested by:* history, scar
	Confirmed by: CXR

Trachea displaced

Palpate with the middle finger, with the index and ring fingers on either side of the trachea. Localize apex beat to see if the lower mediastinum is also displaced.

Some differential diagnoses and typical outline evidence

Scoliosis	*Suggested by:* chest wall deformity and curved spine
	Confirmed by: **spinal X-ray, CXR**
Pulled by ipsilateral pneumothorax	*Suggested by:* reduced breath sounds, reduced tactile vocal fremitus, resonant percussion note
	Confirmed by: **CXR** showing space with absent lung markings "pulling" on mediastinum
Pulled by ipsilateral upper lobe fibrosis, atelectasis, or resection	*Suggested by:* tuberculosis (TB) (chronic), radiation fibrosis (skin changes, tattoo marks), surgery (scar), ankylosing spondylitis, sarcoidosis. Reduced upper chest wall expansion
	Confirmed by: **chest X-ray** or **CT** findings
Pushed by contralateral tension pneumothorax	*Suggested by:* in extremis with high pulse rate and hypotension, reduced breath sounds, reduced tactile vocal fremitus, resonant percussion note
	Confirmed by: **insertion of needle into second intercostal space**
Pushed by contralateral pleural effusion	*Suggested by:* reduced breath sounds, reduced tactile vocal fremitus, stony dull percussion note
	Confirmed by: **CXR** showing large homogenous white opacification "pushing" on mediastinum

Reduced vocal fremitus

Some differential diagnoses and typical outline evidence

Pleural effusion	*Suggested by:* reduced breath sounds, reduced expansion, stony dull percussion noted
	Confirmed by: **CXR, CT,** or **ultrasound of chest**. (see Figs. 19.4, 19.22)
Pneumothorax	*Suggested by:* reduced breath sounds, reduced expansion, resonant percussion note. Trachea and apex displaced
	Confirmed by: **CXR** showing no lung markings next to chest wall, and line of demarcation with lung tissue. Best seen at lung apex (see Fig. 19.20)
Collapsed lobe with no consolidation	*Suggested by:* reduced breath sounds, reduced expansion, normal percussion note
	Confirmed by: **CXR** (see Fig. 19.2; collapse of different lobes will have different patterns radiologically, e.g., showing fan-shaped shadow arising from mediastinum, mediastinal shift, raised hemidiaphragm, displaced horizontal fissure or "sail sign"). **CT thorax** confirms lobar collapse.

Stony dull percussion

This implies pleural effusion (see Fig. 19.4).

Some differential diagnoses and typical outline evidence

Transudates	*Suggested by:* bilateral effusions, underlying clinical cause
	Confirmed by: ↓*protein in effusion* or fluid–serum protein ratio <0.5 (except in treated heart failure)
Left heart failure, SVC obstruction, pericarditis, peritoneal dialysis	*Suggested by:* peripheral edema, raised JVP, basal crackles, third heart sound
	Confirmed by: **CXR, echocardiogram, CT thorax**
Low albumin states, e.g., liver cirrhosis, nephrotic syndrome	*Suggested by:* malnutrition, generalized edema
	Confirmed by: low **serum albumin**
Miscellaneous causes: myxedema, atelectasis	

Exudates	*Suggested by:* unilateral effusion (but may be bilateral)
	Confirmed by: ↑**protein in effusion** or fluid–serum protein ratio >0.5
Infective: bacterial/ empyema, TB, viral, etc.	*Suggested by:* history, fever, pH↓, glucose in pleural fluid ↓. Many lymphocytes in exudates often seen in TB, caseating granuloma on pleural biopsy
	Confirmed by: Gram stain or **ZN stain and cultures of pleural fluid and blood or cultures from pleural biopsy**
Neoplastic: lung primary or secondaries, breast, ovarian, lymphomas, Kaposi's, local chest wall tumors, mesothelioma	*Suggested by:* history, especially weight loss. Signs of local or distal spread
	Confirmed by: **pleural aspiration, biopsy, or other tissue histology** (see Fig. 19.22)
Rheumatoid, SLE, etc.	*Suggested by:* history, other organ-specific involvement, positive rheumatoid factor in fluid, very low fluid glucose
	Confirmed by: **autoantibodies, response to immunosuppression**
Pulmonary infarction	*Suggested by:* history. Sudden onset of pleuritic chest pain, and breathlessness. Associated risk factors. Usually hypoxic. CXR may show other evidence, e.g., Fleischner lines, Hampton's hump, wedge-shaped shadowing
	Confirmed by: helical CT (spiral CT, CT pulmonary angiogram [CTPA])

Dull to percussion but not stony dull

Some differential diagnoses and typical outline evidence

Consolidation	*Suggested by:* reduced breath sounds, bronchial breathing, increased tactile vocal fremitus. Fever, cough (may be productive)
	Confirmed by: air bronchogram on **CXR** and **CT** (see Figs. 19.1a, 19.1b, 19.15)
Pulmonary edema usually due to left ventricular failure	*Suggested by:* displaced apex beat, S3, basal crackles
	Confirmed by: **CXR, echocardiogram** (see Fig. 19.13)
Elevated hemidiaphragm	*Suggested by:* absent breath sounds (asymptomatic).
	Confirmed by: **CXR**
Severe fibrosis or atelectasis	*Suggested by:* reduced breath sounds, crackles, poor expansion, tracheal deviation
	Confirmed by: **CXR, CT thorax** (see Figs 19.2, 19.17)
Mesothelioma or severe pleural thickening	*Suggested by:* chest pain, weight loss, asbestos exposure, clubbing, reduced breath sounds
	Confirmed by: **CT thorax** and **pleural biopsy**

Hyperresonant percussion

Some differential diagnoses and typical outline evidence

Emphysema (also can come under the term COPD)	*Suggested by:* >10 pack-year smoking history, chronic, progressive breathlessness, cough with sputum, reduced breath sounds, hyperresonance, pursed-lip breathing, tracheal tug. Hyperinflation and paucity of lung markings on **CXR**
	Confirmed by: **CT thorax**, obstructive deficit with reduced transfer factor and no reversibility on **lung function** (see Figs. 19.19a, 19.19b)
Large bullae	*Suggested by:* other signs of emphysema
	Confirmed by: **CT thorax** (see Fig. 19.21)
Pneumothorax	*Suggested by:* acute breathlessness, chest pain, **unilateral signs** such as reduced breath sounds, reduced tactile vocal fremitus, poor expansion
	Confirmed by: **CXR** showing no lung markings next to chest wall and line of demarcation with lung tissue (see Fig. 19.20)

Diminished breath sounds

Ensure that the patient breathes with the mouth open, regularly and deeply, and does not vocalize (e.g., groaning).

Some differential diagnoses and typical outline evidence

Poor respiratory effort	*Suggested by:* reduced consciousness or cooperation, any cause of poor chest wall expansion (see p. 192).
	Confirmed by: history, physical exam, **arterial blood gas (ABG)**
Pleural effusion	*Suggested by:* reduced expansion, stony dull percussion, reduced tactile vocal fremitus
	Confirmed by: **CXR, CT,** or **ultrasound** of **chest**. (see Fig. 19.4)
Endobronchial obstruction, e.g., tumor, retained secretions, inhaled foreign body	*Suggested by:* cough, stridor, unilateral dullness to percussion, crackles, and reduced breath sounds
	Confirmed by: **CT thorax, bronchoscopy**
Severe asthma (bronchoconstriction)	*Suggested by:* history, sudden onset, often precipitating factor; wheezing (though may be absent in worst cases). Patient in extremis, reduced consciousness.
	Confirmed by: **peak flow rate** undetectable. **ABG,** very ↑ airway pressure after intubation and mechanical ventilation begun
Emphysema (or COPD)	*Suggested by:* history of COPD, smoking; chronic, progressive breathlessness; cough with sputum; hyperinflation, hyperresonance, pursed-lip breathing. Hyperinflation and paucity of lung markings on CXR
	Confirmed by: **CT thorax**, obstructive deficit with decreased DL_{CO} and no reversibility on **pulmonary function testing** (see Figs. 19.19a, 19.19b)
Mesothelioma or severe pleural thickening	*Suggested by:* chest pain, weight loss, asbestos exposure, clubbing, reduced breath sounds
	Confirmed by: **CT thorax** and **pleural biopsy**
Bullae	*Suggested by:* history or physical findings or pulmonary function test findings of COPD, localized bronchial breathing (if large)
	Confirmed by: **CXR, CT thorax** (see Fig. 19.21)

Consolidation	*Suggested by:* reduced percussion, increased tactile vocal fremitus, bronchial breathing
	Confirmed by: **CXR** (see Figs. 19.1a, 19.1b, 19.15)
Pneumothorax	*Suggested by:* acute breathlessness, chest pain, reduced expansion, hyperresonance
	Confirmed by: **CXR** (see Fig. 19.20)
Elevated hemidiaphragm, phrenic nerve paralysis	*Suggested by:* being asymptomatic. Scar from phrenic nerve surgery or injury
	Confirmed by: **CXR**

Bronchial breathing

There is a prolonged expiration phase with definite silence between inspiration and expiration (the same as the sound heard with the stethoscope bell over the trachea).

Some differential diagnoses and typical outline evidence

Consolidation	*Suggested by:* fever, reduced breath sounds, reduced percussion, crackles, increased tactile vocal fremitus
	Confirmed by: **CXR** (see Figs. 19.1a, 19.1b, 19.15)
Lung cavity	*Suggested by:* localized bronchial breathing, otherwise normal examination
	Confirmed by: **CXR, CT thorax**
Pulmonary fibrosis	*Suggested by:* reduced expansion, normal or reduced percussion, late inspiratory fine crackles, clubbing
	Confirmed by: **HR-CT thorax** (see Fig. 19.17)

Fine inspiratory crackles

Fine crackles resemble the sound made when hair near the ear is rolled between the finger and thumb or by unfastening a Velcro pad.

Some differential diagnoses and typical outline evidence

Incidental	*Suggested by:* late in inspiration, disappears on coughing
	Confirmed by: **CXR** showing normal lung fields
Pulmonary edema	*Suggested by:* crackles late in inspiration, dullness to percussion at lung bases (with associated effusion), third heart sound
	Confirmed by: **CXR** showing fluffy shadows, large heart and linear opacities (Kerley lines) in upper lobes. **Echocardiogram** may show reduced LV contraction, low ejection fraction (EF) (see Fig. 19.13)
Pulmonary fibrosis	*Suggested by:* very fine crackles late in inspiration, reduced chest expansion, finger clubbing.
	Confirmed by: **CXR** and **HR-CT thorax** (see Fig. 19.3, 19.17)
Consolidation	*Suggested by:* early inspiratory crackles, fever, reduced breath sounds, reduced percussion, increased tactile vocal fremitus
	Confirmed by: **CXR** (see Figs. 19.1a, 19.1b, 19.15)

Coarse crackles

These are bubbly crackles.

Some differential diagnoses and typical outline evidence

Bronchiectasis	*Suggested by:* copious amounts of mucopurulent sputum, chest pain, wheezing. Previous chest infections, asthma, surgery, or cystic fibrosis. Crackles not disappearing after coughing, clubbing
	Confirmed by: **CXR, HR-CT thorax** (see Fig. 19.18)

Pleural rub

This sounds like two wet leather surfaces rubbing together (or crunching through snow). It is caused by inflammation of the pleura.

Some differential diagnoses and typical outline evidence

Pleuritic infection with adjacent pneumonia	*Suggested by:* fever, reduced breath sounds, reduced percussion, crackles, increased tactile vocal fremitus
	Confirmed 0062y: **CXR, sputum, blood cultures**
Pulmonary embolus (PE)	*Suggested by:* signs of DVT, loud P2, tachycardia, dyspnea, hypoxia, ↓PaCO$_2$, d-dimer
	Confirmed by: **V/Q, helical CT,** (rarely now) **pulmonary angiogram**
Pleural tumors, e.g., secondaries or mesothelioma	*Suggested by:* history, e.g., asbestos exposure
	Confirmed by: **CT thorax, pleural biopsy**

Stridor ± inspiratory wheeze

Suggests obstruction in or near larynx.

Some differential diagnoses and typical outline evidence

Epiglottitis	*Suggested by:* fever, upper respiratory tract infection (URTI) coryzal symptoms, drooling
	Confirmed by: "thumb sign" on **lateral neck X-ray**, **indirect laryngoscopy** under controlled (anesthetic) conditions
Croup	*Suggested by:* high-pitched cough in infants
	Confirmed by: above presentation and findings
Inhaled foreign body	*Suggested by:* history of inhaling peanut, bead, etc.
	Confirmed by: **CXR, CT thorax, bronchoscopy**
Rapidly progressive laryngomalacia	*Suggested by:* change in voice over months to years.
	Confirmed by: **indirect laryngoscopy, CT thorax.**
Laryngeal papillomas	*Suggested by:* change in voice over weeks to months
	Confirmed by: **indirect laryngoscopy**
Laryngeal edema due to anaphylaxis	*Suggested by:* flushing of face and trunk, urticarial rash, lip and facial swelling, tachycardia, BP↓
	Confirmed by: improvement with adrenaline IM and removal of precipitating allergen

Inspiratory rhonchus or wheeze

This suggests large airway obstruction. A lesion above the carina can be immediately life threatening, as neither lung can be ventilated.

Some differential diagnoses and typical outline evidence

Acute bilateral vocal cord paralysis	*Suggested by:* change in voice, which becomes weaker over minutes to hours
	Confirmed by: **laryngoscopy**
Inhalation of foreign body	*Suggested by:* history of inhaling peanut, bead, or other foreign body
	Confirmed by: **CXR, CT thorax** and **neck, bronchoscopy**
Tracheal tumors or stenosis after ventilation	*Suggested by:* Stridor, over weeks to months, bilateral reduced breath sounds
	Confirmed by: **bronchoscopy**
Extrinsic compression by mediastinal masses	*Suggested by:* neck and chest discomfort ± swelling over weeks to months
	Confirmed by: **CT thorax and neck**
Extrinsic compression by esophageal tumors	*Suggested by:* dysphagia, weight loss over weeks to months
	Confirmed by: **CT thorax and neck**
Tracheal blunt trauma	*Suggested by:* history, pain and swelling, change in voice over minutes or hours after trauma
	Confirmed by: **laryngoscopy, bronchoscopy**
Laryngeal edema due to anaphylaxis	*Suggested by:* flushing of face and trunk, urticarial rash, lip and facial swelling, tachycardia, BP↓
	Confirmed by: improvement with adrenaline IM and removal of precipitating allergen

Expiratory rhonchus

This is large airway obstruction.

Some differential diagnoses and typical outline evidence

Endobronchial carcinoma (benign lesions very rare)	*Suggested by:* smoker, weight loss, cough, chest pain, hemoptysis, clubbing. Unilateral wheeze and reduced breath sounds. Signs of consolidation
	Confirmed by: **bronchoscopy and biopsy**
Acute bilateral vocal cord paralysis	*Suggested by:* change in voice, bilateral reduced breath sounds and wheeze
	Confirmed by: **laryngoscopy**
Inhalation of foreign body	*Suggested by:* history of sudden cough and stridor when eating
	Confirmed by: **CXR, CT thorax and neck, bronchoscopy**
Tracheal tumors	*Suggested by:* cough, hemoptysis
	Confirmed by: **bronchoscopy**
Extrinsic compression by mediastinal masses	*Suggested by:* neck or chest discomfort ± swelling
	Confirmed by: **CT thorax and neck**
Extrinsic compression by esophageal tumors	*Suggested by:* dysphagia, weight loss over weeks to months
	Confirmed by: **CT thorax and neck**
Tracheal blunt trauma	*Suggested by:* history, pain and swelling, change in voice over minutes or hours after trauma
	Confirmed by: **laryngoscopy**

Expiratory polyphonic, high-pitched wheeze

This suggests small airways obstruction.

Some differential diagnoses and typical outline evidence

Bronchial asthma	*Suggested by:* nonproductive cough or white sputum, worse in the morning. Some episodes not related to infection
	Confirmed by: FEV_1 response to bronchodilators
Wheezy bronchitis	*Suggested by:* association with infective episodes of bronchitis alone
	Confirmed by: FEV_1 response to bronchodilators and antibiotics
Anaphylaxis	*Suggested by:* history of allergen exposure, feeling of dread, hypotension, facial or generalized edema, flushed, urticaria
	Confirmed by: above history, ***response to adrenaline and removal of precipitating cause***
Left ventricular failure and pulmonary edema	*Suggested by:* "cardiac asthma": pink frothy sputum, third heart sound, displaced apex beat
	Confirmed by: ***echocardiogram, CXR*** (see Fig. 19.13)

GI symptoms

Severe weight loss over weeks or months

The degree and speed of weight loss is relevant; the more severe, and the more likely is it to be due to a demonstrable cause.

Some differential diagnoses and typical outline evidence

Any advanced malignancy	*Suggested by:* progressive onset over weeks or months of specific symptoms, e.g., neurological deficit, hemoptysis, rectal bleeding, change in bowel habits
	Confirmed by: metastases on **CXR,** metastases on **ultrasound scan of liver,** or leukemic changes on **CBC** or tumor on **bronchoscopy** or **GI endoscopy**
Depression	*Suggested by:* sleep disorders, poor concentration, social withdrawal, lack of interest in usual activities
	Confirmed by: response to antidepressants. Psychotherapy
Thyrotoxicosis	*Suggested by:* heat intolerance, tremor, nervousness, palpitation, frequency of bowel movements, goiter, fine tremor, warm and moist palms
	Confirmed by: TSH↓, ↑FT4, ↑FT3
Uncontrolled diabetes mellitus	*Suggested by:* thirst, polydipsia, polyuria
	Confirmed by: **fasting blood glucose** >125 mg/dL (on two occasions) OR random or GTT blood glucose >200 mgl/dL
Infection, e.g., tuberculosis	*Suggested by:* night sweats, fever, malaise, cough
	Confirmed by: **CXR** showing opacification of pneumonia and presence of **AFB in sputum** on microscopy and culture
Addison's disease	*Suggested by:* lethargy, weakness, dizziness, hyperpigmentation (buccal, scar), hypotension
	Confirmed by: 9 A.M. plasma cortisol ↓ and impaired response to short ACTH stimulation test *(cosyntropin stimulation test)*

Vomiting

Vomiting is not only a feature of GI disorders but is also associated with a wide variety of local and systemic disorders. Therefore, more leads are needed. Ask about the amount, frequency, and nature of vomitus—red blood (hematemesis), "coffee-ground" appearance, and timing in relation to meals. Also ask about weight loss, fever, headache, and abdominal pain.

Try subdividing vomiting into

- Vomiting *with* weight loss
- Vomiting *without* weight loss
- Vomiting *(within hours)* of food
- Vomiting unrelated to food but *with abdominal pain AND fever*
- Vomiting unrelated to food, *with abdominal pain but NO fever* (nonmetabolic)
- Vomiting unrelated to food, *with abdominal pain but NO fever* (metabolic)
- Vomiting unrelated to food *without abdominal pain but with headaches*
- Vomiting unrelated to food and *without abdominal pain or headaches*

Vomiting with weight loss

Some differential diagnoses and typical outline evidence

Esophageal carcinoma	*Suggested by:* dysphagia to solid food first, then semisolid, and, finally, fluid
	Confirmed by: **barium swallow** showing filling defect, **fiber-optic gastroscopy** with mucosal biopsy of visible tumor
Gastric carcinoma	*Suggested by:* satiety after small meal
	Confirmed by: **esophagogastroscopy** showing and allowing biopsy of visible tumor, **barium meal** showing filling defect
Achalasia	*Suggested by:* vomiting after large meals, undigested solid food and fluid, dysphagia to fluid, nocturnal regurgitation
	Confirmed by: **barium swallow** demonstrating absence of peristaltic contractions, **esophagogastroscopy** showing dilatation
Esophageal stricture	*Suggested by:* undigested solid food and fluid in vomitus
	Confirmed by: **barium swallow, esophagogastroscopy** showing food residue and fixed narrowing
Small intestinal tumor, e.g., lymphoma	*Suggested by:* abdominal pain, anorexia
	Confirmed by: **small bowel follow-through, CT abdomen, flexible enteroscopy with biopsy**

Vomiting without weight loss

Some differential diagnoses and typical outline evidence

Pharyngeal pouch	*Suggested by:* no pain, regurgitation of undigested food
	Confirmed by: **barium swallow** showing saccular opacification outside pharynx
Achalasia	*Suggested by:* vomiting after large meals, undigested solid food and fluid, dysphagia to fluid, nocturnal regurgitation
	Confirmed by: **barium swallow** demonstrating absence of peristaltic contractions, **esophagogastroscopy** showing dilatation
Esophagitis and ulceration	*Suggested by:* retrosternal pain, heartburn, dyspepsia, "waterbrash"
	Confirmed by: **esophagogastroscopy** showing inflammation and/or ulceration

Vomiting shortly after food

Some differential diagnoses and typical outline evidence

Gastritis or peptic ulcer disease	*Suggested by:* epigastric pain, dull or burning discomfort (gastric ulcer pain typically exacerbated by food and duodenal ulcer pain relieved by it), "waterbrash"
	Confirmed by: **esophagogastroscopy, barium meal** and **pH study**
Gastroparesis due to diabetes mellitus	*Suggested by:* intermittent vomiting, abdominal fullness or bloating, distended upper abdomen, succussion splash, history of diabetes
	Confirmed by: **esophagogastroscopy, double-contrast barium meal** showing normal mucosa but dilatation
Gastric outlet obstruction e.g., carcinoma, lymphoma, chronic scarring, congenital pyloric stenosis in newborn	*Suggested by:* intermittent vomiting, abdominal fullness or bloating, distended upper abdomen, succussion splash
	Confirmed by: **esophagogastroscopy, double-contrast barium meal** shows structural abnormality
Small intestinal tumor e.g., lymphoma	*Suggested by:* abdominal pain, anorexia, weight loss
	Confirmed by: **small bowel barium meal and follow-through** showing filling defect, **CT abdomen** showing abnormal tumor in wall, **flexible enteroscopy** with biopsy showing abnormal histology
Acute cholecystitis due to cholelithiasis	*Suggested by:* symptoms after fatty food with colicky abdominal pain
	Confirmed by: ↑**serum amylase, ultrasound scan** of biliary tree and gallbladder
Acute pancreatitis	*Suggested by:* severe epigastric or central abdominal pain, jaundice, tachycardia, Cullen's sign (periumbilical discoloration) or Grey Turner's sign (discoloration at the flank)
	Confirmed by: **serum amylase, serum lipase**, ↓Ca^{2+}

Vomiting with abdominal pain and fever

The vomiting is usually unrelated to eating.

Some differential diagnoses and typical outline evidence

Gastroenteritis	*Suggested by:* diarrhea, ↑ bowel sounds
	Confirmed by: **stools for WBC and culture**
Food poisoning	*Suggested by:* associated with diarrhea, eating companions affected
	Confirmed by: **stools for WBC and culture, cultures of vomitus, food, and blood**
Urinary tract infection (UTI)	*Suggested by:* dysuria, frequency, abnormal dipstick
	Confirmed by: **urine microscopy and culture** (ultrasound scan for possible anatomical abnormality)
Acute appendicitis, mesenteric adenitis	*Suggested by:* RLQ pain, anorexia, low-grade fever
	Confirmed by: RLQ guarding or right-sided rectal tenderness
Hepatitis A or B	*Suggested by:* RUQ pain, jaundice
	Confirmed by: alanine transaminase (ALT) ↑↑ and bilirubin ↑, **hepatitis serology**
Toxic shock syndrome	*Suggested by:* use of tampons, high fever, vomiting and profuse watery diarrhea, confusion, skin rash, hypotension, myalgia
	Confirmed by: **cultures of blood, stool, vaginal swab** for *Staphylococcus* and toxin. Thrombocytopenia on CBC. ↑CPK (creatine phosphokinase)
Pneumonia (lower lobe)	*Suggested by:* cough, dyspnea, fever
	Confirmed by: **CXR** shows consolidation. **Sputum and blood cultures. Serology** if atypical
Pelvic inflammatory disease	*Suggested by:* lower abdominal pain, fever, vaginal discharge
	Confirmed by: high vaginal swab, elevated ESR and CRP. FBC: leukocytosis, **pelvic ultrasound**, ± **laparoscopy**
Hemolytic uremic syndrome (HUS)	*Suggested by:* hematuria, fever, confusion
	Confirmed by: FBC: thrombocytopenia, fragmented RBCs on **blood film**, renal failure on blood chemistries
Malaria	*Suggested by:* recent travel to malaria zone, periodic paroxysms of rigors, fever, sweating, nausea
	Confirmed by: *Plasmodium* in **blood smear**.

Vomiting with abdominal pain alone (unrelated to food, no fever)—nonmetabolic causes

This is associated with a wide variety of GI and systemic disorders; it is nonspecific.

Some differential diagnoses and typical outline evidence

Large bowel obstruction, e.g., malignancy, strangulated hernia	*Suggested by:* fecal vomiting, abdominal distension
	Confirmed by: **abdominal X-ray (AXR)** showing bowel dilation, **barium enema, colonoscopy**
Hepatic carcinoma, primary or secondary	*Suggested by:* RUQ pain and mass, jaundice
	Confirmed by: weight loss over weeks to months, **ultrasound or CT of liver** showing hepatic mass
Mesenteric artery occlusion	*Suggested by:* periumbilical pain, diarrhea, melena
	Confirmed by: **mesenteric angiography** showing filling defect
Intussusception	*Suggested by:* child, usually between 6 and 18 months of life, acute onset of colicky, intermittent abdominal pain, "red currant jelly" rectal bleeding, ± sausage-shaped mass in upper abdomen
	Confirmed by: **barium enema**, may reduce with appropriate hydrostatic pressure
Ectopic pregnancy, miscarriage	*Suggested by:* cramping pain, spotting, vaginal bleeding
	Confirmed by: positive pregnancy test, **ultrasound scan of pelvis**
Renal calculi	*Suggested by:* colicky loin pain, hematuria
	Confirmed by: **plain AXR, ultrasound, intravenous urogram (IVU)**
Acute inferior myocardial infarction	*Suggested by:* retrosternal chest pain, sweating, nausea
	Confirmed by: characteristic ST changes on ECG, ↑cardiac enzymes (**Ck-MB** or **troponin**)
Congestive cardiac failure (and liver congestion)	*Suggested by:* dyspnea, orthopnea, PND, liver enlargement and tenderness, leg edema
	Confirmed by: **CXR** and **echocardiogram**

Vomiting with abdominal pain alone (unrelated to food, no fever)—metabolic causes

This is associated with a wide variety of GI and systemic disorders. It is nonspecific.

Some differential diagnoses and typical outline evidence

Drugs overdose, e.g., digoxin	*Suggested by:* drug history
	Confirmed by: **serum drug levels**
Diabetic ketoacidosis	*Suggested by:* polyuria, dehydration, and ± Kussmaul respiration
	Confirmed by: ↑**blood glucose, ↓pH, ketonuria** or **plasma bicarbonate** <15 mmol/L
Hypercalcemia	*Suggested by:* lethargy, confusion, constipation, muscle weakness, polydipsia, and polyuria
	Confirmed by: ↑**serum Ca^{2+}**
Acute intermittent porphyria	*Suggested by:* family history, constipation, peripheral neuropathy, hypertension, psychoses, urine darkens on standing
	Confirmed by: elevated **urinary aminolevulinic acid** and **porphobilinogen, plasma porphyrins**
Lead poisoning	*Suggested by:* anorexia, personality changes, headaches, metallic taste
	Confirmed by: elevated whole **blood lead concentration** >2.4 μmol/L
Vitamin A intoxication	*Suggested by:* ↑ intracranial pressure, headache, irritability
	Confirmed by: symptoms and signs disappearing within 1–4 weeks after stopping vitamin A ingestion
Pheochromocytoma	*Suggested by:* headache, sweating, palpitations, pallor, nausea, hypertension (intermittent or persistent), tachycardia
	Confirmed by: 24-hour urinary metanephrines ↑serum catecholamines (epinephrine, norepinephrine), CT abdomen, MRI scan

Vomiting with headache alone (unrelated to food, no abdominal pain)

Some differential diagnoses and typical outline evidence

Migraine	*Suggested by:* throbbing headache with preceding visual auras or other transient sensory symptoms and "trigger" factors, e.g., premenstrual, stress, particular foods
	Confirmed by: history, but if in doubt, **MRI scan** to exclude anatomical abnormalities
Raised intracranial pressure	*Suggested by:* being worse in morning, on coughing and leaning forward, papilledema
	Confirmed by: **CT scan head** showing flattening of sulci and darkening of brain tissue
Meningitis (viral or bacterial)	*Suggested by:* photophobia, fever, neck stiffness
	Confirmed by: **CT scan**: no signs of ↑ intracranial pressure, and **lumbar puncture (LP)**: ↑ lymphocytes in viral, ↑ neutrophils in bacterial meningitis, with organisms on staining and culture
Hemorrhagic stroke	*Suggested by:* sudden onset of headache, hemiparesis, sparing of upper face, dysarthria ± dysphasia, extensor plantar response
	Confirmed by: **CT brain scan**: high attenuation area representing hemorrhage
Severe hypertension	*Suggested by:* continuous throbbing headache (non-severe hypertension is usually asymptomatic) but headache ± visual disturbance in malignant hypertension
	Confirmed by: **serial BP measurement**: usually >140 mmHg diastolic and/or >240 mmHg systolic
Epilepsy	*Suggested by:* aura, altered consciousness, abnormal movement
	Confirmed by: EEG result: spikes and waves over focus
Acute glaucoma	*Suggested by:* blurred vision, painful red eye, colored halos
	Confirmed by: ↑ intraocular pressure on measurement
Addison's disease	*Suggested by:* lethargy, weakness, dizziness, pigmentation (buccal, scar), hypotension
	Confirmed by: 9 A.M. plasma cortisol ↓ and impaired response to short ACTH stimulation test (Cortrosyn stimulation test)

Vomiting alone (unrelated to food, without abdominal pain or headaches)

Some differential diagnoses and typical outline evidence

Gastroenteritis	*Suggested by:* diarrhea, decreased bowel sounds
	Confirmed by: **stools for WBC and culture**
Sliding hiatus hernia	*Suggested by:* occasional chest pain precipitated by heavy meals, lying flat
	Confirmed by: **barium meal** showing reflux
Acute viral labyrinthitis	*Suggested by:* vertigo, nystagmus
	Confirmed by: being self-limiting over days
Ménière's disease	*Suggested by:* vertigo, tinnitus, deafness
	Confirmed by: **audiometry**: sensory hearing loss
Pregnancy	*Suggested by:* being worse soon after waking, amenorrhea
	Confirmed by: pregnancy test positive
Anaphylaxis	*Suggested by:* bronchospasm, laryngeal edema, flushing, urticaria, angioedema
	Confirmed by: relief with antihistamines or steroids
Renal failure (CRF)	*Suggested by:* fatigue, pruritus, anorexia, nausea, lemon-tinged skin
	Confirmed by: ↑**serum creatinine, ↓creatinine clearance**. If chronic renal failure (CRF): Hb low, small kidneys on **renal ultrasound**.
Addison's disease	*Suggested by:* lethargy, weakness, dizziness, pigmentation (buccal mucosa, scars), hypotension
	Confirmed by: 9 A.M. plasma cortisol low ↓ and impaired response to short ACTH stimulation test (Cortrosyn stimulation test)
Drugs, e.g., antibiotics, cytotoxics, any overdose, excessive alcohol ingestion	*Suggested by:* history of drug ingestion
	Confirmed by: response of symptoms to avoidance of drug
Functional	*Suggested by:* vomiting during or soon after a meal ± other psychological disturbance and no symptoms and physical signs of organic disease
	Confirmed by: response to psychotherapy

Jaundice

This can be a symptom reported by the patient or a physical sign. It is confirmed by ↑ bilirubin in the plasma. Yellow sclerae and skin usually become visible when the serum bilirubin level is >35 μmol/L, so urine tests may provide the first clue.

First subdivide investigation into the five leads below. Remember that hemolysis causes ↑ urinary urobilinogen and ↓ serum haptoglobin. Hepatic failure causes ↑ serum unconjugated bilirubin, but intrahepatic or extrahepatic biliary obstruction results in ↑ serum conjugated bilirubin.

Some differential diagnoses and typical outline evidence

Carotinemia	*Suggested by:* onset over months. Skin yellow with white sclerae, normal stools and normal urine. Diet rich in yellow vegetables and fruits
	Confirmed by: no bilirubin, no **urobilinogen** in the urine, and normal **serum bilirubin**. Normal **liver function tests (LFTs)**. Response to diet change
Prehepatic jaundice due to hemolysis	*Suggested by:* jaundice and anemia (the combination seen as lemon or pale yellow). Normal dark stools and normal-looking urine
	Confirmed by: ↑ (unconjugated and thus insoluble) **serum bilirubin** but normal (conjugated and soluble) bilirubin, thus no ↑ bilirubin in urine. ↑ **urobilinogen in urine** and ↓**serum haptoglobin**. Normal liver function tests. ↑**Reticulocyte count, ↓Hb**
Hepatic jaundice due to congenital enzyme defect	*Suggested by:* Normal-looking stools and urine
	Confirmed by: ↑**serum bilirubin** (unconjugated), but no (conjugated) bilirubin in urine. No **urobilinogen in urine** and **normal haptoglobin**. Normal **LFTs**
Hepatocellular jaundice (hepatic with element of obstructive jaundice)	*Suggested by:* onset of jaundice over days or weeks, stools pale or normal but *dark* urine
	Confirmed by: ↑**serum** (conjugated) **bilirubin** and thus ↑**urine bilirubin**. Normal urine urobilinogen. Liver function tests all abnormal, especially ↑↑ALT
Obstructive jaundice	*Suggested by:* onset of jaundice over days or weeks with pale stools and dark urine. Bilirubin ↑ (i.e., conjugated and thus soluble) in urine
	Confirmed by: ↑ serum conjugated bilirubin and thus ↑urine bilirubin but no ↑ urobilinogen in urine. Markedly ↑ alkaline phosphatase, but less abnormal LFTs and ↑GGT

Prehepatic jaundice due to hemolysis

This is suggested by coexisting jaundice and anemia. Stools are normally dark and urine looks normal. There is ↑ unconjugated serum bilirubin but normal conjugated bilirubin and bilirubinuria. Evidence of hemolysis includes ↑ urinary urobilinogen and serum lactate dehydrogenase (LDH), ↓serum haptoglobin, and ↑ reticulocyte count. Other liver function tests are normal, and Hb is decreased.

Some differential diagnoses and typical outline evidence

Hereditary hemolytic anemia	*Suggested by:* family history, anemia, splenomegaly, and leg ulcers
	Confirmed by: above evidence of hemolysis, ↑osmotic fragility; enzyme deficiency, e.g., **glucose-6-phosphate dehydrogenase (G6PD), pyruvate kinase**
Acquired hemolytic anemia	*Suggested by:* sudden onset, in later life, and on medication
	Confirmed by: above evidence of hemolysis, **blood film**, positive **Coombs' test** in autoimmune type
Septicemic hemolysis due to pneumonia, UTI, etc.	*Suggested by:* fever, ± shock symptoms, and signs of infection
	Confirmed by: evidence of hemolysis, **blood culture** positive
Malaria	*Suggested by:* recent travel to malaria zone, periodic paroxysms of rigors, fever, sweating, and nausea
	Confirmed by: Plasmodium in **blood smear**

Hepatic jaundice due to congenital enzyme defect

This is suggested by jaundice, normal-looking stools, and normal-looking urine. It is confirmed by ↑ unconjugated bilirubin, but no (conjugated) bilirubin in urine, no urobilinogen in urine, normal haptoglobin, reticulocyte count, and other liver function tests.

Some differential diagnoses and typical outline evidence

Gilbert's syndrome (normal lifespan)	*Suggested by:* above evidence of impaired conjugation, asymptomatic
	Confirmed by: demonstration of unconjugated hyperbilirubinemia with normal LFT, no hemolysis. Rise in **bilirubin when fasting and after nicotinic acid**
Crigler–Najjar syndrome (type I: severe, neonatal, and often fatal; type II: normal lifespan)	*Suggested by:* above evidence of impaired conjugation
	Confirmed by: unconjugated hyperbilirubinemia with otherwise normal LFT, no hemolysis. No rise in **bilirubin when fasting or after nicotinic acid**

Hepatocellular jaundice (due to hepatitis or very severe liver failure)

This condition is suggested by the onset of jaundice over days or weeks, stools pale or dark, but dark urine. It is confirmed by ↑ conjugated bilirubin and urine bilirubin, and normal urine urobilinogen. Liver function tests are all increasingly abnormal, especially ↑↑ALT.

Some differential diagnoses and typical outline evidence

Acute (viral) hepatitis A	*Suggested by:* tender hepatomegaly
	Confirmed by: presence of **hepatitis A IgM antibody** suggests acute infection
Acute hepatitis B	*Suggested by:* history of IV drug user, blood transfusion, needle punctures, tattoos, tender hepatomegaly
	Confirmed by: presence of **HBsAg in serum**
Acute hepatitis C	*Suggested by:* history of IV drug use, blood transfusion, tender hepatomegaly
	Confirmed by: presence of **anti-HCV antibody, hepatitis C virus by polymerase chain reaction (HCV-PCR)**
Alcoholic hepatitis	*Suggested by:* history of drinking, presence of spider nevi and other signs of chronic liver disease. **AST:ALT** ratio >2
	Confirmed by: resolution with abstinence
Drug-induced hepatitis e.g., paracetamol halothane	*Suggested by:* drug history, recent surgery
	Confirmed by: drug levels improvement after stopping the offending drug
Primary hepatoma	*Suggested by:* weight loss, abdominal pain, RUQ mass
	Confirmed by: ultrasound/CT liver, liver biopsy, ↑α-fetoprotein
Right heart failure	*Suggested by:* ↑JVP, hepatomegaly, ankle edema
	Confirmed by: CXR: large heart. **Echocardiogram:** dilated right ventricle
Infectious mononucleosis	*Suggested by:* cervical lymphadenopathy, enlarged liver, ± splenomegaly, ± jaundice
	Confirmed by: Paul-Bunnell, positive heterophil antibody test

Obstructive jaundice

This is suggested by jaundice with *pale* stools and *dark* urine. There is bilirubin in the urine (i.e., conjugated and thus soluble). It is confirmed by ↑*serum conjugated bilirubin* and thus *urine bilirubin* but no ↑ urobilinogen in the urine. There is markedly ↑ *alkaline phosphatase*, but less abnormal (↑) liver function test and ↑γGT.

Some differential diagnoses and typical outline evidence

Common bile duct stones	*Suggested by:* pain in RUQ ± Murphy's sign
	Confirmed by: **ultrasound liver**: dilatation of biliary ducts
Cancer of head of pancreas	*Suggested by:* progressive, painless jaundice, palpable gallbladder (Courvoisier's law), weight loss
	Confirmed by: **ultrasound liver**: dilatation of biliary ducts. **CT pancreas, endoscopic retrograde (ERCP)** or **magnetic resonance cholangiopancreatography (MRCP)**: obstruction within head of pancreas
Sclerosing cholangitis	*Suggested by:* progressive fatigue, pruritus
	Confirmed by: ↑ALP. **Ultrasound liver**: no gallstones. ERCP: beading of the intra- and extrahepatic biliary ducts
Primary biliary cirrhosis	*Suggested by:* scratch marks, non-tender hepatomegaly, ± splenomegaly, xanthelasmata and xanthomas, arthralgia
	Confirmed by: positive **antimitochondrial antibody,** ↑↑**serum IgM**: infiltrate around hepatic bile ducts and cirrhosis on **liver biopsy**
Drug-induced	*Suggested by:* drug history of oral contraceptive pill, phenothiazines, anabolic steroids, erythromycin, etc.
	Confirmed by: symptoms receding when drug discontinued

Pregnancy (last trimester)	*Suggested by:* jaundice during pregnancy
	Confirmed by: resolution following delivery
Alcoholic hepatitis or cirrhosis	*Suggested by:* history of excess alcohol intake, presence of spider nevi and other signs of chronic liver disease
	Confirmed by: **ultrasound** or **CT liver, liver biopsy**, improvement with abstinence
Dubin–Johnson syndrome (decreased excretion of conjugated bilirubin)	*Suggested by:* intermittent jaundice, and associated pain in the right hypochondrium. No hepatomegaly
	Confirmed by: normal ALP, normal LFT. ↑**urinary bilirubin**. Pigment granules on **liver biopsy**

Dysphagia for solids that stick

The patient is often able to point to a specific point where the food sticks.

Some differential diagnoses and typical outline evidence

Esophageal stricture	*Suggested by:* history of gastroesophageal reflux, ingestion of corrosives, radiation or trauma
	Confirmed by: **barium swallow and meal, fiber-optic endoscopy** showing necrotic mucosa ± ulceration
Carcinoma of esophagus	*Suggested by:* progressive dysphagia, weight loss
	Confirmed by: **barium swallow** showing filling defect, **fiber-optic endoscopy** with biopsy of mass
Carcinoma of cardia of stomach	*Suggested by:* weight loss, epigastric pain, vomiting
	Confirmed by: **barium swallow** shows filling defect, **fiber-optic endoscopy** with biopsy of mass
External esophageal compression	*Suggested by:* few other GI symptoms
	Confirmed by: **barium swallow** shows filling defect, **endoscopy** shows normal mucosa, **CT thorax** shows extrinsic mass from retrosternal goiter, neoplasms (lung or mediastinal tumors, lymphoma); aortic aneurysm

Dysphagia for solids (that do not stick) > for fluids

It is important to distinguish from odynophagia—painful swallowing.

Some differential diagnoses and typical outline evidence

Pharyngeal pouch (pharyngoesophageal diverticulum)	*Suggested by:* regurgitation of undigested food, sensation of a lump in the throat, halitosis, neck bulge on drinking, aspiration into lungs
	Confirmed by: **barium swallow** shows extraluminal collection (esophagoscopy avoided)
Xerostomia	*Suggested by:* dryness of mouth, elderly, occurs especially in females
	Confirmed by: clinical appearance of atrophic, dry oral mucosa
Post-cricoid web congenital, or Plummer–Vincent or Paterson–Kelly syndrome	*Suggested by:* untreated severe iron deficiency anemia
	Confirmed by: **barium swallow** shows a thin, horizontal shelf; **endoscopy** to exclude malignancy
Globus pharyngeus	*Suggested by:* feeling of a lump in the throat which needs to be swallowed, may be associated with anxiety
	Confirmed by: normal **barium swallow, endoscopic resolution** with reassurance and/or **psychotherapy**

Sore throat

With odynophagia—painful swallowing.

Some differential diagnoses and typical outline evidence

Viral pharyngitis	*Suggested by:* sore throat, pain on swallowing, fever, cervical lymphadenopathy and injected pharynx. ↑lymphocytes, leukocytes normal in WBC
	Confirmed by: negative **throat swab** for bacterial culture, self-limiting: resolution within days
Acute follicular tonsillitis (streptococcal)	*Suggested by:* severe sore throat, pain on swallowing, fever, enlarged tonsils with white patches (like strawberries and cream). Cervical lymphadenopathy, especially in angle of jaw. Fever, ↑ leukocytes in WBC
	Confirmed by: **throat swab** for culture and sensitivities of organisms
Infectious mononucleosis (glandular fever) due to Epstein–Barr virus	*Suggested by:* very severe throat pain with enlarged tonsils covered with creamy membrane. Petechiae on palate. Profound malaise. Generalized lymphadenopathy, splenomegaly
	Confirmed by: ↑ atypical lymphocytes in WBC. **Paul–Bunnel** test positive. **Viral titers**
Candidiasis of buccal or esophageal mucosa	*Suggested by:* painful dysphagia, white plaque, history of immunosuppression, diabetes, or recent antibiotics
	Confirmed by: **esophagoscopy** showing erythema and plaques, **brush cytology ± biopsy** shows spores and hyphae
Agranulocytosis	*Suggested by:* sore throat, background history of taking a drug or contact with noxious substance
	Confirmed by: low or absent neutrophil count
Meningococcal meningitits	*Suggested by:* headache, photophobia, vomiting, sore throat, red pharynx without purulent patches, neck stiffness. High blood neutrophil count
	Confirmed by: lumbar puncture showing pus or neutrophil count and organisms on microscopy or culture

Dysphagia for fluids > solids

This implies that there is a neuromuscular and not an obstructive cause.

Some differential diagnoses and typical outline evidence

Myasthenia gravis	*Suggested by:* difficult start to swallowing movement, cough (inhalation) precipitated by swallowing
	Confirmed by: inhalation on **Gastrografin swallow**. Response to **Tensilon test,** ↑*anti-acetylcholine receptor antibody*
Pseudobulbar palsy due to brain stem stroke, multiple sclerosis, motor neuron disease	*Suggested by:* nasal, Donald Duck—like speech, small spastic tongue
	Confirmed by: inhalation of **Gastrograffin**, clinical features of brain stem stroke, multiple sclerosis, motor neuron disease, etc.
Bulbar palsy	*Suggested by:* nasal, quiet or hoarse speech, flaccid, fasciculating tongue
	Confirmed by: clinical features of motor neuron disease, Guillain–Barré syndrome, brain stem tumor, syringobulbia, pontine demyelination
Motor neurone disease	*Suggested by:* combination of upper and lower motor neuron signs
	Confirmed by: **EMG** and **nerve conduction studies**
Achalasia (progressive)	*Suggested by:* dysphagia with almost every meal, regurgitation (postural and effortless, contains undigested food)
	Confirmed by: **barium swallow, esophageal manometry, and esophagoscopy** demonstrate absence of progressive peristalsis
Diffuse esophageal spasm (intermittent)	*Suggested by:* intermittent crushing, retrosternal pain
	Confirmed by: **barium swallow**—sometimes "corkscrew esophagus," **esophageal manometry** showing abnormal pressure profiles
Scleroderma	*Suggested by:* reflux symptoms: cough and inhalation of fluids, tight skin, hooked nose, mouth rugae
	Confirmed by: **barium swallow**—diminished or absent peristalsis, **esophageal manometry**—subnormal or absent lower esophageal sphincter tone

Acute pain in the upper abdomen

Attempts to localize pain in the upper abdomen to the right, left, or middle may be difficult for the patient.

Some differential diagnoses and typical outline evidence

Esophagitis	*Suggested by:* retrosternal pain, heartburn
	Confirmed by: **esophagogastroscopy**
Acute coronary syndrome (unstable angina or infarction)	*Suggested by:* chest tightness or pain on exertion
	Confirmed by: **exercise ECG ± coronary angiography** if troponin normal, or later if troponin ↑
Hiatus hernia	*Suggested by:* heartburn, worsens with stooping or lying, relieved by antacids
	Confirmed by: **esophagogastroscopy, barium meal**
Gastritis	*Suggested by:* epigastric pain, dull or burning discomfort, nocturnal pain
	Confirmed by: **esophagogastroscopy, barium meal and pH study**
Gallstone colic (with no acute inflammation or infection)	*Suggested by:* jaundice, biliary colic, pain in epigastrium or RUQ radiating to right lower scapula. No fever or ↑WBC
	Confirmed by: **ultrasound of gallbladder and biliary ducts**
Acute cholecystitis	*Suggested by:* fever, guarding and positive Murphy's sign (abrupt stopping of inspiration when the palpating hand meets the inflamed gallbladder descending with the liver from behind the subcostal margin on the right side—but not on the left side). ↑WBC
	Confirmed by: **ultrasound of gallbladder and biliary ducts**

Duodenal ulcer	*Suggested by:* epigastric pain, dull or burning discomfort, typically relieved by food, nocturnal pain
	Confirmed by: **esophagogastroscopy, barium meal and pH study** (*Helicobacter pylori* often present in mucosa or by serology)
Gastric ulcer	*Suggested by:* epigastric pain, dull or burning discomfort, typically exacerbated by food, nocturnal pain
	Confirmed by: **esophagogastroscopy, barium meal and pH study**
Gastric carcinoma	*Suggested by:* marked anorexia, fullness, pain, Troisier's sign (a Virchow's node, i.e., large lymph node in the left supraclavicular fossa)
	Confirmed by: **upper GI endoscopy with biopsy**
Pancreatitis	*Suggested by:* pain radiating straight through to the back, better on sitting up or leaning forward
	Confirmed by: **↑serum amylase, CT pancreas**

Acute central abdominal pain

Some differential diagnoses and typical outline evidence

Small bowel obstruction	*Suggested by:* vomiting, constipation with complete obstruction
	Confirmed by: **AXR** shows small bowel loops and fluid levels
Crohn's disease	*Suggested by:* chronic diarrhea with abdominal pain, weight loss, palpable RLQ mass or fullness, mouth ulcers
	Confirmed by: **colonoscopy with biopsy, barium studies** showing "skip lesions," string sign in advanced cases
Mesenteric artery occlusion	*Suggested by:* vomiting, bowel urgency, melena, diarrhea
	Confirmed by: **mesenteric angiography, exploratory laparotomy**
Abdominal aortic dissection	*Suggested by:* tearing pain ± shock ± hypotension and peripheral cyanosis
	Confirmed by: **ultrasound** or **CT of abdomen**

Acute lateral abdominal pain

Some differential diagnoses and typical outline evidence

Pyelonephritis	*Suggested by:* pain in loin (upper lateral), rigors, fever, vomiting, frequency of micturition, renal-angle tenderness
	Confirmed by: FBC: leukocytosis. Urinalysis: pyuria, urine culture and sensitivities
Renal calculus	*Suggested by:* renal colic mainly in loin (upper lateral), hematuria
	Confirmed by: **urinalysis, renal ultrasound, IVU, CT/MRI**
Ureteral calculus	*Suggested by:* renal colic, moving from loin (upper lateral) down to RLQ, hematuria
	Confirmed by: **urinalysis, renal ultrasound, IVU, CT/MRI**
Appendicitis	*Suggested by:* pain initially central, then radiating to RLQ, anorexia, low-grade fever, constipation. RLQ tenderness and guarding
	Confirmed by: Inflamed appendix at laparotomy
Salpingitis	*Suggested by:* fever, nausea, vomiting, mucopurulent cervical discharge, irregular menses. Bilateral lower abdominal tenderness and guarding
	Confirmed by: FBC: leukocytosis. **High vaginal swab, laparoscopy**

Acute lower central (hypogastric) abdominal pain

Some differential diagnoses and typical outline evidence

Infective or ulcerative colitis	*Suggested by:* abdominal pain, diarrhea with blood and mucus
	Confirmed by: **stool microscopy and culture, colonoscopy**
Large bowel obstruction	*Suggested by:* severe distension, late vomiting, visible peristalsis, resonant percussion, increased bowel sounds. Supine **AXR** showing peripheral abdominal large bowel shadow (with haustra partly crossing the lumen). Fluid levels on erect film
	Confirmed by: **abdominal ultrasound and laparotomy findings**
Cystitis	*Suggested by:* frequency, urgency, dysuria, ± hematuria
	Confirmed by: urine for microscopy and culture
Pelvic inflammatory disease	*Suggested by:* vaginal discharge, dysuria, dyspareunia, pelvic tenderness on moving cervix, ↑ESR and CRP. WBC: leukocytosis
	Confirmed by: **High vaginal swab, pelvic ultrasound, ± laparoscopy**
Pelvic endometriosis	*Suggested by:* dysmenorrhea, ovulation pain, dyspareunia, infertility, pelvic mass
	Confirmed by: **laparoscopy**
Ectopic pregnancy	*Suggested by:* constant unilateral pain ± referred shoulder pain, amenorrhea, vaginal bleeding (usually less than normal period), faintness with an acute rupture
	Confirmed by: pregnancy test positive, bimanual examination reveals slightly enlarged uterus, **pelvic ultrasound** shows empty uterus with thickened decidua

Sudden diarrhea, fever, and vomiting

Sudden diarrhea can occur with fever, ± malaise, colicky abdominal pain, and vomiting.

Some differential diagnoses and typical outline evidence

Antibiotic-induced bacterial opportunist: *Clostridium difficile*	*Suggested by:* diarrhea with a history of recent antibiotic therapy, ↑WBC *Confirmed by:* C. difficile toxin in **stool**
Viral gastroenteritis: Rotavirus	*Suggested by:* diarrhea in children <5 years, symptoms resolve in a week
Norwalk virus	*Suggested by:* diarrhea in older children and adults, symptoms resolve in 2 weeks
Food poisoning or toxins: Staphylococcus aureus	*Suggested by:* eating "doubtful" meat, incubation period <6 hours, marked vomiting *Confirmed by:* isolation of Staph. aureus from **examination of suspected food**
Bacillus cereus	*Suggested by:* eating "doubtful" rice, incubation period <6 hours, marked vomiting *Confirmed by:* **stool microscopy** and culture
Vibrio para hemolyticus	*Suggested by:* "doubtful" seafood, incubation period 16–72 hours *Confirmed by:* **stool microscopy and culture**
Clostridium perfringens	*Suggested by:* eating "doubtful" meat, incubation period 8–16 hours, abdominal cramps, little vomiting *Confirmed by:* organism **isolation from feces or suspected food**
Botulism	*Suggested by:* eating "doubtful" canned food, incubation period 18–36 hours, but may vary from 4 hours to 8 days. Abdominal cramps, dry mouth, diplopia, progressive paralysis *Confirmed by:* C. botulinum toxin in serum or feces. C. botulinum toxin isolation from suspected food
Salmonella typhimurium	*Suggested by:* eating "doubtful" meat, egg, or poultry. Fever (with relative bradycardia), headache, dry cough *Confirmed by:* stool microscopy and culture

Recurrent diarrhea with blood ± mucus—bloody flux

Recurrent diarrhea with blood-stained stools ± mucus or fever.

Some differential diagnoses and typical outline evidence

Crohn's disease	*Suggested by:* chronic diarrhea with abdominal pain, weight loss, RLQ mass or fullness, mouth ulcers
	Confirmed by: **colonoscopy with biopsy, barium studies** showing "skip lesions," string sign (in advanced cases)
Ulcerative colitis	*Suggested by:* lower abdominal cramps, ↑ urgency to defecate, severe diarrhea, ↑ fever in acute attack. **CBC** showing ↑WBC
	Confirmed by: **colonoscopy with biopsy, barium studies** show loss of haustration, mucosal edema, ulceration
Colonic carcinoma	*Suggested by:* alternate diarrhea and constipation
	Confirmed by: **barium enema** showing filling defect, **colonoscopy with biopsy** shows mass and malignant histology
Colorectal carcinoma	*Suggested by:* sensation of incomplete evacuation.
	Confirmed by: **sigmoidoscopy with biopsy** showing mass and malignant histology, **barium enema** shows filling defect
Diverticular disease or diverticulitis	*Suggested by:* middle-aged or elderly patient, diarrhea, left iliac fossa pain, abdominal and rectal mass
	Confirmed by: **barium enema** showing opaque filling diverticula, **colonoscopy** showing inflammatory foci

Acute bloody diarrhea ± mucus— "dysentery"

Some differential diagnoses and typical outline evidence

Shigella (bacillary) dysentery	*Suggested by:* blood and mucus, fever, abdominal pain
	Confirmed by: **stool microscopy** revealing red cells, pus cells, and appearance of organism
Campylobacter enteritis	*Suggested by:* associated severe abdominal pain
	Confirmed by: **stool microscopy** and **culture** of organism
Enteroinvasive *Escherichia coli*	*Suggested by:* fever, watery diarrhea
	Confirmed by: **stool microscopy** and **culture** of organism
Enterohemor-rhagic type 0157 *E. coli*	*Suggested by:* bloody diarrhea ± hemolytic uremic syndrome (HUS)
	Confirmed by: **stool microscopy and culture** of organism
Entameba histolytica (amebic) dysentery	*Suggested by:* abdominal discomfort, flatulence, frequent watery, bloody diarrhea
	Confirmed by: **stool microscopy** and **culture** of organism
First episode of cause of recurrent "bloody flux" (see p. 236)	*Suggested by:* no specific features
	Confirmed by: **barium enema** and **colonoscopy** showing evidence of chronic cause after acute episode

Watery diarrhea

Note that diarrhea can result in severe dehydration.

Some differential diagnoses and typical outline evidence

Traveler's diarrhea	*Suggested by:* recent travel, no obvious ingestion of contaminated water or food
	Confirmed by: rapid resolution or response to ciprofloxacin
Enterotoxigenic *E. coli* (most common)	*Suggested by:* incubation period 12–72 hours in relation to contact to others with similar features
	Confirmed by: **stool microscopy and culture**
Vibrio cholera	*Suggested by:* incubation period from a few hours to 5 days, profuse watery diarrhea, fever, vomiting
	Confirmed by: **stool microscopy and culture**
Rotavirus	*Suggested by:* diarrhea in children <5 years, symptoms resolve in a week
Norwalk virus	*Suggested by:* diarrhea in older children and adults, symptoms resolve in 2 weeks

Recurrent diarrhea with no blood in the stools, no fever

Some differential diagnoses and typical outline evidence

Irritable bowel syndrome	*Suggested by:* no weight loss, intermittent daytime diarrhea, pain relieved by defecation, abdominal distension, mucus but no blood in the stool
	Confirmed by: normal **colonoscopy and barium studies**
HIV infection	*Suggested by:* weight loss, other opportunistic infection, lympadenopathy, Kaposi's sarcoma
	Confirmed by: **HIV serology, stool microscopy and cultures** showing *Cryptosporidium*, microsporidia, *Isospora belli*, enteropathy, etc.
Malabsorption due to celiac disease, lactose intolerance, pancreatic disease, Whipple's disease	*Suggested by:* pale, bulky offensive stools, weight loss, signs of nutritional deficiencies
	Confirmed by: **celiac screen, small bowel biopsy; or lactose tolerance test; intestinal biopsy** shows foamy macrophages containing periodic acid Schiff (PAS)-positive glycoprotein in Whipple's disease
Drug -induced	*Suggested by:* history of laxative abuse, magnesium alkalis, antibiotics, hypotensive agents, alcohol
	Confirmed by: resolution on withdrawing drug
Fecal impaction with overflow	*Suggested by:* elderly patient and hard feces on rectal examination
	Confirmed by: **AXR** may show fecal impaction. Response to suppositories or removal of feces
Diabetic autonomic neuropathy	*Suggested by:* intermittent diarrhea, postural hypotension, impotence, urinary retention, history of diabetes
	Confirmed by: lying and standing BP, loss of **beat-to-beat variation** during slow deep breathing
Thyrotoxicosis	*Suggested by:* heat intolerance, tremor, nervousness, palpitation, frequent bowel movements, goiter
	Confirmed by: ↓↓TSH, ↑FT4 or ↑FT3
Carcinoid syndrome	*Suggested by:* facial flushing ± wheeze, abdominal pain
	Confirmed by: ↑24-hour **urinary 5-HIAA**

Change in bowel habit

This may be an increase in constipation or diarrhea or both alternating.

Some differential diagnoses and typical outline evidence

Colonic carcinoma	*Suggested by:* alternate diarrhea and constipation, anemia or weight loss
	Confirmed by: **colonoscopy with biopsy, barium enema**
Change in diet	*Suggested by:* history of ↓ diet fiber, ↓ fluid intake
	Confirmed by: normal **endoscopy** and response to diet change
Drug induced	*Suggested by:* constipating drugs (opioids, hypotensive agents, aluminum alkalis, etc.), purgative dependence
	Confirmed by: normal **endoscopy** and response to withdrawal of suspected agent
Depression	*Suggested by:* sleep disorders, social withdrawal, lack of interest in usual activities
	Confirmed by: normal **endoscopy** and response to lifting of depression
Immobility	*Suggested by:* history
	Confirmed by: normal **endoscopy** and history
Cerebral or spinal cord lesion	*Suggested by:* neurological symptoms and signs ± abnormal sphincter tone and anal sensation
	Confirmed by: **CT** or **MRI**
Metabolic disturbances: hypothyroidism, hyperthyroidism, hypercalcemia, hypokalemia	*Suggested by:* symptoms of metabolic disturbance or absence of anatomical abnormality
	Confirmed by: **thyroid function tests (TFT), serum calcium, potassium**, etc.

Hematemesis ± melena

Vomiting of bright red blood and/or passage of black tarry motions. This implies bleeding usually from the upper GI tract: esophagus, stomach, and duodenum.

Some differential diagnoses and typical outline evidence

Bleeding duodenal ulcer	*Suggested by:* epigastric pain and tenderness, nausea
	Confirmed by: **esophagogastroscopy** showing bleeding ulcer
Gastric erosion	*Suggested by:* history of NSAIDs or alcohol ingestion, epigastric pain, dull or burning discomfort, nocturnal pain
	Confirmed by: appearance of erosion on **esophagogastroscopy** and **pH study** showing hyperacidity
Gastric ulcer	*Suggested by:* epigastric pain, dull or burning discomfort, nocturnal pain
	Confirmed by: appearance of ulcer on **esophagogastroscopy** and **pH study** showing hyperacidity
Mallory–Weiss tear	*Suggested by:* preceding marked vomiting, later bright red blood
	Confirmed by: **esophagogastroscopy** showing tear
Gastroesophageal reflux	*Suggested by:* heartburn worse when lying flat, anorexia, nausea, ± regurgitation of gastric content
	Confirmed by: appearance of erosion on **esophagoscopy, barium meal** and **pH study** showing hyperacidity
Hiatus hernia	*Suggested by:* heartburn, worse with stooping, relieved by antacids
	Confirmed by: herniation of stomach into chest on plain (X-ray or barium meal), appearance of erosion on **esophagoscopy** and **pH study** showing hyperacidity

False hematemesis	*Suggested by:* swallowed nose bleed or hemoptysis
	Confirmed by: normal **esophagogastroscopy** and **bleeding** source identified in nose
Esophageal carcinoma	*Suggested by:* progressive dysphagia with solids, which sticks, weight loss
	Confirmed by: **barium swallow, fiber-optic gastroscopy with mucosal biopsy** showing malignant tissue
Gastric carcinoma	*Suggested by:* marked anorexia, fullness, pain, Troisier's sign (enlarged left supraclavicular lymph [Virchow's] node)
	Confirmed by: **esophagogastroscopy with biopsy** showing malignant tissue
Ingestion of corrosives	*Suggested by:* history of ingestion
	Confirmed by: **esophagogastroscopy** showing severe erosions
Esophageal varices	*Suggested by:* liver cirrhosis, splenomegaly, prominent upper abdominal veins
	Confirmed by: **esophagogastroscopy** showing varicose mucosa and blood distally and in stomach
Meckel's diverticulum	*Suggested by:* no hematemesis, usually asymptomatic, anemia, rectal bleeding
	Confirmed by: **technetium-labeled red blood cell scan**, showing isotopes in gut lumen and laparotomy
Other causes: angiodysplasia, bleeding disorders	

Passage of blood per rectum (hematochezia)

This may only be discovered on rectal examination.

Some differential diagnoses and typical outline evidence

Bleeding hemorrhoids	*Suggested by:* pain, discharge, pruritus, staining of toilet paper following defecation
	Confirmed by: physical and digital rectal examination, proctoscopy
Anal fissure	*Suggested by:* skin tag, pain on defecation, staining of toilet paper following defecation, exquisite anal tenderness
	Confirmed by: history and clinical examination
Diverticulitis	*Suggested by:* bloody splash in the pan, abdominal pain, usually LIF, diarrhea and constipation
	Confirmed by: **colonoscopy, barium enema**
Carcinoma rectum	*Suggested by:* rectal bleeding with defecation
	Confirmed by: **sigmoidoscopy with biopsy**
Colonic carcinoma	*Suggested by:* red blood mixed with stool and alternate diarrhea and constipation
	Confirmed by: **flexible colonoscopy with biopsy**
Ulcerative colitis	*Suggested by:* lower abdominal pain, ↑ urgency to defecate, severe bloody diarrhea, ↑ fever in acute attack.
	Confirmed by: **colonoscopy with biopsy, barium studies** show loss of haustration, mucosal edema, ulceration
Meckel's diverticulum	*Suggested by:* usually asymptomatic, anemia, rectal bleeding
	Confirmed by: **technetium-labeled red blood cell scan, laparotomy**

Crohn's disease	*Suggested by:* chronic diarrhea with abdominal pain, weight loss, palpable RLQ mass or fullness, mouth ulcers
	Confirmed by: **colonoscopy with biopsy, barium studies** show "skip lesions," string sign in advanced cases
Massive upper GI bleed	*Suggested by:* bright or dark red, maroon-colored stool
	Confirmed by: **upper GI endoscopy**
Trauma (in children, possible non-accidental injury)	*Suggested by:* fresh blood, sometimes external signs of trauma.
	Confirmed by: sensitive and careful history, possible surveillance etc.
Intussusception	*Suggested by:* child in first 6–18 months of life, acute onset of colicky intermittent abdominal pain, red currant "jelly" PR bleed, ± a sausage shape mass in upper abdomen
	Confirmed by: **barium enema**, ±reduction of intussusception with appropriate hydrostatic pressure

Tenesmus

In tenesmus there is the sensation of needing to defecate, but no stool is produced.

Some differential diagnoses and typical outline evidence

Rectal inflammation (proctitis)	*Suggested by:* rectal bleeding, mucus discharge
	Confirmed by: proctoscopy or **sigmoidoscopy reveals** inflamed rectal mucosa
Rectal tumor	*Suggested by:* rectal bleeding with defecation, blood limited to surface of stool
	Confirmed by: **sigmoidoscopy with rectal biopsy**
Tumor of descending colon	*Suggested by:* alternate diarrhea and constipation
	Confirmed by: **colonoscopy with biopsy, barium enema**
Pelvic inflammatory disease	*Suggested by:* lower abdominal pain, fever, vaginal discharge, dysuria, elevated ESR and CRP, leukocytosis
	Confirmed by: **high vaginal swab, pelvic ultrasound, ± laparoscopy**

Anorectal pain

Some differential diagnoses and typical outline evidence

Anal fissure	*Suggested by:* skin tag, pain on defecation, staining of toilet paper following defecation
	Confirmed by: physical zexamination of anal region
Hemorrhoids	*Suggested by:* rectal bleeding following defecation, perianal protrusion with pain
	Confirmed by: digital rectal examination
Perianal abscess	*Suggested by:* tender lump, redness
	Confirmed by: digital rectal examination
Proctitis	*Suggested by:* rectal bleeding, mucus discharge
	Confirmed by: proctoscopy or **sigmoidoscopy** revealing inflamed rectal mucosa
Prostatitis	*Suggested by:* rigor, ↑ fever, urinary frequency and urgency, dysuria, hemospermia
	Confirmed by: tender prostate gland on rectal examination, **urine microscopy**
Proctalgia fugax, coccydynia	*Suggested by:* fleeting pain in rectum or coccyx that may be related to sitting, but not defecation
	Confirmed by: physical examination, tenderness of levator muscle

GI signs

General examination checklist

Preliminary findings should have been discovered during the general examination. These include jaundice, anemia, clubbing, xanthelasma, or gynecomastia; abnormalities of the lips, buccal mucosa, throat, and tongue; the presence of supraclavicular lump(s).

Distended abdomen

Inspect the abdomen from a sitting position next to the bed or couch. Consider the general shape, then look at the skin. Next, consider movement of the abdomen. The causes are the traditional 6 *F*'s: Fat, Fluid, Flatus, Feces, Fibroids, and Fetus.

Some differential diagnoses and typical outline evidence

Fat (obese)	*Suggested by:* usually sunken umbilicus, dullness to percussion throughout
	Confirmed by: **CT abdomen**
Fluid (ascites)	*Suggested by:* bilateral bulging flanks, shifting dullness, fluid thrill
	Confirmed by: **ultrasound liver and abdomen**
Flatus (gas) due to normal dietary variation	*Suggested by:* tympanic sound throughout. Often associated with constipation
	Confirmed by: **AXR** shows normal gas shadow
Small bowel obstruction ("flatus" again)	*Suggested by:* mild distension, early vomiting, central and high abdominal pain, resonant percussion, and increased bowel sounds. Supine **AXR** showing central gas but no peripheral abdominal large-bowel shadow (i.e., without haustra partly crossing) but valvulae conniventes of small intestine entirely crossing the lumen. Fluid levels on erect film
	Confirmed by: **abdominal ultrasound and laparotomy findings**
Large bowel obstruction	*Suggested by:* severe distension, late vomiting, visible peristalsis, resonant percussion, and increased bowel sounds. Supine **AXR** showing peripheral abdominal large-bowel shadow (with haustra partly crossing the lumen). Fluid levels on erect film
	Confirmed by: **abdominal ultrasound and laparotomy findings**
Fecal impaction	*Suggested by:* paucity of bowel movement and constipation. **AXR** shows stippled pattern of fecal loading
	Confirmed by: digital exam, resolution of distension with evacuation
Fibroids, large ovarian cyst	*Suggested by:* mass in pelvis in middle-aged female
	Confirmed by: **abdominal ultrasound**
Fetus	*Suggested by:* amenorrhea and mass in pelvis (cannot get below it)
	Confirmed by: positive **urine pregnancy test** or ↑*plasma β-hCG*. Also **abdominal ultrasound**

Distended abdominal veins

Some differential diagnoses and typical outline evidence

Portal hypertension	*Suggested by:* veins radiating out from umbilicus (caput medusa), ± ascites, ± splenomegaly, other stigmata of chronic liver disease, venous hum over collaterals
	Confirmed by: **ultrasound scan** appearance of liver, which is small cirrhotic with dilated portal veins
Inferior vena cava obstruction	*Suggested by:* distended veins with blood flow up from groin toward chest when compressed and one end released
	Confirmed by: **CT abdomen**
Superior vena cava obstruction	*Suggested by:* distended veins with blood flow from chest toward groin when compressed and one end released
	Confirmed by: **CT thorax**

Abdominal bruising

Also consider the general causes of bruising as indicated in the general examination findings.

Some differential diagnoses and typical outline evidence

Retroperitoneal hemorrhage e.g., in acute pancreatitis	*Suggested by:* abdominal tenderness and rigidity and bruises in and around the umbilicus (Cullen's sign) or on one or both flanks (Grey Turner's sign)
	Confirmed by: ↑*serum amylase, CT abdomen*
Ruptured or dissecting abdominal aortic aneurysm	*Suggested by:* hypotension and abdominal pain, tenderness, and rigidity, and bruises in and around the umbilicus (Cullen's sign) or on one or both flanks (Grey Turner's sign). Expansive pulsatile mass >3 cm diameter and can hear bruit over the mass
	Confirmed by: **abdominal ultrasound** or **CT abdomen**

Poor abdominal movement

From the sitting position, watch and ask about any areas of tenderness and begin furthest away, palpating gently while looking at the patient's face to see if there is any reaction. "Rigidity" is when there is no initial lack of resistance but reflex rigidity from the outset.

Some differential diagnoses and typical outline evidence

Small bowel obstruction ("flatus" again)	*Suggested by:* mild distension, early vomiting, central and high abdominal pain, resonant percussion, and increased bowel sounds. Supine **AXR** shows central gas but no peripheral abdominal large bowel shadow (i.e., without haustra partly crossing) but valvulae conniventes of small intestine crossing the entire lumen. Fluid levels on erect film
	Confirmed by: **abdominal ultrasound and laparotomy findings**
Large bowel obstruction ("flatus" again)	*Suggested by:* severe distension, late vomiting, visible peristalsis, resonant percussion, and increased bowel sounds. Supine **AXR** shows peripheral abdominal large-bowel shadow (with haustra partly crossing the lumen). Fluid levels on erect film
	Confirmed by: **abdominal ultrasound and laparotomy findings**
Peritonitis from perforated stomach, duodenum, diverticulum; intraperitoneal hemorrhage, or bowel infarction	*Suggested by:* decreased or absent abdominal movement, generalized tenderness and rigidity, absent bowel sounds, and board-like rigidity
	Confirmed by: **erect AXR or CXR** showing free gas under diaphragm and laparotomy

Localized tenderness in the hypogastrium (suprapubic area)

Some differential diagnoses and typical outline evidence

Acute bladder distension (due to prostatic hypertrophy in males)	*Suggested by:* suprapubic mass (cannot get below), dull to percussion *Confirmed by:* **bladder ultrasound scan, urethral catheterization** and drainage of high volume of urine (e.g., >1 liter)
Cystitis	*Suggested by:* frequency of urine, dysuria, turbid urine, hematuria on dipstick *Confirmed by:* excess **WBC** and organisms on microscopy and growth of significant bacterial colonies on **urine culture**

Localized tenderness in the right upper quadrant (RUQ)

Guarding is when there is reflex rigidity on palpation.

Some differential diagnoses and typical outline evidence

Acute cholecystitis	*Suggested by:* fever, guarding and positive Murphy's sign (abrupt stopping of inspiration when the palpating hand meets the inflamed gallbladder descending with the liver from behind the subcostal margin on the right side—but not on the left side)
	Confirmed by: **ultrasound gallbladder and biliary ducts**
Acute alcoholic hepatitis	*Suggested by:* history of recent drinking binge, tender hepatomegaly, jaundice
	Confirmed by: rise and fall in liver function tests to coincide with binge, negative **hepatitis serology**
Acute viral hepatitis A	*Suggested by:* negative history of recent binge drinking, fever, tender hepatomegaly, jaundice
	Confirmed by: positive **hepatitis serology A, B C, D, or E**
Acute liver congestion	*Suggested by:* tender hepatomegaly, ↑JVP, leg edema
	Confirmed by: **CXR showing large heart, liver ultrasound showing distension**

Localized tenderness in the left upper quadrant (LUQ)

Some differential diagnoses and typical outline evidence

Pyelonephritis	*Suggested by:* fever, rigor, vomiting, groin pain, tenderness at costovertebral angle (CVA), ↑**WBC** proteinuria, hematuria, leukocytes on **urine testing**
	Confirmed by: above clinical picture and significant growth of organisms on **urine culture**. Ultrasound scan for possible anatomical abnormality
Splenic rupture	*Suggested by:* history of trauma, plain **AXR** showing loss of left psoas shadow, **peritoneal tap** demonstrates free blood
	Confirmed by: **CT scan** and laparotomy
Splenic infarct	*Suggested by:* presence of predisposing cause, especially sickle cell disease and crisis
	Confirmed by: **CT** abdomen

Localized tenderness in the epigastrium or central abdomen

Some differential diagnoses and typical outline evidence

Gastritis	*Suggested by:* epigastric pain, dull or burning discomfort, nocturnal pain
	Confirmed by: **esophagogastroscopy, barium meal and pH study**
Duodenal ulcer	*Suggested by:* epigastric pain, dull or burning discomfort, typically relieved by food, nocturnal pain
	Confirmed by: esophagogastroscopy, barium meal and pH study. **Helicobacter pylori** present in mucosa or **serology**
Gastric ulcer	*Suggested by:* epigastric pain, dull or burning discomfort, typically exacerbated by food
	Confirmed by: **esophagogastroscopy, barium meal and pH study**
Pancreatitis	*Suggested by:* rigidity or guarding ± bruises, e.g., Cullen or Grey Turner's signs
	Confirmed by: **↑serum amylase, CT pancreas** showing enlargement by cyst or pseudocyst
Small bowel infarction	*Suggested by:* abdominal distension, absent bowel sounds. Predisposing cause, e.g., atrial fibrillation, extensive atheroma in diabetes
	Confirmed by: **AXR** showing dilated loop of small bowel with valvulae conniventes but no large bowel (with haustra, etc.)
Ruptured or dissecting abdominal aortic aneurysm	*Suggested by:* hypotension and abdominal pain, tenderness and rigidity, bruises in and around the umbilicus (Cullen's sign) and on one or both flanks (Grey Turner's sign). Expansive pulsatile mass >3 cm in diameter and can hear bruit over the mass
	Confirmed by: **abdominal ultrasound** or **CT abdomen**

Localized tenderness in the left or right loin

Some differential diagnoses and typical outline evidence

Pyelonephritis	*Suggested by:* fever, rigor, vomiting, groin pain, tenderness at renal angle, ↑*WBC* proteinuria, hematuria, leukocytes on **urine testing**
	Confirmed by: clinical picture and significant growth of organisms on **urine culture**. Ultrasound scan for possible anatomical abnormality
Renal calculus	*Suggested by:* colicky pain beginning in loin and radiating down to lower abdomen. Tenderness at renal angle
	Confirmed by: hematuria, dilated ureter on **renal ultrasound**, filling defect on **IVU**
Ruptured or dissecting abdominal aortic aneurysm	*Suggested by:* hypotension and abdominal pain, tenderness and rigidity, bruises in and around the umbilicus (Cullen's sign) and on one or both flanks (Grey Turner's sign). Expansive pulsatile mass >3 cm in diameter, bruit over the mass
	Confirmed by: **abdominal ultrasound** or **CT abdomen**

Localized tenderness in left or right lower quadrant

Some differential diagnoses and typical outline evidence

Appendicitis	*Suggested by:* abdominal pain, then localized to right (rarely left in situs inversus) lower quadrant, fever, guarding, positive Rovsing's sign (tenderness on contralateral side), psoas sign (pain from passive extension of right hip), adductor pain (pain on passive internal rotation of flexed thigh); anterior tenderness on rectal examination
	Confirmed by: macroscopic and microscopic appearances at *laparotomy*
Diverticulitis	*Suggested by:* left iliac fossa tenderness ± tender mass
	Confirmed by: flexible sigmoidoscopy, barium enema
Ureteric calculus	*Suggested by:* colicky pain with radiation to lower abdomen, microscopic or frank hematuria
	Confirmed by: ureteric dilation on *renal ultrasound*, filling defect on *IVU*
Mesenteric adenitis	*Suggested by:* symptoms and signs similar to those for early appendicitis but without guarding or rectal tenderness
	Confirmed by: clinical findings or made at laparotomy or laparoscopy
Salpingitis	*Suggested by:* severe adnexal tenderness, cervical motion tenderness, cervical discharge
	Confirmed by: *cervical swab culture, laparoscopy*
Ectopic pregnancy	*Suggested by:* enlarged uterus (but often small for dates), vaginal bleeding, faintness or shock in acute rupture
	Confirmed by: pregnancy test positive, mass on bimanual examination. *Pelvic ultrasound* shows empty uterus with thickened decidua

Hepatomegaly—smooth and tender

Some differential diagnoses and typical outline evidence

Right heart failure from pulmonary hypertension acutely due to pulmonary embolus	*Suggested by:* ↑JVP, leg edema *Confirmed by:* large heart on **CXR** and associated large pulmonary arteries or pulmonary edema if congestive heart failure (CHF)
Alcoholic hepatitis	*Suggested by:* history of drinking binge, ↑MCV, jaundice *Confirmed by:* abnormal **liver function tests**: ↑AST: ↑ALP, **liver biopsy** later
Infectious hepatitis	*Suggested by:* sharp edge, no or slight splenomegaly, jaundice *Confirmed by:* abnormal liver function tests, hepatitis A serology positive
Glandular fever (infectious mononucleosis)	*Suggested by:* cervical lymphadenopathy, sharp edge, ± splenomegaly, ± jaundice *Confirmed by:* **Paul–Bunnell**, positive **heterophil antibody** test
Right heart failure due to tricuspid regurgitation	*Suggested by:* pulsatile liver, ± jaundice, ↑JVP with prominent v waves, systolic murmur louder on inspiration *Confirmed by:* **echocardiography**

Hepatomegaly—smooth but not tender

Some differential diagnoses and typical outline evidence

Cirrhosis of the liver (early + fatty change)	*Suggested by:* firm, round edge, ± splenomegaly, other stigmata of chronic liver disease (e.g., spider nevi)
	Confirmed by: small liver with abnormal parenchyma on **liver ultrasound and biopsy** appearance
Lymphoma	*Suggested by:* generalized lymphadenopathy, splenomegaly
	Confirmed by: **lymph node biopsy, bone marrow biopsy, CT thorax/abdomen**
Leukemia	*Suggested by:* anemia, lymphadenopathy, splenomegaly
	Confirmed by: abnormal **WBC** on blood film, **bone marrow examination**
Hemochromatosis	*Suggested by:* bronze skin pigmentation, evidence of diabetes mellitus, cardiac failure, arthropathy
	Confirmed by: elevated **serum ferritin** (>500 µg/L), **liver biopsy with hepatic iron measurement**
Primary biliary cirrhosis	*Suggested by:* xanthelasmata and xanthomas, scratch marks, arthralgia, ± splenomegaly
	Confirmed by: positive **antimitochondrial antibody,** ↑**serum IgM, liver biopsy**
Amyloidosis primary or secondary to chronic inflammation	*Suggested by:* evidence of underlying chronic infective disease if secondary
	Confirmed by: **biopsy of rectal mucosa,** stained with Congo red dye

Hepatomegaly—irregular, not tender

Some differential diagnoses and typical outline evidence

Metastatic carcinoma	*Suggested by:* hard, ± nodular, cachexia.
	Confirmed by: **liver ultrasound ± biopsy**
Hepatoma	*Suggested by:* firm, nodular edge, ± arterial bruit ↑serum AFP
	Confirmed by: α-fetoprotein ↑, **liver ultrasound** and **biopsy**
Hydatid cyst	*Suggested by:* sometimes hard, nodular
	Confirmed by: **liver ultrasound** showing cyst and daughter cysts inside, eosinophilia, **serology** (*Echinococcus granulosus*), **Casoni intradermal test**.

Splenomegaly—slight (< 3 fingers)

The spleen enlarges diagonally downward toward the RLQ. Begin there so as not to miss the edge of massive enlargement.

Some differential diagnoses and typical outline evidence

Glandular fever	*Suggested by:* cervical lymphadenopathy, hepatomegaly with sharp edge
	Confirmed by: **Paul–Bunnell, positive heterophil antibody test (monospot)**
Brucella	*Suggested by:* occupation, e.g., farmer, hepatomegaly
	Confirmed by: **Brucella serology**
Hepatitis A, B, C, or D	*Suggested by:* jaundice, tender hepatomegaly, lymphadenopathy
	Confirmed by: abnormal **liver function tests, hepatitis A, B, C, and D serology**
Bacterial endocarditis	*Suggested by:* splinter hemorrhages, heart murmur, anemia, microscopic hematuria
	Confirmed by: **blood cultures, transesophageal echocardiography**
Amyloidosis primary or secondary to chronic inflammation	*Suggested by:* evidence of underlying chronic infective disease if secondary
	Confirmed by: **biopsy of rectal mucosa**, stained with Congo red dye
Hemolytic anemia	*Suggested by:* anemia, jaundice
	Confirmed by: **CBC** showing reticulocytosis, anemia, **liver function tests** showing ↑ unconjugated bilirubin, haptoglobin

Splenomegaly—moderate (3–5 fingers)

Some differential diagnoses and typical outline evidence

Lymphoma	*Suggested by:* generalized lymphadenopathy, non-tender hepatomegaly
	Confirmed by: **lymph node biopsy, bone marrow biopsy, CT thorax/abdomen**
Chronic leukemia	*Suggested by:* lymphadenopathy, non-tender hepatomegaly
	Confirmed by: abnormal **CBC** and **blood film, bone marrow examination**
Cirrhosis ± portal hypertension	*Suggested by:* hard, round edge, ± hepatomegaly, other stigmata of chronic liver disease
	Confirmed by: small nodular **liver** on **ultrasound** ± **biopsy**

Splenomegaly—massive (> 5 fingers)

The spleen enlarges diagonally downward toward the RLQ. Begin there so as not to miss the edge of massive enlargement.

Some differential diagnoses and typical outline evidence

Chronic myeloid leukemia	*Suggested by:* variable hepatomegaly, bruising, anemia
	Confirmed by: presence of **Philadelphia chromosome,** BCR-ABL fusion mRNA or BCR-ABL protein
Myelofibrosis	*Suggested by:* anemia, ± hepatomegaly, ± lymphadenopathy
	Confirmed by: **bone marrow tap** is usually dry, **bone marrow biopsy** shows fibrosis
Malaria	*Suggested by:* anemia, jaundice, hepatomegaly, paroxysmal rigors
	Confirmed by: **thick and thin blood films** showing Plasmodium
Kala-azar (visceral leishmaniasis)	*Suggested by:* pancytopenia, hepatomegaly
	Confirmed by: demonstration of Leishmania donovani in **Giemsa-stained smears**, specific **serological test**

Bilateral masses in upper abdomen

The lower half of a normal right kidney is often palpable. A renal mass is bimanually ballotable and moves slightly downward on inspiration.

Some differential diagnoses and typical outline evidence

Polycystic renal disease	*Suggested by:* masses are bimanually ballotable, hypertension
	Confirmed by: **ultrasound/CT kidneys**
Amyloidosis, primary or secondary to chronic inflammation	*Suggested by:* evidence of underlying chronic infective disease
	Confirmed by: **biopsy of kidney or rectal mucosa,** stained with Congo red dye
Bilateral hydronephroses	*Suggested by:* masses bimanually ballotable, renal impairment
	Confirmed by: dilated ureters ± renal calyces on **abdominal ultrasound**

Unilateral mass in right or left upper quadrant

Some differential diagnoses and typical outline evidence

Renal carcinoma	*Suggested by:* hematuria, fever of unknown origin (FUO), ± polycythemia
	Confirmed by: **renal ultrasound/CT with biopsy**
Unilateral hydronephrosis	*Suggested by:* no other symptoms and signs except bimanually ballotable mass
	Confirmed by: unilateral dilated ureter ± renal calyx on **abdominal ultrasound**
Renal cyst	*Suggested by:* tense, fluctuant feel
	Confirmed by: cyst on **abdominal ultrasound**
Distended gall bladder (on right side)	*Suggested by:* right-sided pear-shaped, rounded mass that continues with the liver above (Courvoisier's sign—implies extrahepatic biliary obstruction)
	Confirmed by: **ultrasound of gallbladder and biliary ducts**

Mass in epigastrium (± umbilical area)

Some differential diagnoses and typical outline evidence

Gastric carcinoma	*Suggested by:* anorexia, weight loss over weeks to months, hard, irregular mass, left supraclavicular node (Virchow's node giving Troisier's sign)
	Confirmed by: **gastroscopy with biopsy**
Carcinoma of pancreas	*Suggested by:* progressive painless jaundice ± abdominal or back pain later
	Confirmed by: **ERCP** or **MRCP**
Aortic aneurysm	*Suggested by:* >3 cm in diameter, pulsatile swelling with bruit
	Confirmed by: **abdominal ultrasound** or **CT abdomen**

Mass in right lower quadrant (RLQ)

Some differential diagnoses and typical outline evidence

Appendix mass	*Suggested by:* recent history of fever and right iliac fossa (RIF) pain
	Confirmed by: **ultrasound** or **CT abdomen and finding at laparotomy**
Crohn's granuloma	*Suggested by:* aphthous ulcers, wasting, anemia, tender mass, scars of previous surgery, anal fissures, fistulae
	Confirmed by: **barium follow-through** and **small bowel enema, colonoscopy with biopsy**
Carcinoma of cecum	*Suggested by:* asymptomatic RIF mass, iron-deficiency anemia
	Confirmed by: **colonoscopy with biopsy**
Transplanted kidney	*Suggested by:* obvious history of transplant and scar over mass, usually in iliac fossa
	Confirmed by: **abdominal ultrasound**
Other causes: intussusception, carcinoma of ascending colon, cecal volvulus	

Mass in hypogastrium (suprapubic region)

Some differential diagnoses and typical outline evidence

Distended bladder	*Suggested by:* suprapubic dullness, resonance in flank, tender mass, and acute retention of urine
	Confirmed by: mass disappears on **bladder ultrasound scan and catheterization, abdominal/pelvic ultrasound**
Pregnant uterus	*Suggested by:* suprapubic dullness, resonance in flank
	Confirmed by: pregnancy test positive, bimanual examination, **abdominal/pelvic ultrasound scan**
Uterine fibroid	*Suggested by:* asymptomatic, hard, rounded, non-tender mass on bimanual palpation
	Confirmed by: **pelvic examination and ultrasound**
Uterine neoplasm	*Suggested by:* postmenopausal bleeding, blood-stained vaginal discharge, irregular bleeding
	Confirmed by: pelvic examination and **pelvic ultrasound**
Ovarian cyst	*Suggested by:* tense, fluctuant feel, fluid thrill if cyst is large
	Confirmed by: pelvic examination and **ultrasound of ovary**

Mass in left lower quadrant (LLQ)

Some differential diagnoses and typical outline evidence

Diverticular abscess	*Suggested by:* fever, tender mass
	Confirmed by: ultrasound or **CT abdomen/pelvis**
Carcinoma of descending or sigmoid colon	*Suggested by:* hard mass, not tender
	Confirmed by: **barium enema, colonoscopy with biopsy**
Fecal impaction	*Suggested by:* paucity of bowel movement and constipation. **AXR** shows stippled pattern of fecal loading
	Confirmed by: resolution of swelling with evacuation or partly with flatus tube

Central dullness, resonance in flank

Some differential diagnoses and typical outline evidence

Distended bladder	*Suggested by:* suprapubic mass, tender in acute retention of urine
	Confirmed by: mass disappears on **bladder ultrasound scan and catheterization**
Pregnant uterus	*Suggested by:* suprapubic mass
	Confirmed by: ↑ serum or urine β-hCG, **pelvic or abdominal ultrasound**
Massive ovarian cyst	*Suggested by:* tense, fluctuant feel, fluid thrill
	Confirmed by: **pelvic or abdominal ultrasound**

Shifting dullness

This implies ascites.

Some differential diagnoses and typical outline evidence

Carcinomatosis with spread to peritoneum	*Suggested by:* cachexia
	Confirmed by: **diagnostic paracentesis** including **cytology, liver ultrasound with biopsy**
Cirrhosis	*Suggested by:* stigmata of chronic liver disease, ± splenomegaly
	Confirmed by: **paracentesis, liver ultrasound with biopsy**
Congestive cardiac failure	*Suggested by:* ↑JVP, leg edema, ± tender hepatomegaly
	Confirmed by: **liver function tests, FBC, diagnostic paracentesis, CXR**
Nephrotic syndrome	*Suggested by:* generalized edema including face on rising from bed
	Confirmed by: **proteinuria, hypoalbuminemia**
TB peritonitis	*Suggested by:* fever, history of tuberculosis, generalized tenderness
	Confirmed by: **diagnostic paracentesis including microscopy, bacterial and AFB cultures**
Peritoneal dialysis	*Suggested by:* renal failure, continuous ambulatory peritoneal dialysis (CAPD)
	Confirmed by: elevated **serum creatinine**

Silent abdomen with no bowel sounds

Some differential diagnoses and typical outline evidence

Peritonitis e.g., due to bowel perforation	*Suggested by:* decreased or absent abdominal movement, generalized tenderness with board-like rigidity
	Confirmed by: **AXR,** erect **CXR** show gas under diaphragm
Bowel infarction	*Suggested by:* decreased or absent abdominal movement, generalized tenderness with board-like rigidity
	Confirmed by: **AXR,** erect **CXR** show no gas under diaphragm

High-pitched bowel sounds

Some differential diagnoses and typical outline evidence

Small bowel obstruction	*Suggested by:* mild distension, early vomiting, central, high abdominal pain, resonant percussion, increased bowel sounds. Supine *AXR* showing central gas but no peripheral abdominal large-bowel shadow (i.e., without haustra partly crossing) but valvulae conniventes of small intestine entirely crossing the lumen. Fluid levels on erect film
	Confirmed by: **abdominal ultrasound and laparotomy findings**
Large bowel obstruction	*Suggested by:* severe distension, late vomiting, resonant percussion, increased bowel sounds. Supine *AXR* showing peripheral abdominal large-bowel shadow (with haustra partly crossing the lumen). Fluid levels on erect film
	Confirmed by: **abdominal ultrasound and laparotomy findings**
Adhesions of bowel	*Suggested by:* scars, **signs of bowel obstruction**
	Confirmed by: **abdominal ultrasound and laparotomy findings**
Tumor in bowel	*Suggested by:* palpable abdominal mass, **signs of bowel obstruction**
	Confirmed by: **abdominal ultrasound and laparotomy findings**
Hernial orifice strangulation	*Suggested by:* hernia visible, not reducible, very ill, peritonism, **signs of bowel obstruction**
	Confirmed by: **laparotomy findings**
Sigmoid volvulus	*Suggested by:* **signs of severe bowel obstruction**. Supine *AXR* showing U-shaped gas shadow
	Confirmed by: **sigmoidoscopy and reduction with flatus tube and laparotomy findings**
Irritable bowel syndrome	*Suggested by:* slight distension, history of abdominal pain, and small, hard motions
	Confirmed by: abdominal ultrasound and spontaneous resolution
Fecal impaction	*Suggested by:* paucity of bowel movement and constipation. Hard feces on rectal examination. *AXR* shows stippled pattern of fecal loading
	Confirmed by: resolution of swelling with evacuation or partly with flatus tube

Abdominal or groin bruit

Some differential diagnoses and typical outline evidence

Aortic aneurysm	*Suggested by:* systolic bruit in the epigastrium (over mass), expansive pulsatile swelling
	Confirmed by: **ultrasound/CT abdomen**
Renal artery stenosis	*Suggested by:* systolic bruit in the right upper quadrant, hypertension
	Confirmed by: **renal arteriography—digital subtraction angiography**
Dissecting aorta	*Suggested by:* tearing abdominal pain radiating to back and hypotension. Brachial–ankle gradient and pulse delay
	Confirmed by: urgent **ultrasound/CT abdomen**

Lump in the groin

Some differential diagnoses and typical outline evidence

Inguinal hernia	*Suggested by:* origin horizontally just above and medial to pubic tubercle, impulse on coughing or bearing down, reducible
	Confirmed by: above clinical examination and surgery
Femoral hernia	*Suggested by:* origin horizontally just below and lateral to pubic tubercle, cough impulse rarely detectable, usually irreducible (because of narrow femoral canal)
	Confirmed by: above clinical examination and surgery
Strangulated hernia	*Suggested by:* irreducible, tense and tender, red, followed by symptoms and signs of bowel obstruction
	Confirmed by: above clinical examination and surgery
Lymph node inflammation	*Suggested by:* enlarged, tender, mobile, nodes, usually multiple
	Confirmed by: above clinical examination
Lymphoma or secondary tumor	*Suggested by:* fixed nodes when infiltrated by tumor
	Confirmed by: **ultrasound, exploration of groin**
Femoral artery aneurysm	*Suggested by:* lump lies below the midpoint of the inguinal ligament, expansive pulsation
	Confirmed by: above clinical examination. **Duplex ultrasound scan**
Saphena varix (dilatation of long saphenous vein in the groin)	*Suggested by:* soft and diffuse swelling that lies below inguinal ligament, empties with minimal pressure and refills on release, disappears on lying down, cough impulse
	Confirmed by: above clinical examination
Cold abscess of psoas sheath	*Suggested by:* fluctuant tender swelling arising below the inguinal ligament
	Confirmed by: **ultrasound, exploration of groin**

Anal appearance

The rectal examination (with a chaperone) begins with an examination of the anus by parting the buttocks with the patient lying in the left lateral position with knees flexed.

Some differential diagnoses and typical outline evidence

Prolapsed internal hemorrhoids	*Suggested by:* segmental, plum-colored rectal protrusion
	Confirmed by: proctoscopy
Acute anal fissure	*Suggested by:* acute pain during defecation, exquisite anal tenderness. Mucosal fissure with skin tag if chronic (sentinel pile)
	Confirmed by: above history and clinical **examination under anesthesia**
Spontaneous perianal hematoma	*Suggested by:* blue-black lump in the skin near the anal margin
	Confirmed by: above history and examination
Perianal abscess	*Suggested by:* tender, fluctuant, perianal mass
	Confirmed by: above clinical examination
Rectal prolapse	*Suggested by:* smooth, elongated rectal protrusion continuous with anal skin
	Confirmed by: above clinical examination

Melena on finger

The rectal examination ends by inspecting the fecal smear on the examining gloved finger for color, especially bright red blood or tarry melena.

Some differential diagnoses and typical outline evidence

Bleeding duodenal ulcer	*Suggested by:* epigastric pain and tenderness, nausea
	Confirmed by: **esophagogastroscopy**
Gastric erosion	*Suggested by:* history of NSAIDs or alcohol ingestion, epigastric pain, dull or burning discomfort, and nocturnal pain
	Confirmed by: **esophagogastroscopy, barium meal and pH study**
Gastric ulcer	*Suggested by:* epigastric pain, dull or burning discomfort, and nocturnal pain
	Confirmed by: **esophagogastroscopy, barium meal and pH study**
Mallory–Weiss tear	*Suggested by:* preceding marked vomiting and later bright red blood
	Confirmed by: **esophagogastroscopy**
Gastroesoph-ageal reflux	*Suggested by:* heartburn, anorexia, nausea, and ± regurgitation of gastric content
	Confirmed by: **esophagogastroscopy, barium meal and esophageal pH study**
Hiatus hernia	*Suggested by:* heartburn, worsens with stooping or lying, and relieved by antacids
	Confirmed by: **esophagogastroscopy, barium meal**
False (pseudo) hematemesis	*Suggested by:* epistaxis or hemoptysis
	Confirmed by: normal **esophagogastroscopy and ENT endoscopy**
Esophageal carcinoma	*Suggested by:* progressive dysphagia with solids, which sticks, and weight loss
	Confirmed by: **barium swallow, fiber-optic gastroscopy with mucosal biopsy**
Gastric carcinoma	*Suggested by:* marked anorexia, fullness, pain, Troisier's sign (enlarged left supraclavicular lymph node [Virchow's node])
	Confirmed by: **esophagogastroscopy with biopsy**
Ingestion of corrosives	*Suggested by:* history of ingestion, etc.
	Confirmed by: **esophagogastroscopy later**

Esophageal varices	*Suggested by:* liver cirrhosis, splenomegaly, prominent upper abdominal veins
	Confirmed by: **esophagogastroscopy**
Bleeding diathesis	*Suggested by:* symptoms or signs of bleeding elsewhere (or bruising), history of warfarin use, etc.
	Confirmed by: abnormal clotting screen and/or low platelets and/or improvement on withdrawal of a potentially causal drug (but consider possibility of another cause)

Fresh blood on finger on rectal examination

This is usually suggestive of lower GI bleeding but occasionally from massive upper GI bleeding passing through rapidly without alteration.

Some differential diagnoses and typical outline evidence

Hemorrhoids	*Suggested by:* rectal bleeding follows defecation, perianal protrusion with pain
	Confirmed by: anal inspection and **proctoscopy** (hemorrhoids drop over edge of proctoscope as it is withdrawn)
Rectal carcinoma	*Suggested by:* rectal bleeding with defecation, blood often limited to surface of stool
	Confirmed by: **sigmoidoscopy with rectal biopsy**
Colonic carcinoma	*Suggested by:* alternate diarrhea and constipation with red blood
	Confirmed by: **colonoscopy with biopsy, barium enema**
Ulcerative colitis	*Suggested by:* loose blood-stained stools, anemia, arthropathy, uveitis and iritis
	Confirmed by: **colonoscopy with biopsy, barium studies**
Crohn's disease	*Suggested by:* aphthous ulcers, anemia, tender mass, scars of previous surgery, anal fissures, fistulae
	Confirmed by: **colonoscopy with biopsy, barium studies**
Angiodysplasia	*Suggested by:* chronic, recurrent GI bleeding
	Confirmed by: **endoscopy, mesenteric angiography**
Diverticulitis	*Suggested by:* history of red "splash" in the toilet bowl, LIF tenderness ± tender mass
	Confirmed by: **flexible sigmoidoscopy, barium enema**
Ischemic colitis	*Suggested by:* left-sided abdominal pain, loose stools, dark clots
	Confirmed by: **barium enema** (may show "thumb-printing" sign), **colonoscopy**
Meckel's diverticulum	*Suggested by:* usually asymptomatic, anemia, rectal bleeding
	Confirmed by: **technetium-labeled red blood cell scan, laparotomy**

Intussusception (in children or elderly)	*Suggested by:* child, usually between 6 and 18 months of life, acute onset of colicky, intermittent abdominal pain, "red currant jelly" rectal bleed, and ± a sausage-shaped mass in upper abdomen
	Confirmed by: **barium or air enema**, may reduce the intussusceptions with appropriate hydrostatic pressure
Mesenteric infarction (acute occlusion)	*Suggested by:* acute abdominal pain, generalized tenderness, shock, and profuse diarrhea (patient often in atrial fibrillation)
	Confirmed by: **mesenteric angiography, exploratory laparotomy**
Massive upper GI bleed	*Suggested by:* hypotension or associated hematemesis
	Confirmed by: **esophagogastroscopy**
Trauma	*Suggested by:* pain, history or physical signs of trauma (e.g., sexual assault)
	Confirmed by: sigmoidoscopy

Neurological symptoms

Headache—acute, new onset

Onset is over seconds to hours.

Some differential diagnoses and typical outline evidence

Meningitis viral or bacterial	*Suggested by:* photophobia, fever, neck stiffness, vomiting, Kernig's sign. Petechial or purpuric rash (in meningococcal meningitis)
	Confirmed by: **CT brain** if neurological signs present, **Lumbar puncture**—viral meningitis: cerebrospinal fluid (CSF) clear, ↑ lymphocytes, ↑ protein, normal glucose. Bacterial meningitis: CSF with ↑ neutrophils, ↑ protein, ↓glucose, ↑ visible bacteria on Gram stain
Low CSF pressure	*Suggested by:* worsening or recurrence of headache after lumbar puncture (usually for suspected meningitis) made worse by sitting up
	Confirmed by: spontaneous resolution after a few days
Subarachnoid hemorrhage	*Suggested by:* sudden occipital headache (often described as "like a blow to the head" or "worst headache of my life"), variable degree of consciousness, ± neck stiffness, subhyaloid hemorrhage, ± focal neurological signs
	Confirmed by: **CT or MRI brain scan. Lumbar puncture:** blood-stained CSF that does not clear in successive bottles, presence of xanthochromia in CSF (up to 2 weeks after the hemorrhage)
Intracranial hemorrhage	*Suggested by:* focal neurological signs
	Confirmed by: **CT/MRI** brain scan
Head injury with cerebral contusion	*Suggested by:* history of trauma, cuts or bruises, reduced conscious level, lucid period, amnesia
	Confirmed by: **skull X-ray, CT head** normal or showing edema but no subdural hematoma or extradural hemorrhage
Acute angle-closure glaucoma	*Suggested by:* red eyes, haloes, reduced visual acuity due to corneal clouding, pupil abnormality
	Confirmed by: raised **intraocular pressure**
Sinusitis	*Suggested by:* fever, facial pain, mucopurulent nasal discharge, tender over sinuses ± upper respiratory infection (URI)
	Confirmed by: **X-ray of sinuses or CT scan:** mucosal thickening, air-fluid level or opacification

Tension headache	*Suggested by:* generalized or bilateral, continuous, tight band-like, worsens as the day progresses, associated with stress or tension, ± aggravated by eye movement
	Confirmed by: spontaneous improvement with simple analgesia
Bilateral migraine	*Suggested by:* bilateral, throbbing, ± vomiting, aura ± visual or other neurological disturbances with precipitating factor, e.g., premenstrual
	Confirmed by: resolution over hours in a dark room and analgesics, helped by sleep

Headache—subacute onset

Onset is over hours to days.

Some differential diagnoses and typical outline evidence

Raised intracranial pressure due to tumor, hydrocephalus, cerebral abscess, etc.	*Suggested by:* dull headache, worse on waking, vomiting, aggravated by, e.g., cough, sneezing, bending, look for papilledema, ↑BP, ↓ pulse rate, progressive focal neurological signs
	Confirmed by: CT/MRI brain scan
Encephalitis	*Suggested by:* fever, confusion, reduced conscious level
	Confirmed by: CSF microscopy, serology or PCR
Temporal/giant cell or cranial arteritis	*Suggested by:* scalp tenderness, jaw claudication, loss of temporal arterial pulsation, sudden loss of vision. ↑↑ESR
	Confirmed by: **temporal artery biopsy** (may be done shortly after starting corticosteroids)

Headache—chronic and recurrent

Onset is over weeks to months.

Some differential diagnoses and typical outline evidence

Tension headache	*Suggested by:* generalized or bilateral, continuous, tight band-like, worsens as the day progresses, associated with stress or tension, often aggravated by eye movement
	Confirmed by: spontaneous improvement with simple analgesia
Migraine	*Suggested by:* typically unilateral, throbbing, ± vomiting, aura ± visual disturbances, precipitating factors
	Confirmed by: resolution over hours in a dark room and analgesics, helped by sleep
Cluster headache	*Suggested by:* episodic, typically nightly pain in one eye for weeks
	Confirmed by: episodes resolving over hours (like migraine)
Cervical root headache	*Suggested by:* occipital and back of the head, temples, vertex and frontal regions, worse on neck movement or restricted neck movements
	Confirmed by: **cervical X-ray** showing degenerative changes (or normal) and response to NSAIDs
Eye strain	*Suggested by:* headaches worse after reading. Refractory error
	Confirmed by: improvement with appropriate eye glasses
Drug side effect	*Suggested by:* drug history (e.g., nitrates)
	Confirmed by: improvement on drug withdrawal

Stroke

This is a sudden onset of a neurological deficit.

Some differential diagnoses and typical outline evidence

Cerebral infarction	*Suggested by:* onset over minutes to hours of hemiparesis or major neurological defect that lasts >24 hours
	Confirmed by: **CT scan** findings appearing after days
Transient cerebral ischemic attack due to carotid artery stenosis, etc. (see below)	*Suggested by:* onset over seconds to minutes of a neurological deficit that is improving already
	Confirmed by: deficit resolving within 24 hours
Cerebral embolus due to atheroma, atrial fibrillation, myocardial infarction	*Suggested by:* onset over seconds of hemiparesis or other neurological defect that lasts >24 hours
	Confirmed by: **CT scan** and **lumbar puncture** showing little change originally. Evidence of a potential source for an embolus
Cerebral hemorrhage due to atheromatous degeneration, cerebral tumor	*Suggested by:* onset over seconds of hemiparesis or major neurological defect that lasts >24 hours
	Confirmed by: **CT** showing high attenuation ± surrounding low attenuation (edema) area ± high density (blood) in ventricles
Subdural hemorrhage (or hematoma) due to blunt head injury	*Suggested by:* onset over hours, days, or weeks of a fluctuating hemiparesis following history of head injury or fall, especially in elderly or alcoholic
	Confirmed by: **CT** showing low attenuation parallel to skull if chronic but high attenuation if acute
Extradural hemorrhage due to skull fracture lacerating middle meningeal artery	*Suggested by:* onset over minutes or hours of confusion, disturbed consciousness, and hemiparesis after lucid interval of hours following head injury
	Confirmed by: **CT head** showing high attenuation adjacent to skull ± hyperdensity ± dark (edema) ± midline shift

Subarachnoid hemorrhage from berry aneurysm	*Suggested by:* sudden onset over seconds of headache ± disturbance of consciousness (usually under 45 years of age), neck stiffness
	Confirmed by: **CT head** showing high-attenuation area on surface of brain. **Lumbar puncture** showing blood
Cerebellar stroke	*Suggested by:* sudden onset of ataxia
	Confirmed by: **MRI scan** (CT head poorly visualizes hind brain)
Pontine stroke	*Suggested by:* sudden loss of consciousness. Cheyne–Stokes breathing (cycles of tachypnea [rapid breathing] and bradypnea [slowing breathing), pin-point pupils, hemiparesis and eyes deviated toward paresis
	Confirmed by: above clinical findings ± MRI scan

Dizziness

Dizziness is often nonspecific and no cause is found, but one of the following will be discovered in a proportion of patients. Distinguish between dizziness and vertigo (which has a sensation of movement), the latter being more specific for an identifiable lesion.

Some differential diagnoses and typical outline evidence

Panic attacks and hyperventilation	*Suggested by:* associated anxiety and claustrophobia. Finger and lip paresthesia of hyperventilation. Resting tachypnea, no hypoxia
	Confirmed by: **ABGs:** PO_2 normal or ↑, ↓CO_2; **CXR:** normal, *spirometry* normal Response to anxiolytics and psychotherapy
Postural hypotension due to drugs to lower BP, loss of circulating volume, dehydration, diabetic autonomic neuropathy, old age + heavy meal, dopamine agonists, Addison's disease	*Suggested by:* associated palpitations, loss of consciousness. Supine and standing BP after 1 minute: >10 mm drop
	Confirmed by: response of BP changes to treatment of cause
Anemia	*Suggested by:* subconjunctival pallor (± face, nail, and hand pallor)
	Confirmed by: **CBC:** ↓Hb
Hypoxia	*Suggested by:* blue hands and tongue (central cyanosis), restlessness, confused, drowsy, or unconscious
	Confirmed by: **ABG:** ↓PaO_2 <60 mmgH on blood gas analysis or *pulse oximetry* of <90% saturation (mild) or <80% (severe)

Carotid sinus hypersensitivity	*Suggested by:* onset on head turning or shaving neck
	Confirmed by: reproduction of symptoms while turning neck or pressure on carotid sinus
Epilepsy	*Suggested by:* aura followed by other positive neurological symptoms
	Confirmed by: **EEG** findings
Drug effect	*Suggested by:* history of taking sedative or hypotensive drug, including alcohol
	Confirmed by: resolution of symptom after stopping drug

Vertigo

Vertigo is a sensation of movement of self ± the environment, especially rotation or oscillation.

Some differential diagnoses and typical outline evidence

Vertibrobasilar insufficiency (brain stem ischemia)	*Suggested by:* visual disturbances, other signs of cerebral ischemia, e.g., dysarthria, faint
	Confirmed by: **carotid Doppler** evidence of arterial disease. MRA of brain and neck vessels
Benign positional vertigo	*Suggested by:* attacks with duration of minutes only
	Confirmed by: **head tilt test:** nystagmus after 5 seconds, lasting a minute. Shorter duration when repeated
Ménière's disease	*Suggested by:* attacks with duration of up to 24 hours. Progressive deafness (especially in older age groups)
	Confirmed by: **audiometry:** hearing loss with loudness recruitment
Vestibular neuronitis	*Suggested by:* sudden, single prostrating attack, usually with nystagmus, with resolution over weeks
	Confirmed by: **caloric testing**
Middle ear disease	*Suggested by:* painful ear, recurrent attacks, or persistent vertigo and nystagmus
	Confirmed by: **audiometry:** conductive deafness. Otoscopic appearance of otitis media or cholesteotoma
Reversible drug toxicity	*Suggested by:* vertigo, slurring of speech and nystagmus with suggestive drug history, e.g., alcohol, barbiturates, phenytoin
	Confirmed by: resolution on withdrawal of drug. Drug levels if in doubt
Wernicke's encephalopathy (due to thiamine deficiency, usually in alcoholism)	*Suggested by:* persistence of vertigo, slurring of speech and nystagmus despite withdrawal of alcohol
	Confirmed by: resolution or improvement on thiamine treatment

Ototoxic drugs	*Suggested by:* recurrent attacks or persistent vertigo and little nystagmus, history of streptomycin, gentamycin, kanamycin, phenytoin, quinine, or salicylates, etc.
	Confirmed by: bilateral loss of response to **caloric tests.** No signs of disease in brain stem, ears, or cerebellum
Brain stem ischemia	*Suggested by:* sudden onset, and associated with peripheral vascular disease
	Confirmed by: associated cranial nerve abnormalities, long tract signs
Posterior fossa tumor	*Suggested by:* mild vertigo of onset over months and slight nystagmus. Bilateral papilledema. Ipsilateral absent corneal reflex. Cranial nerve lesions V, VI, VII, X, and XI. Ipsilateral cerebellar and contralateral pyramidal signs
	Confirmed by: **MRI scan** showing tumor
Multiple sclerosis (MS)	*Suggested by:* sudden onset and central-type nystagmus (occurs equally in both directions and sometimes vertically) in young person, other neurological disturbances, scanning speech, optic atrophy
	Confirmed by: other similar neurological episodes disseminated in time and space and multiple, enhancing lesions in various parts of nervous system on **MRI scan**
Migraine	*Suggested by:* associated headache (vertigo instead of visual aura)
	Confirmed by: resolution and recurrence consistent with natural history of migraine
Temporal lobe epilepsy	*Suggested by:* associated temporal lobe symptoms, e.g., odd taste, smells, visual hallucinations
	Confirmed by: **EEG** findings
Ramsay Hunt syndrome	*Suggested by:* associated ear pain, lower motor neuron (LMN) facial palsy
	Confirmed by: zoster vesicles at the external auditory meatus or pharynx

Seizure

There is often a history of aura, loss of consciousness, and tonic and clonic movements.

Some differential diagnoses and typical outline evidence

Febrile convulsion	*Suggested by:* young age, especially in childhood and associated with a febrile illness
	Confirmed by: normal **EEG** and **CT scan** and no subsequent recurrence without febrile illness on follow-up
Idiopathic epilepsy—new presentation	*Suggested by:* young age, especially in teens
	Confirmed by: abnormal or normal **EEG** and normal **CT scan** but subsequent recurrence
Known idiopathic epilepsy	*Suggested by:* history of previous seizures
	Confirmed by: PMH of past investigations and on treatment
Brain tumor	*Suggested by:* older age (but any age), headaches, papilledema.
	Confirmed by: **CT** or **MRI scan** showing cerebral mass
Epilepsy due to meningitis	*Suggested by:* fever, neck stiffness
	Confirmed by: CT scan and lumbar puncture
Epilepsy due to old brain scar tissue	*Suggested by:* past history of serious head injury, or stroke
	Confirmed by: abnormal **EEG, CT** or **MRI brain scan**
Alcohol withdrawal	*Suggested by:* recent heavy alcohol intake (usually superimposed on habitually high intake)
	Confirmed by: subsequent episodes in similar circumstances
Hypoglycemia from too much insulin in a diabetic, or insulinoma	*Suggested by:* sweating, hunger ± known diabetic on insulin or medication
	Confirmed by: blood glucose ↓ (<40 mg/dL) during episode
Sudden severe hypotension (especially cardiac arrest)	*Suggested by:* peripheral and central cyanosis, no pulse or BP
	Confirmed by: **ECG** shows asystole or ineffectual fast or slow rhythm (or electromechanical dissociation)

Severe electrolyte disturbance due to very high or low sodium, calcium, magnesium, etc.	*Suggested by:* abnormality on serum biochemistry *Confirmed by:* no recurrence of seizures after metabolic abnormality treated
"Functional" seizure (pseudo-seizure)	*Suggested by:* always occurring in front of audience, eyes closed during episode *Confirmed by:* normal EEG when episode documented on video recording. Normal CT scan

Transient neurological deficit

There is sudden dysphasia, with facial or limb weakness resolving within 24 hours.

Some differential diagnoses and typical outline evidence

Transient cerebral ischemic attack TIA from thromboembolus or due to carotid artery stenosis or vasculitic process	*Suggested by:* onset over minutes and then immediate improvement with prospect of complete resolution within 24 hours ± carotid bruit
	Confirmed by: resolution within 24 hours, absence of previous seizure, no throbbing migrainous headache, no chest pain, normal **ECG** and **troponin** after 12 hours, normal **plasma sodium**, normal **blood sugar**, no witnessed seizures and normal **CT** or **MRI scan**. **Doppler ultrasound** of carotids (to seek operable stenosis). **ESR** or **CRP** ↑ (if there is a vasculitic process, e.g., cranial arteritis)
Atrial fibrillation with cerebral embolus	*Suggested by:* Irregularly irregular pulse
	Confirmed by: irregularly irregular QRS complexes, no P wave on **ECG**
Intracerebral space–occupying lesion: tumor, aneurysm hematoma, arteriovenous malformation	*Suggested by:* associated headache
	Confirmed by: **CT** or **MRI scan** appearance
Transient hypotension due to arrhythmia or myocardial infarction	*Suggested by:* history of chest pain or PMH of IHD
	Confirmed by: **ECG:** ST changes. ↑**Troponin**. **24-hour ECG:** recurrence of arrhythmia
Todd's paralysis (following seizure)	*Suggested by:* witness's history of seizure
	Confirmed by: **EEG** changes

Migraine	*Suggested by:* associated headache (neurological deficit instead of visual aura)
	Confirmed by: resolution consistent with other features of migraine
Hypoglycemic episode	*Suggested by:* a known diabetic and associated sudden hunger, sweating, confusion
	Confirmed by: **blood glucose** <40 mg/dL
Hyponatremia	*Suggested by:* ↓↓ sodium concentration (e.g. <120 mmol/L) and ↓ serum osmolality. Associated confusion
	Confirmed by: resolution of deficit as **sodium concentration** and **osmolality** abnormality corrected
Multiple sclerosis (MS)	*Suggested by:* sudden-onset and central-type nystagmus (occurs equally in both directions and sometimes vertically) in young person, other neurological disturbances, scarring speech, optic atrophy
	Confirmed by: other similar neurological episodes disseminated in time and space and multiple, enhancing lesions in various parts of nervous system on **MRI scan**
Psychological (no neurological deficit)	*Suggested by:* past history of similar episodes from young (<30 years) age
	Confirmed by: absence of any objective evidence of physical cause of deficit on follow-up

Fatigue, "tired all the time"

This is generally a poor lead, but consider the following.

Some differential diagnoses and typical outline evidence

Depression	*Suggested by:* early-morning wakening, fatigue worse in the morning that never goes away during the day, anhedonia, poor appetite
	Confirmed by: response to psychotherapy or antidepressants
Sleep apnea syndrome	*Suggested by:* frequent awakening at night, snoring and breathing pauses during sleep (history from a sleeping partner), and sleepiness during the day
	Confirmed by: multiple dips in PO_2 or O_2 saturation while asleep during home or sleep lab monitoring
Drug-induced	*Suggested by:* taking sedating drug, including antiepileptic treatment
	Confirmed by: improvement by stopping or changing drug
Postviral fatigue	*Suggested by:* history of recent viral illness, especially glandular fever
	Confirmed by: resolution after weeks or months
Diabetes mellitus	*Suggested by:* thirst, polyuria, polydipsia, family history (but all may be absent)
	Confirmed by: **fasting blood glucose** ≥140 mg/dL on two occasions OR fasting, **random,** or **GTT glucose** ≥200 mg/dL in combination with symptoms
Chronic fatigue syndrome (CFS)	*Suggested by:* (1) impaired memory and concentration unrelated to drugs or alcohol use, (2) unexplained muscle pain, (3) polyarthralgia, (4) unrefreshing sleep, (5) postexertional malaise lasting over 24 hours, (6) persisting sore throat not caused by glandular fever, (7) unexplained tender cervical or axillary nodes
	Confirmed by: 4/7 or more of the above present for >6 months
Poor sleep habit	*Suggested by:* long work hours, little sleep, insomnia
	Confirmed by: sleep diary and improvement with better sleep habits
Parasomnias	*Suggested by:* restless legs, cataplexy, narcolepsy, and day-time somnolescence
	Confirmed by: response of symptoms to stimulant medication

Neurological signs

Examining the nervous system

If there are no symptoms at all suggestive of neurological disease, it is customary to perform a quick examination of the nervous system, and if this examination is normal, then the nervous system is not examined further.

At this point, you will have had an opportunity to note the patient's posture and gait in the consulting room (or as the patient moves around the bed on the ward). If the patient's face looks normal and moves normally during speech, then there is unlikely to be a cranial nerve abnormality. Ask the patient to hold both arms out to assess posture, perform a finger–nose test, tap each hand on the other in turn, show the motion used to unscrew lightbulbs, and tap each foot on the floor (or the examiner's hand if in bed); then do a heel–shin test with each leg.

Finally, test the reflexes in the arms and legs. If all of these are normal (and, as emphasized already, there are no symptoms of neurological disorder), then there is no need to examine the nervous system further. If there is a symptom or sign of neurological disorder, the nervous system has to be examined carefully, perhaps beginning with the territory under suspicion.

Disturbed consciousness

Consciousness is assessed using the Glasgow Coma Scale (GCS), which is based on adding scores for (a) best motor response (p. 304), (b) best verbal response (p. 305), and (c) eye opening (p. 305).

Some differential diagnoses and typical outline evidence

Probably no current brain damage	*Suggested by:* GCS = >15 (patient complying with all requests, oriented in time and place, opening eyes spontaneously)
	Confirmed by: neurological observation
Probable minor brain injury	*Suggested by:* GCS of 13–15
	Confirmed by: neurological observation or CT or MRI scan appearance
Probable moderate brain injury	*Suggested by:* GCS of 9–12
	Confirmed by: neurological observation or CT or MRI scan appearance
Probable severe brain injury	*Suggested by:* GCS of 3–8
	Confirmed by: neurological observation or CT or MRI scan appearance
Probable very severe brain injury	*Suggested by:* GCS =<3 (no response to pain, no verbalization, and no eye opening)
	Confirmed by: neurological observation or CT or MRI scan appearance

Best motor response

This is used to compute the GCS score.

Differential diagnosis

Carrying out verbal requests: score 6	*Confirmed by:* doing simple things that you ask (ignore grasp reflex)
Localizing response to pain: score 5	*Confirmed by:* purposeful movement in response to pressure on fingernail, supraorbital ridges, and sternum
Withdraws to pain: score 4	*Confirmed by:* pulling limb away from painful stimulus
Flexor response to pain decorticate posture: score 3	*Confirmed by:* flexion of limbs to painful stimulus
Extensor response to pain decerebrate posture: score 2	*Confirmed by:* pain causing adduction and internal rotation of shoulder and pronation of forearm
No response to pain: score 1	*Confirmed by:* no response to painful stimulus

Best verbal response

This is used to compute the GCS score.

Differential diagnosis

Oriented: score 5	*Confirmed by:* knowing own name, the place, why there, year, season, and month
Confused conversation: score 4	*Confirmed by:* conversation but does not know name, nor place, nor why there, nor year, season, or month
Inappropriate speech: score 3	*Confirmed by:* no conversation but random speech or shouting
Incomprehensible speech: score 2	*Confirmed by:* moaning but no words
No speech at all: score 1	*Confirmed by:* silence

Eye opening

This is used to compute the GCS score.

Differential diagnosis

Spontaneous eye opening: score 4	*Confirmed by:* eyes open and fixing on objects
Eye opening in response to speech: score 3	*Confirmed by:* response to specific request or a shout
Eye opening in response to pain: score 2	*Confirmed by:* response to pain
No eye opening at all: score 1	*Confirmed by:* no response to pain

Speech disturbance

Inability to converse can result from a disturbance in any part of the process such as deafness, poor attention, receptive dysphasia, motor dysphasia, dysarthria, dysphonia, aphonia, or combinations of these factors.

Some differential diagnoses and typical outline evidence

Deafness due to ear disease or eighth cranial nerve lesions	*Suggested by:* no reaction to speech or noises (e.g., startling) *Confirmed by:* features of ear disease
Inattention due to dementia, depression, etc.	*Suggested by:* normal reaction (e.g., startling) to noise or speech but no interest in source of noise or speech *Confirmed by:* features of causal condition, e.g., dementia or depression
Sensory dysphasia due to lesions in Wernicke's area	*Suggested by:* inability to understand or comprehend speech (as if a foreign language is being spoken to patient). Worse for vocabulary or language acquired later in life *Confirmed by:* CT or MRI scan showing lesion in Wernicke's area in dominant temporal lobe
Motor dysphasia (or aphasia) due to lesion in dominant frontal-parietal lobe	*Suggested by:* inability to find words or names of things (nominal dysphasia) *Confirmed by:* CT or MRI scan showing lesion in Broca's area in frontal lobe
Dysarthria (or anarthria) due to cerebellar connections, upper or lower motor neuron lesion	*Suggested by:* inability to coordinate speech, with slurring, mumbling, and failure to initiate or sustain speech *Confirmed by:* associated features of weakness or in coordination of oral muscles
Dysphonia (or aphonia) due to vocal cord dysfunction	*Suggested by:* hoarseness, voice loss or weakness, inability to cough properly *Confirmed by:* indirect laryngoscopy (using mirror) to show vocal cord dysfunction or paresis

Dysarthria

This is difficulty with articulation, and incoordination of speech muscles.

Some differential diagnoses and typical outline evidence

Cortical cerebral lesion (due to bleed, infarction, or tumor)	*Suggested by:* slow, stiff speech (and dysphasia if extensive lesion in dominant hemisphere, i.e., most dextrous hand is also affected) and other cortical signs *Confirmed by:* CT or MRI scan of brain
Internal capsule cerebral lesion (due to bleed, infarction, or tumor)	*Suggested by:* slow, stiff speech and other internal capsule signs (e.g., spastic hemiparesis) *Confirmed by:* CT or MRI scan of brain
Upper motor neuron brain stem (pseudobulbar palsy due to ischemia, motor neuron disease, multiple sclerosis [MS])	*Suggested by:* slow, stiff speech, nasal quality, slurring, other brain stem signs (e.g., spastic hemiparesis, dysphagia) *Confirmed by:* MRI scan of brain stem
Lower motor neuron brain stem (bulbar) palsy (due to ischemia, motor neuron disease, polio syringobulbia, MS)	*Suggested by:* nasal quality, other brain stem signs (e.g., spastic hemiparesis, dysphagia) *Confirmed by:* MRI scan of brain stem
Extrapyramidal dysarthria (due to Parkinson's disease)	*Suggested by:* difficulty in initiating speech, which is slow with other signs of Parkinsonian syndrome *Confirmed by:* response to dopaminergic drugs
Cerebellar lesion (due to MS, ischemia, tumor, hereditary ataxias)	*Suggested by:* staccato, undulating speech, broken flow, slurring, and other cerebellar signs (e.g., ataxia) *Confirmed by:* MRI scan of cerebellum
Drug effect (e.g., alcohol, sedatives)	*Suggested by:* dysarthria (slurred speech) and other drug effects *Confirmed by:* response to removal of drug

Anosmia (absent sense of smell)

This is not tested routinely, but ask the patient if there is anything abnormal about his or her sense of smell or taste. This is tested using bottles with familiar scents.

Some differential diagnoses and typical outline evidence

Coryza (common cold)	*Suggested by:* running nose, fever, headache, sporadic perhaps with contact history
	Confirmed by: history and nasal speculum examination
Nasal allergy	*Suggested by:* running nose, fever, headache, recurrent and recognizable precipitant
	Confirmed by: history and nasal speculum examination
Skull fracture	*Suggested by:* history of facial or head injury
	Confirmed by: history or skull X-ray in acute phase
Frontal lobe tumor	*Suggested by:* personality change, features of dementia, recent epilepsy
	Confirmed by: CT or MRI scan of brain
Kallman's syndrome (anosmia and hypogonadism)	*Suggested by:* delayed puberty or poor secondary sexual characteristics and libido, infertility. Primary amenorrhea in women
	Confirmed by: low estrogen or testosterone and low FSH and LH

Abnormal ophthalmoscopy

Start with high positive (+) numbers for the eye surface and use the lowest light level possible. Look for the red reflex and zoom in to the eye until the red reflex fills the field of view.

Examine the retina by rotating down to negative (−) numbers. Start with the disc, found by looking toward the patient's midline, and then follow the four main arteries out and back.

Examine the macula by asking the patient to look at the light.

Some differential diagnoses and typical outline evidence

Corneal opacity in quiet eye (old ulcer due to past trauma, trachoma—tropical countries)	*Suggested by:* gray opacity in the clear cornea without dilated blood vessels, gradual loss of vision *Confirmed by:* absence of staining with fluorescine
Cataract (due to aging [75%], diabetes, trauma, steroids, radiation, intra-uterine rubella or toxoplasmosis, or rubella, hypo-calcemia, etc.)	*Suggested by:* history of gradual onset of visual blurring and lens opacity visible during the red reflex examination with the ophthalmoscope. Usually >65 years of age or history of underlying condition (often already known and cataract develops later) *Confirmed by:* ophthalmoscopic appearance
Optic nerve swelling or (eventually) atrophy (due to papillitis from MS, or papilledema or optic nerve infarction in temporal arteritis and retinal artery occlusion)	*Suggested by:* raised pink optic disc with blurred margins ± distended capillaries, and adjacent streak hemorrhages progressing to pale white disc with pale margins. Gradual loss of vision after initial disturbance *Confirmed by:* visual field mapping. Ophthalmoscopic appearance
Peripheral retinal damage (laser therapy for diabetic retinopathy)	*Suggested by:* irregular pale patches of depigmentation with central black areas of pigment clumping *Confirmed by:* ophthalmoscopic appearance and history

Age-related macular degeneration (usually senile)	*Suggested by:* gradual loss of central vision, large, central, yellowish white scar or hemorrhage when patient looks at ophthalmoscope light
	Confirmed by: ophthalmoscopic appearance
Retinal vein occlusion	*Suggested by:* sudden vision loss often in upper or lower half only
	Confirmed by: extensive superficial retinal hemorrhages following the nerve fiber layer which may be in only the upper or lower half of the retina
Retinal artery occlusion	*Suggested by:* sudden loss of vision. May be total or partial upper or lower field
	Confirmed by: in the first few days, retinal pallor. Later, a white, thready, thin artery
Primary optic atrophy (prior inflammation not seen—due to MS or optic nerve infarction)	*Suggested by:* gradual visual loss in a quiet eye and pale disc with sharp margins
	Confirmed by: ophthalmoscopic appearance of pale white, featureless disc and may have thin, thready vessels
Glaucoma	*Suggested by:* gradual loss of vision, deeply cupped disc
	Confirmed by: ophthalmoscopic appearance of deep cupping with visible cribriform plate and nasal displacement of vessels. Loss of peripheral field. Raised intraocular pressure
Retinitis pigmentosa	*Suggested by:* loss of peripheral and night vision
	Confirmed by: visual-field mapping. Pale disc, thin, thready blood vessels, and fine, star-shaped pigment without patches of depigmentation. Visual-field mapping
Choroidoretinitis	*Suggested by:* gradual loss of vision or blurring (in acute phases), and patchy visual loss—scotoma
	Confirmed by: visual-field mapping showing irregular, patchy areas of visual loss. Corresponding areas in the eye of irregular depigmentation with dense areas of pigment in the center.
	Tests results for underlying cause: CXR, serology, sputum, lung biopsy

Ophthalmoscopic findings in the diabetic patient

The red-free or green light of the ophthalmoscope is very useful for detecting retinopathy. Use serial visual-acuity measurements to detect early maculopathy.

Some differential diagnoses and typical outline evidence

Diabetic cataract	*Suggested by:* gradual visual loss in a diabetic
	Confirmed by: ophthalmoscopic appearance
Diabetic glaucoma	*Suggested by:* pale, deeply cupped disc with sharp margins
	Confirmed by: ophthalmoscopic appearance and visual-field test. Raised intraocular pressure
Diabetic microaneurysm and bleeding into retina	*Suggested by:* **dots** (microaneurysms or deep hemorrhages) and **blots or flames** (deep and superficial hemorrhages)
	Confirmed by: regular retinal photography for progress
Venous irregularity preceding hemorrhage	*Suggested by:* localized widening of veins (e.g., sausage-shaped veins)
	Confirmed by: regular retinal photography for progress
Diabetic hard exudates	*Suggested by:* round and small pale area (after a single serous leak), circular with central red dot (indicating a continuous leak), enlarging circle with time
	Confirmed by: regular retinal photography for progress
Diabetic macular exudates (leading to visual loss)	*Suggested by:* star-shaped pallor (as the exudates follow the radial nerve fiber arrangement) and loss of visual acuity
	Confirmed by: regular retinal photography for progress

Diabetic soft exudates (nerve fiber infarct preceding new vessels)	*Suggested by:* pale gray area with indistinct margins
	Confirmed by: regular retinal photography for progress
Diabetic new vessel formation (leads to hemorrhage)	*Suggested by:* "frond" growing forward into the vitreous (seen by adjusting focus) or like a net growing on the surface of the retina, arising from disc or larger peripheral veins
	Confirmed by: three-dimensional clinical appearance
Retinal hemorrhage and detachment	*Suggested by:* subhyaloid hemorrhage obscuring underlying vessels, often forming nest shape—flat top and round bottom
	Confirmed by: three-dimensional clinical appearance
Vitreous hemorrhage	*Suggested by:* sudden loss of vision in a diabetic and a poor red reflex on ophthalmoscopy
	Confirmed by: retinal photography
Retinal vein occlusion	*Suggested by:* sudden vision loss, often in upper or lower half only
	Confirmed by: extensive superficial retinal hemorrhages following the nerve fiber layer, which may be in only the upper or lower half of the retina

Ophthalmoscopic findings in the hypertensive patient

Some differential diagnoses and typical outline evidence

Grade I hypertensive retinopathy	*Suggested by:* raised blood pressure on 3 occasions, typically >90 mmHg diastolic or >140 mmHg systolic
	Confirmed by: segmental narrowing and tortuosity of arteries
Grade II hypertensive retinopathy	*Suggested by:* moderately raised blood pressure on 3 occasions, typically >100 mmHg diastolic or >160 mmHg systolic
	Confirmed by: segmental narrowing and tortuosity of arteries and arteriovenous (AV) nicking
Grade III hypertensive retinopathy	*Suggested by:* severely raised blood pressure on 3 occasions, typically >120 mmHg diastolic or >180 mmHg systolic
	Confirmed by: segmental narrowing and tortuosity of arteries and AV nicking and hemorrhages and exudates
Grade IV hypertensive retinopathy	*Suggested by:* severely raised blood pressure, typically >140 mmHg diastolic or >200 mmHg systolic
	Confirmed by: segmental narrowing and tortuosity of arteries and AV nicking and hemorrhages and exudates and papilledema

Loss of central vision and acuity only

Visual acuity is tested in each eye with a Snellen chart at 20 feet: 20/20 = 100% acuity (actually, a reference point, not "normal"), and 20/40 = 50% acuity (letters readable by a person with 20/20 acuity at 20 feet only visible at 10 feet).

Fields are tested by facing patient and having the patient close matching eyes. Wag your finger, moving in from the periphery horizontally and diagonally, changing hands. Test for scotoma with red marker-pen top, moving horizontally and asking for change of color and disappearance. The rate of onset is important; sudden loss of vision is an emergency.

Acute onset of visual loss

Optic nerve swelling or (eventually) atrophy	*Suggested by:* raised pink optic disc with blurred margins ± distended capillaries, and adjacent streak hemorrhages progressing to pale white disc with pale margins. Gradual loss of vision after initial disturbance
(due to papillitis from MS, or papilledema or optic nerve infarction in temporal arteritis and retinal artery occlusion)	*Confirmed by:* visual-field mapping. Ophthalmoscopic appearance
Temporal/giant cell or cranial arteritis	*Suggested by:* scalp tenderness, jaw claudication, loss of temporal arterial pulsation, sudden loss of vision, ↑↑ESR
	Confirmed by: **temporal artery biopsy** (may be done shortly after starting corticosteroids)
Retinal artery occlusion	*Suggested by:* sudden loss of vision. May be total or partial upper or lower field
	Confirmed by: in the first few days, retinal pallor. Later, a white, thready, thin artery
Retinal vein occlusion	*Suggested by:* sudden vision loss, often in upper or lower half only
	Confirmed by: extensive superficial retinal hemorrhages following the nerve fiber layer, which may be in only the upper or lower half of the retina
Vitreous hemorrhage	*Suggested by:* sudden loss of vision in a diabetic and a poor red reflex on ophthalmoscopy
	Confirmed by: retinal photography

Gradual onset of visual loss

Cataract (due to ageing [75%], diabetes, trauma, steroids, radiation, intrauterine rubella or toxoplasmosis, or rubella, hypocalcemia)	*Suggested by:* gradual onset of visual blurring and lens opacity visible during red reflex examination with the ophthalmoscope. Usually >65 years of age or history of underlying condition (often already known and cataract develops later) *Confirmed by:* opthalmoscopic appearance
Macular degeneration (age-related)	*Suggested by:* gradual loss of central vision, large, central, yellowish white scar or hemorrhage when patient looks at ophthalmoscope light *Confirmed by:* ophthalmoscopic appearance
Choroidoretinitis	*Suggested by:* gradual loss of vision, or blurring (in acute phases), and patchy visual loss—scotomata *Confirmed by:* visual-field mapping showing irregular patchy areas of visual loss. Corresponding areas in the eye of irregular depigmentation with dense areas of pigment in the center. Tests results for underlying cause: CXR, serology, sputum, lung biopsy
Glaucoma	*Suggested by:* gradual loss of vision, deeply cupped disc *Confirmed by:* ophthalmoscopic appearance of deep cupping with visible cribriform plate and nasal displacement of vessels. Loss of peripheral field. Raised intraocular pressure
Primary optic atrophy (prior inflammation not seen; due to MS or optic nerve infarction)	*Suggested by:* gradual visual loss in a quiet eye and pale disc with sharp margins *Confirmed by:* ophthalmoscopic appearance of pale white, featureless disc and may have thin, thready vessels

Peripheral visual-field defect

An upper or lower half defect is due to ocular pathology. Lesions between eye and chiasm cause unilateral defects but those from chiasm to brain are homonymous, i.e., affecting same area in each eye.

Some differential diagnoses and typical outline evidence

Psychogenic field defect	*Suggested by:* tunnel vision (same diameter at all distances). Normal optic disc, visual acuity and color vision
	Confirmed by: no progression on follow-up
Retinitis pigmentosa	*Suggested by:* tunnel vision with good visual acuity in light, but inability to navigate around objects and virtually blind in the dark
	Confirmed by: pale, atrophic disc, thin, thready vessels, and asterisk or reticular type pigment in the retina without pale patches of depigmentation. Visual-field mapping
Choroiditis (choroidoretinitis) (due to TB, sarcoid toxoplasmosis, toxacara)	*Suggested by:* gradual loss vision or blurring (in acute phases), gray–white raised patch on retina, vitreous opacities, muddiness in the anterior chamber, then white patch with pigmentation around on retina (choroidoretinal scarring)
	Confirmed by: tests results for underlying cause: CXR, serology, sputum, lung biopsy
Optic chiasm lesion (due to pituitary tumor, craniopharyngioma, aneurysm)	*Suggested by:* bitemporal hemianopia (or sometimes bitemporal upper quadrantinopia from tumor pushing up)
	Confirmed by: visual-field mapping. CT or MRI scan appearance
Optic tract lesion (due to middle cerebral artery thrombosis of contralateral side)	*Suggested by:* homonymous hemianopia
	Confirmed by: visual-field mapping. MRI scan appearance
Visual cortex lesion (due to posterior cerebral artery occlusion, tumor)	*Suggested by:* homonymous hemianopia or, occasionally, quadrantanopia. May have macular sparing (visual acuity normal). Tunnel vision if bilateral
	Confirmed by: visual-field mapping. CT or MRI scan appearance

Ptosis (drooping of one or both upper eyelids)

Some differential diagnoses and typical outline evidence

Oculomotor (third-nerve) lesion due to pituitary tumor, intracavernous or posterior communicating artery aneurysm, meningioma, tentorial pressure cone diabetes mellitus, syphilis, and brain stem ischemia	*Suggested by:* ptosis, diplopia, and squint maximal on looking up and in. But in total loss, eye looks down and out. *Dilated pupil (except in diabetes mellitus, syphilis, and brain stem ischemia when pupil not dilated);* other cranial nerve lesions that form pattern (see p. 332) *Confirmed by:* CT or MRI scan appearance
Horner's syndrome due to neck trauma or tumors, cervical rib, Pancoast tumor (in lung apex) syringo-myelia (in cervical spine), lateral medullary syndrome (in brain stem), hypothalamic lesion	*Suggested by:* ptosis and constricted (miotic) pupil, recessed globe of the eye, and diminished sweating on same side of face *Confirmed by:* history of trauma or onset over week or months suggestive of tumor, or years suggestive of MS or syrinx. Other cranial nerve signs that form pattern of cervical plexus lesion or brain stem lesion. X-ray of upper chest, ribs, or neck. CT of neck or upper chest or MRI scan of brain stem
Myasthenia gravis	*Suggested by:* bilateral partial ptosis worsening as day progresses *Confirmed by:* eyes begin to droop after 15 minutes of up-gaze. Positive Tensilon test (edrophonium results in improvement in ptosis)

Myopathy (dystrophia myotonica)	*Suggested by:* bilateral partial ptosis with evidence of weakness in other muscle groups. Frontal balding, inability to release hand grip
	Confirmed by: biopsy histology of other affected muscle
Congenital ptosis	*Suggested by:* unilateral or bilateral partial ptosis present since birth. Compensatory head posture
	Confirmed by: absence of other neurological signs

Large (mydriatic) pupil with no ptosis

Some differential diagnoses and typical outline evidence

Holmes–Adie pupil due to ciliary ganglion degeneration	*Suggested by:* dilated pupil (often widely) that only reacts slowly to light by constricting in well-lit room after 30 minutes. Reacts to accommodation. Usually unilateral. Absent knee jerks. Usually in females
	Confirmed by: benign outcome with no action necessary
Traumatic iridoplegia	*Suggested by:* **history of direct trauma**. Dilated, fixed, irregular pupil that does not accommodate or react to light
	Confirmed by: slit-lamp examination of anterior eye chamber
Drug effect due to cocaine, amphetamines, tropicamide, atropine	*Suggested by:* bilateral pupil dilation
	Confirmed by: drug history, and resolution with withdrawal
Severe brainstem dysfunction (or brain death)	*Suggested by:* bilateral pupil dilation with no reaction to light, comatose, long tract pyramidal signs
	Confirmed by: absent corneal reflex response, no vestibulo-ocular reflexes, no cranial motor response to stimulation, no gag reflex, insufficient respiratory effort when PCO_2 >50 mm Hg to prevent further ↑ of PCO_2 and ↓PO_2

Small (miotic) pupil with no ptosis

Some differential diagnoses and typical outline evidence

Argyll Robertson pupil (due to syphilis and diabetes mellitus, rarely)	*Suggested by:* unilateral, small, irregular pupil that accommodates by constricting when focusing on near finger but does not react to light
	Confirmed by: syphilis serology or fasting blood glucose ≥7 mmol/L and random GTT glucose ≥11.0 mmol/L. Positive syphilis serology or abnormal blood glucose suggesting diabetes mellitus
Anisocoria normal variation	*Suggested by:* unilateral, small, miotic pupil that reacts normally to light and accommodation
	Confirmed by: no change with time, benign outcome with no action necessary
Age-related miosis due to autonomic degeneration	*Suggested by:* bilateral, small, miotic pupils that react normally to light and accommodate normally
	Confirmed by: discovery in old age, no change with time, benign outcome with no action
Drug effect due to opiates, pilocarpine	*Suggested by:* bilateral, small pupils. Not reacting to light
	Confirmed by: drug history, and resolution with withdrawal
Pontine hemorrhage	*Suggested by:* bilateral, small, miotic pupils that react to light. Patient comatose, bilaterally or unilaterally hyperreflexic, with high or fluctuating temperature.
	Confirmed by: evolution of signs to localize to brain stem. MRI scan

Squint and diplopia: ocular palsy

This is elicited by asking the patient to follow the examiner's finger and asking if this results in seeing double, and looking for development of a convergent or divergent squint.

For a cover test, have the patient fix focus in the distance and alternately cover either eye in quick succession. As the cover is lifted observe the eye. If the uncovered eye now moves in, this indicates a divergent squint. If the eye moves out, this indicates a convergent squint.

Some differential diagnoses and typical outline evidence

Oculomotor (third-nerve) paresis intracavernous or posterior communicating artery aneurysm, meningioma, tentorial pressure cone, DM, syphilis, and brain stem ischemia	*Suggested by:* ptosis, diplopia and squint maximal on looking up and in; but therefore in total loss eye looks down and out. **Dilated pupil (except in diabetes mellitus, syphilis and brain stem ischemia when pupil not dilated)** *Confirmed by:* other cranial nerve lesions that form a pattern (see p. 332), skull X-ray posterior–anterior (P-A) and lateral, CT or MRI scan appearance
Trochlear (fourth cranial nerve) paresis	*Suggested by:* diplopia and squint maximal on looking down and in. Double vision for reading and walking down stairs *Confirmed by:* other cranial nerve lesions that form pattern (see p. 332). MRI scan appearance
Abducent (sixth cranial nerve) paresis	*Suggested by:* **double vision when looking in direction of the affected muscle**. Head turn in direction of affected muscle *Confirmed by:* other cranial nerve lesions that form pattern (see p. 332). MRI scan appearance
Myasthenia gravis, Graves' disease, orbital cellulitis, or tumor	*Suggested by:* diplopia and squint in all directions of gaze *Confirmed by:* CT or MRI scan of orbit or positive Tensilon test (edrophonium results in less diplopia and squint in myasthenia)
Internuclear ophthalmoplegia from lesion in medial longitudinal bundle, usually due to MS or sometimes vascular	*Suggested by:* impaired conjugate gaze (slowness of adducting eye and nystagmus in abducting eye) *Confirmed by:* other signs of brain stem lesion

Loss of facial sensation

Some differential diagnoses and typical outline evidence

Ophthalmic branch of trigeminal nerve lesion	*Suggested by:* absent corneal reflex (present corneal reflex excludes lesion) with diminished touch and pain sensation in upper face above the line of the eye
	Confirmed by: other cranial nerve lesions that form pattern (see p. 332). MRI scan appearance
Maxillary branch of trigeminal nerve lesion	*Suggested by:* diminished touch and pain sensation in mid-face between line of mouth and line of eye
	Confirmed by: other cranial nerve lesions that form pattern (see p. 332). MRI scan appearance
Mandibular branch of trigeminal nerve lesion	*Suggested by:* diminished touch and pain sensation in lower face below line of mouth
	Confirmed by: other cranial nerve lesions that form pattern (see p. 332). MRI scan appearance

Jaw muscle weakness

Some differential diagnoses and typical outline evidence

Motor branch of trigeminal nerve (fifth cranial): lower motor neuron type on same (ipsilateral) side	*Suggested by:* weakness of jaw movement. Deviation of jaw when opening against resistance and poor contraction of masseter on clenching. ***Decreased*** jaw jerk
	Confirmed by: other cranial nerve lesions that form pattern (see p. 332). MRI scan appearance
Motor branch of trigeminal nerve (fifth cranial): *upper motor neuron type on other (contralateral) side*	*Suggested by:* weakness of jaw movement. Deviation of jaw when opening against resistance and poor contraction of masseter on clenching. ***Increased*** jaw jerk
	Confirmed by: other cranial nerve lesions that form pattern (see p. 332). MRI scan appearance

Facial muscle weakness

Distinguish between upper (forehead muscles movement preserved) and lower (forehead movement weak) motor neuron type.

Some differential diagnoses and typical outline evidence

Facial nerve palsy (seventh cranial): upper motor neuron type, other (contralateral) side due to internal capsule lesion—cerebrovascular accident, tumor	*Suggested by: **able** to raise eyebrows and close eye, but **unable** to grimace or smile symmetrically; other cranial nerve lesions that form pattern (see p. 332) *Confirmed by:* MRI scan
Facial nerve palsy (seventh cranial): lower motor neuron type, same (ipsilateral) side (see below for causes)	*Suggested by:* inability to raise eyebrows nor close eye (rolls upwards to hide iris revealing the white of the eye) nor grimace nor smile symmetrically; other cranial nerve lesions that form pattern (see p. 332) *Confirmed by:* MRI scan
Bell's palsy	*Suggested by:* lower motor neuron seventh-nerve palsy. Prior ache behind ear. No other physical signs (corneal reflex present and no deafness or vertigo) *Confirmed by:* above clinical features
Ramsey Hunt syndrome	*Suggested by:* lower motor neuron seventh-nerve palsy. Taste diminished on same side. Vesicles in external auditory meatus *Confirmed by:* above clinical features
Facial nerve palsy from parotid swelling	*Suggested by:* lower motor neuron seventh-nerve palsy. Swelling in mid-face on same side *Confirmed by:* above clinical features and MRI scan

Cerebellopontine lesion (e.g., tumor)	*Suggested by:* lower motor neuron seventh-nerve palsy. Associated fifth (loss of corneal reflex) and seventh cranial nerve lesion
	Confirmed by: above clinical features. MRI scan appearance
Cholesteatoma	*Suggested by:* lower motor neuron seventh-nerve palsy. Also deafness and vertigo
	Confirmed by: above clinical features. MRI scan appearance
Facial nerve palsy from demyelination	*Suggested by:* lower motor neuron seventh-nerve palsy. Other focal neurological signs and symptoms disseminated in time and space
	Confirmed by: above clinical features. MRI scan appearance
Facial nerve palsy from brain stem ischemia	*Suggested by:* lower motor neuron seventh-nerve palsy. Signs of adjacent dysfunction, e.g., nystagmus, long tract signs, e.g., spastic hemiparesis
	Confirmed by: above clinical features. MRI scan appearance

Loss of hearing

The patient is unable to hear whispering or a ticking watch. Test hearing with a tuning fork held near the ear; test both air and bone conduction.

Some differential diagnoses and typical outline evidence

Eighth-nerve conduction defect on side X due to wax, foreign body, otitis externa, recurrent otitis media, injury to tympanic membrane, otosclerosis, cholesteatoma	*Suggested by:* forehead vibration heard louder on side X than on side Y (Weber's test), and mastoid vibration on side X louder than for air (Rinne's test) *Confirmed by:* auroscope appearance, formal audiometry, and other cranial nerve lesions that form pattern (see p. 332). MRI scan appearance
Sensorineural (eighth cranial) lesion on side Y due to old age, noise trauma, Paget's disease, Menier's disease, drugs, viral infections (e.g., measles), con-genital rubella, meningitis, acoustic neuroma, meningioma	*Suggested by:* forehead vibration heard louder on side X than on side Y (Weber's test), and mastoid vibration same for both sides (Rinne's test) *Confirmed by:* other cranial nerve lesions that form pattern (see p. 332), formal audiometry, and MRI scan appearance

Abnormal tongue, uvula, and pharyngeal movement

This implies ninth, tenth (not eleventh), and twelfth cranial nerve lesions.

Some differential diagnoses and typical outline evidence

Glossopharyngeal (ninth cranial) nerve lesion	*Suggested by:* loss of gag reflex and taste on posterior 1/3 of tongue; other cranial nerve lesions that form pattern (see p. 332) *Confirmed by:* MRI scan
Vagus (tenth cranial) nerve lesion due to jugular foramen lesion, bulbar palsy	*Suggested by:* deviation of uvula away from affected side when saying "ah"; nasal regurgitation of water. Dysarthria; other cranial nerve lesions that form pattern (see p. 332) *Confirmed by:* MRI scan
Lower motor neuron hypoglossal (twelfth cranial) nerve lesion on same (ipsilateral) side of deviation	*Suggested by:* deviation of tongue to side of lesion on protrusion. Fasciculation and wasting; other cranial nerve lesions that form pattern (see p. 332) *Confirmed by:* MRI scan
Upper motor neuron hypoglossal (twelfth cranial) nerve lesion on other (contralateral) side of deviation	*Suggested by:* deviation of tongue to one side on protrusion. Small, stiff tongue and cortical or internal capsule signs *Confirmed by:* CT or MRI scan

Multiple cranial nerve lesions

Some differential diagnoses and typical outline evidence

Pituitary tumor	*Suggested by:* optic tract or chiasm lesion. Third cranial nerve lesion
	Confirmed by: CT or MRI scan appearance
Anterior communicating artery aneurysm due to pituitary tumor or cerebral artery aneurysm	*Suggested by:* optic nerve lesion, third and fourth cranial nerve lesions
	Confirmed by: CT or MRI scan appearance
Posterior carotid artery aneurysm	*Suggested by:* Fourth and fifth cranial nerve lesions
	Confirmed by: CT or MRI scan appearance
Gradenigo's syndrome (lesion in petrous temporal bone)	*Suggested by:* fifth and sixth cranial nerve lesions
	Confirmed by: MRI scan appearance
Facial canal lesion, e.g., cholesteatoma	*Suggested by:* seventh and eighth cranial nerve lesions alone (no fifth or sixth)
	Confirmed by: CT or MRI scan appearance
Cerebellopontine angle lesion, e.g., tumor	*Suggested by:* fifth, seventh, and eighth ± sixth cranial nerve lesions
	Confirmed by: CT or MRI scan appearance
Jugular foramen syndrome	*Suggested by:* ninth, tenth, and eleventh cranial nerve lesions
	Confirmed by: MRI scan appearance
Lateral medullary syndrome	*Suggested by:* vertigo, nystagmus, fifth cranial nerve lesion, Horner's syndrome, contralateral spinothalamic loss on trunk
	Confirmed by: above clinical features. MRI scan appearance
Weber's syndrome	*Suggested by:* ipislateral third cranial nerve lesion and contralateral hemiparesis
	Confirmed by: above clinical features. MRI scan appearance

Odd posture of arms and hands at rest

Some differential diagnoses and typical outline evidence

Internal capsule lesion or pre-central gyrus and connections, or lower pyramidal tract (upper motor neuron)	*Suggested by:* arms flexed at elbow and wrist, and weak. Increased tone and reflexes. Upper motor neuron facial weakness *Confirmed by:* brain CT or MRI scan appearance
T1 anterior root lesion	*Suggested by:* **claw hand**, wasting of all small muscles of the hand. Loss of sensation in ulnar 1.5 fingers and ulnar border of forearm *Confirmed by:* Nerve conduction study result
Ulnar nerve lesion (below elbow)	*Suggested by:* **claw hand**, wasting of hypothenar eminence and dorsal guttering, especially first. Weakness of finger abduction and adduction. Loss of sensation in ulnar 1.5 fingers
Radial nerve lesion (or C7 anterior root lesion)	*Suggested by:* **wrist drop**. Inability to extend wrist and grip. Loss of sensation over first dorsal interosseous muscle *Confirmed by:* nerve conduction study

Fine tremor of hands

This is elicited by asking the patient to hold the arms out straight in front and then placing a sheet of paper on them (to amplify fine tremor).

Some differential diagnoses and typical outline evidence

Thyrotoxicosis	*Suggested by:* fine tremor, anxiety, tachycardia, sweating, weight loss, goiter, increased reflexes
	Confirmed by: ↑FT4 or FT3 and ↓↓TSH
Anxiety state	*Suggested by:* fine tremor, anxiety, tachycardia, sweating, weight loss, goiter, increased reflexes
	Confirmed by: normal thyroid function tests. Improvement with sedation, psychotherapy, etc.
Alcohol withdrawal	*Suggested by:* fine or coarse tremor, history of high alcohol intake and recent withdrawal, anxiety
	Confirmed by: improvement with sedation, etc.
Sympathomimetic drugs	*Suggested by:* fine tremor, drug history
	Confirmed by: improvement with withdrawal of drug
Benign essential tremor	*Suggested by:* usually coarse tremor, long history, no other symptoms or signs
	Confirmed by: normal thyroid test results. Improvement with beta blocker

Coarse tremor of hands

This is elicited by asking the patient to hold the arms out straight in front and extending the wrists (for asterixis or flap). Then ask the patient to first touch his own nose and then the examiner's finger, with the arm extended, repetitively (for intention tremor).

Some differential diagnoses and typical outline evidence

Hepatic failure	*Suggested by:* flapping tremor (asterixis) aggravated when wrists extended. Spider nevi. Jaundice
	Confirmed by: abnormal liver function tests and prolonged prothrombin time
Carbon dioxide retention	*Suggested by:* flapping tremor (asterixis), aggravated when wrists extended. Muscle twitching, bounding pulse, warm peripheries
	Confirmed by: blood gases show ↑pCO_2
Cerebellar disease	*Suggested by:* intention tremor (past pointing) when patient attempts to touch examiner's finger
	Confirmed by: MRI scan
Parkinsonism due to Parkinson's disease, drugs (chlorpromazine, haloperidol, metoclopramide, prochlorperazine); multisystem atrophy, Alzheimer's disease; postencephalitis, normal-pressure hydrocephalus	*Suggested by:* **resting** coarse tremor (pill-rolling); lead-pipe rigidity; expressionless face, paucity of movement, small hand writing, rapid, shuffling gait with small steps
	Confirmed by: clinical findings, e.g. persistent blinking when forehead tapped (e.g. glabellar tap). Clinical improvement with appropriate treatment
Benign essential tremor	*Suggested by:* usually coarse tremor, long history, no other symptoms or signs
	Confirmed by: normal thyroid test results. Improvement with beta blocker

Wasting of some small muscles of hand

Intermetacarpal grooves are prominent due to muscle wasting.

Some differential diagnoses and typical outline evidence

Median nerve palsy usually due to carpal tunnel syndrome	*Suggested by:* wasting of thenar eminence. Weakness of thumb flexion, abduction and opposition. *Unable* to lift thumb with palm upward but *able* to press with index finger. Loss of sensation over palmar aspect of radial 3.5 fingers of hand
	Confirmed by: nerve conduction study results
Ulnar nerve lesion from elbow (high) to wrist (low)	*Suggested by:* wasting of hypothenar eminence. *Able* to lift thumb with palm upward but *unable* to press with index finger. Weakness of finger abduction and adduction. Loss of sensation in ulnar aspect 1.5 fingers of hand. Claw hand (in lower lesions)
	Confirmed by: nerve conduction study results
T1 lesion: anterior horn cell or root lesion	*Suggested by:* wasting of all small muscles of hand. *Unable* to lift thumb with palm upward but *unable* to press with index finger
	Confirmed by: nerve conduction study results. MRI scan appearance around T1 level
Motor neuron disease	*Suggested by:* **signs of T1 lesion,** prominent fasciculation, spastic paraparesis, wasted fasciculating tongue, no sensory signs
	Confirmed by: clinical presentation and absence of structural abnormality on MRI scan appearance
Syringomyelia	*Suggested by:* **signs of T1 lesion,** fasciculation *not* prominent, burn scars, dissociated sensory loss, Horner's syndrome, nystagmus. History over months to years
	Confirmed by: MRI scan appearances
Any prolonged systemic illness	*Suggested by:* global muscle wasting, general weight loss
	Confirmed by: improvement in muscle wasting if primary disease treatable

Cervical spondylosis compressing nerve root	*Suggested by:* **signs of T1 lesion**, neck pain and stiffness, and referred pain
	Confirmed by: MRI scan showing root canal compression
Tumor compressing nerve root	*Suggested by:* **signs of T1 lesion**, referred pain. Progressing over months
	Confirmed by: MRI scan showing root canal compression
Brachial plexus lesion	*Suggested by:* **signs of T1 lesion** and history of trauma to shoulder area or birth injury
	Confirmed by: nerve conduction study results
Cervical rib	*Suggested by:* **signs of T1 lesion** aggravated by movement or posture
	Confirmed by: X-ray: presence of cervical rib. Relief by surgery
Pancoast tumor	*Suggested by:* **signs of T1 lesion**, Horner's syndrome, features of lung cancer (clubbing, chest signs, lymph nodes, etc.)
	Confirmed by: CXR and CT scan appearances

Wasting of arm and shoulder

Loss of the rounded contour of the deltoid and biceps muscle occurs. Fasciculation is localized twitching of the muscle. Note the patient's facial expression.

Some differential diagnoses and typical outline evidence

Progressive muscular atrophy	*Suggested by:* bilateral wasting of hand, arm, and shoulder girdle with fasciculation
	Confirmed by: EMG results
Motor neuron disease (amyotrophic lateral sclerosis) with anterior horn cell degeneration	*Suggested by:* initially unilateral wasting of shoulder abductor and biceps. Weakness of speech, swallowing. No sensory signs
	Confirmed by: EMG results
Primary muscle disease	*Suggested by:* bilateral wasting of shoulder abductor and biceps
	Confirmed by: EMG findings or muscle biopsy

Abnormalities of arm tone

This is elicited by supporting the patient's elbow in one hand and asking the patient to allow you to flex and extend the arm at the elbow without assistance.

Some differential diagnoses and typical outline evidence

Cerebellar lesion	*Suggested by:* **tone diminished**, no wasting. Diminished reflexes. Past pointing, truncal ataxia, nystagmus
	Confirmed by: CT or MRI scan appearance of cerebellum
Primary muscle disease	*Suggested by:* **tone diminished** with wasting ± fasciculation
	Confirmed by: EMG findings or muscle biopsy
Upper motor neuron	*Suggested by:* **tone increased**. Brisk reflexes below lesion
	Confirmed by: CT or MRI scan of brain or spinal cord
Parkinson's disease	*Suggested by:* **tone increased** with cogwheel effect (superimposed tremor). Poor facial movement, shuffling, hesitant gait, coarse temor
	Confirmed by: Response to drug therapy

Weakness around the shoulder and arm without pain

This is elicited by asking the patient to flex and extend the wrist and elbow against resistance and to abduct, adduct, flex, and extend the shoulder against resistance. Compare both sides.

Some differential diagnoses and typical outline evidence

C4–5 root lesion	*Suggested by:* weakness of abduction at the shoulder only (not elbow or wrist)
	Confirmed by: nerve conduction studies and MRI scan of neck
C5–6 root lesion Erb's palsy	*Suggested by:* weakness of flexion at the shoulder and elbow but not wrist. Arm externally rotated and adducted behind the back (note porter's tip position). History of birth trauma
	Confirmed by: nerve conduction studies and MRI scan of neck
C7 root lesion	*Suggested by:* wrist drop or weakness of grip and extension at the **elbow and wrist**
	Confirmed by: nerve conduction studies and MRI scan of neck
Radial nerve lesion	*Suggested by:* wrist drop or weakness of grip and extension at the wrist but **not** at the elbow
	Confirmed by: nerve conduction studies and history of trauma
C8–T1 root lesion (Klumpke's paralysis)	*Suggested by:* arm held in adduction, paralysis or paresis of the small muscles of the hand, loss of sensation over ulnar border of the hand. History of birth trauma
	Confirmed by: nerve conduction studies and MRI scan of neck

Incoordination on rapid wrist rotation or hand tapping (dysdiadochokinesis)

This is often used as a screening test (i.e., if it isnormal, you can discount any significant neuromuscular condition of the upper limbs in the absence of other symptoms or signs).

Some differential diagnoses and typical outline evidence

Upper motor neuron paresis	*Suggested by:* spastic weakness (i.e., with increased tone) in upper limb
	Confirmed by: CT scan of brain or MRI scan of neck
Lower motor neuron paresis	*Suggested by:* flaccid weakness (i.e., with decreased tone) in upper limb
	Confirmed by: nerve conduction studies and MRI scan of neck
Cerebellar lesion	*Suggested by:* ataxia, past-pointing, difficulty with finger-to-nose or heel-to-shin testing
	Confirmed by: CT or MRI scan of cerebellum
Loss of proprioreception	*Suggested by:* loss of joint position sense and vibration sense
	Confirmed by: nerve conduction studies

Muscle wasting

This must be assessed in the context of the bulk of other muscles.

Some differential diagnoses and typical outline evidence

Adjacent bone, joint, or muscle disease	*Suggested by:* wasting, with pain and limitation of movement. Visible swelling or deformity of bone or joint
	Confirmed by: X-ray of affected part. EMG
Lower motor neuron lesion	*Suggested by:* wasting and fasciculation. Tone decreased. Weakness and diminished reflexes
	Confirmed by: nerve conduction studies
Muscle disease	*Suggested by:* wasting. Tone decreased. Weakness and diminished reflex
	Confirmed by: EMG

Weakness around one lower limb joint

These weaknesses may point strongly to one nerve root lesion. Test by asking the patient to perform the movement against your resistance.

Some differential diagnoses and typical outline evidence

L1/2 root lesion or femoral nerve	*Suggested by:* weakness of hip flexion alone
	Confirmed by: X-ray of lumbar spine and sacrum. Nerve conduction studies. MRI scan where lesion is localized clinically
L2/3 root lesion or obturator nerve	*Suggested by:* weakness of hip adduction alone
	Confirmed by: X-ray of lumbar spine and sacrum. Nerve conduction studies. MRI scan where lesion is localized clinically
L3/4 root lesion or femoral nerve	*Suggested by:* weakness of knee extension alone
	Confirmed by: X-ray of lumbar spine and sacrum. Nerve conduction studies. MRI scan where lesion is localized clinically
L4/5 root lesion or tibial nerve	*Suggested by:* weakness of foot dorsiflexion and inversion at the ankle
	Confirmed by: X-ray of lumbar spine and sacrum. Nerve conduction studies. MRI scan where lesion is localized clinically
L5/S1 root lesion or common peroneal nerve	*Suggested by:* weakness of knee flexion alone
	Confirmed by: X-ray of lumbar spine and sacrum. Nerve conduction studies. MRI scan where lesion is localized clinically
S1/2 root lesion or sciatic nerve	*Suggested by:* weakness of toe flexion alone
	Confirmed by: X-ray of lumbar spine and sacrum. Nerve conduction studies. MRI scan where lesion is localized clinically
Lateral popliteal nerve palsy (usually traumatic)	*Suggested by:* flaccid foot drop, with weakness of eversion and dorsiflexion of the foot and a sensory loss over lateral aspect of leg
	Confirmed by: nerve conduction study result

Bilateral weakness of all foot movements

Some differential diagnoses and typical outline evidence

Guillain–Barré syndrome	*Suggested by:* onset over days, preceding viral illness.
	Confirmed by: high CSF protein. Progressive course then variable recovery
Lead poisoning	*Suggested by:* gradual onset over weeks to months
	Confirmed by: nerve conduction studies, and history of exposure
Porphyria	*Suggested by:* onset over months to years. Usually known to have porphyria
	Confirmed by: EMG and ↑urine or fecal porphobilinogens
Charcot–Marie–Tooth disease	*Suggested by:* onset over years. Associated with foot drop and peroneal atrophy, upper limbs affected later
	Confirmed by: EMG

Spastic paraparesis

Bilateral lower limb paresis with increased tone. This is a *medical emergency* if acute.

Some differential diagnoses and typical outline evidence

Prolapsed disc (anteriorly, thus compressing spinal cord)	*Suggested by:* sudden onset often associated with change in spinal posture *Confirmed by:* MRI scan appearance
Traumatic vertebral displacement or fracture	*Suggested by:* sudden onset associated with violent injury *Confirmed by:* MRI scan appearance
Collapsed vertebra (due to secondary carcinoma or myeloma)	*Suggested by:* sudden onset over minutes or hours. Other symptoms suggestive of neoplasia over months *Confirmed by:* nerve conduction studies. MRI scan appearance
Spondylitic bone formation compressing spinal cord	*Suggested by:* onset over months to years. Often past history of spondylitic back pain *Confirmed by:* MRI scan appearance
Multiple sclerosis affecting spinal cord	*Suggested by:* this and other intermittent neurological symptoms disseminated in site and time *Confirmed by:* MRI scan appearance
Infective space occupying lesion e.g., TB or abscess	*Suggested by:* onset over days or weeks with fever from low grade to spiking *Confirmed by:* MRI scan and findings at surgery, histology and microbiology
Glioma or ependymoma in spinal cord	*Suggested by:* gradual onset over months *Confirmed by:* MRI scan and findings at surgery, histology
Parasaggital cerebral meningioma or other tumor	*Suggested by:* gradual onset over months *Confirmed by:* MRI scan and findings at surgery, histology

Hemiparesis (affecting arm and leg)

Some differential diagnoses and typical outline evidence

Occlusion of upper branch of middle cerebral artery with infarction including Broca's area	*Suggested by:* expressive dysphasia and contralateral lower face and arm weakness *Confirmed by:* MRI or CT scan appearance
Occlusion of perforating branch of middle cerebral artery with lacunar infarction	*Suggested by:* hemiparesis alone with subsequent spasticity (or receptive dysphasia alone or hemi-anesthesia alone) *Confirmed by:* MRI or CT scan appearance
Total middle cerebral artery territory infarction (usually embolic)	*Suggested by:* contralateral flaccid hemiplegia (with little subsequent spasticity) and hemi-anesthesia with deviation of head to side of lesion. Also homonymous hemianopia with aphasia if dominant hemisphere affected or neglect if nondominant hemisphere affected *Confirmed by:* MRI or CT scan appearance
Posterior cerebral artery infarction	*Suggested by:* contralateral homonymous hemianopia or upper quadrantanopia, mild contralateral hemiparesis and sensory loss, ataxia and involuntary movement, memory loss, dyslexia, and ipsilateral third-nerve palsy *Confirmed by:* MRI or CT scan appearance
Anterior cerebral artery infarction	*Suggested by:* paresis of contralateral leg, rigidity, perseveration, grasp reflex in opposite hand, urinary incontinence, and dysphasia if in dominant hemisphere *Confirmed by:* MRI or CT scan appearance

Disturbed sensation in upper limb

This is elicited by testing touch (with a piece of cotton wool), heat (with a cold metal object), and pain (through pinprick with a sterile needle) in each dermatome distribution. Note any discrepancy between these modalities of sensation.

In the palm, examine the radial 3.5 fingers and the ulnar 1.5 fingers. Test joint position sense (by holding digits at their sides) and vibration with a tuning fork over bony prominences. Then use a two-pointed device (2-point discrimination), placing objects in the patient's hand and asking them to guess what they are with eyes closed, e.g., a quarter (stereognosis), and drawing figures on the palm (graphesthesia).

Consider if you have discovered any of the patterns described below.

Some differential diagnoses and typical outline evidence

Contralateral cortical (pre-central gyrus) lesion	*Suggested by:* asteregnosis, diminished 2-point discrimination, and graphesthesia
	Confirmed by: CT or MRI scan of brain
Peripheral neuropathy	*Suggested by:* loss of touch and pinprick sensation worse in hand, progressing upwards
	Confirmed by: Nerve conduction studies
Spinothalamic tract damage (no dorsal column loss) due to syringomyelia in cervical cord	*Suggested by:* loss of pinprick and temperature sensation, normal or disturbed touch but normal joint position and vibration sense in hand
	Confirmed by: Nerve conduction studies. MRI of cervical cord
Cervical or thoracic nerve root lesion	*Suggested by:* loss of sensation in dermatome distribution in hand or forearm or upper arm
	Confirmed by: nerve conduction studies. X-ray and MRI scan of neck
Peripheral nerve lesions in arm	*Suggested by:* loss of sensation localized to the forearm, upper arm, or radial 3.5 fingers or ulnar 1.5 fingers in the palm
	Confirmed by: nerve conduction studies

Diminished sensation in arm dermatome

Some differential diagnoses and typical outline evidence

C5 posterior root lesion	*Suggested by:* loss of sensation of **lateral aspect of upper arm**
	Confirmed by: nerve conduction studies. MRI scan appearance
C6 posterior root lesion	*Suggested by:* loss of sensation of **lateral forearm and thumb**
	Confirmed by: nerve conduction studies. MRI scan appearance
C8 posterior root lesion	*Suggested by:* loss of sensation of **palmar and dorsal aspect of ulnar 1.5 fingers** and the ulnar border of the wrist
	Confirmed by: nerve conduction studies. MRI scan appearance
T1 posterior root lesion	*Suggested by:* loss of sensation of **ulnar border of the forearm**
	Confirmed by: nerve conduction studies. MRI scan appearance
T2 posterior root lesion	*Suggested by:* loss of sensation of **inner aspect of upper arm and breast**
	Confirmed by: nerve conduction studies. MRI scan appearance

Diminished sensation in the hand

Some differential diagnoses and typical outline evidence

Median nerve lesion due to carpal tunnel syndrome, oral contraceptives, pregnancy, hypothyroidism, acromegaly, rheumatoid arthritis or nerve trauma	*Suggested by:* loss of sensation of **palmar aspect of radial 3.5 fingers** (in carpal tunnel syndrome, also discomfort in forearm and tingling if front of wrist tapped). If nerve severed, wasting of thenar eminence and thumb opposition *Confirmed by:* X-ray wrist and elbow. Nerve conduction studies, and thyroid function tests, rheumatoid factor etc.
Ulnar nerve lesion due to compression of deep palmar branch from trauma or ulnar groove at elbow from trauma or osteoarthritis	*Suggested by:* loss of sensation of **palmar and dorsal aspect of ulnar 1.5 fingers** but *not* the ulnar border of the wrist *Confirmed by:* nerve conduction studies. X-ray wrist and elbow
Radial nerve lesion due to local compression (e.g., arm left hanging over a chair)	*Suggested by:* loss of sensation of **dorsal aspect of radial 3.5 fingers** *Confirmed by:* nerve conduction studies
C7 posterior root lesion due to cervical osteophytes	*Suggested by:* loss of sensation of **middle finger alone** *Confirmed by:* nerve conduction studies. MRI scan appearances
C8 posterior root lesion due to cervical osteophytes	*Suggested by:* loss of sensation of **palmar and dorsal aspect of ulnar 1.5 fingers** *and* the ulnar border of the wrist *Confirmed by:* nerve conduction studies. MRI scan appearances

Disturbed sensation in lower limb

Look for specific patterns, as indicated below.

Some differential diagnoses and typical outline evidence

Contralateral cortical (pre-central gyrus) lesion	*Suggested by:* graphesthesia
	Confirmed by: CT or MRI scan of brain
Peripheral neuropathy (due to diabetes mellitus, carcinoma, vitamin B_{12} deficiency, drugs therapy, heavy-metal or chemical exposure	*Suggested by:* loss of touch and pinprick sensation, worse in foot (e.g., stocking distribution), progressing upward
	Confirmed by: nerve conduction studies. MRI scan appearance
Spinothalamic tract damage (no dorsal column loss) due to contralateral hemisection of the cord	*Suggested by:* loss of pinprick and temperature sensation, normal or disturbed touch, but normal joint position and vibration sense in foot
	Confirmed by: nerve conduction studies. MRI of cervical cord
Dorsal column loss due to vitamin B_{12} deficiency, ipsilateral hemisection of the cord, rarely tabes dorsalis	*Suggested by:* loss of joint position and vibration sense in foot. Pinprick and temperature sensation normal
	Confirmed by: nerve conduction studies. B_{12} levels
L1 posterior root lesion	*Suggested by:* loss of sensation in ***inguinal region***
	Confirmed by: nerve conduction studies. X-ray of lumbar spine and sacrum

L2/3 posterior root lesion	*Suggested by:* loss of sensation in **anterior thigh**
	Confirmed by: nerve conduction studies. X-ray of lumbar spine and sacrum
L4/5 posterior root lesion	*Suggested by:* loss of sensation in **anterior shin**
	Confirmed by: nerve conduction studies. X-ray of lumbar spine and sacrum
S1 posterior root lesion	*Suggested by:* loss of sensation in **lateral border of foot**
	Confirmed by: nerve conduction studies. X-ray of lumbar spine and sacrum

Brisk reflexes

Some differential diagnoses and typical outline evidence

Thyrotoxicosis	*Suggested by:* brisk reflexes in all limbs with normal **flexor** plantar responses
	Confirmed by: ↑FT4 and ↓↓TSH levels
High level pyramidal tract lesion (cervical cord, brain stem, bilateral internal capsule or diffuse bilateral cortical lesion)	*Suggested by:* brisk reflexes in all limbs with **extensor** plantar responses
	Confirmed by: normal FT4 and TSH levels. MRI scan appearances
Contralateral pyramidal tract lesion in internal capsule, primary cortex, brain stem, or cervical cord	*Suggested by:* unilateral brisk reflexes in upper and lower limb
	Confirmed by: MRI of brain or cervical cord

Diminished reflexes

Some differential diagnoses and typical outline evidence

Sensory neuropathy	*Suggested by:* diminished reflexes, most marked peripherally. Normal muscle power. Normal *flexor* plantar responses
	Confirmed by: nerve conduction studies
Motor neuropathy	*Suggested by:* diminished reflexes, muscle wasting, fasciculation, and weakness
	Confirmed by: nerve conduction studies and normal EMG
Primary muscle disease	*Suggested by:* diminished reflexes, muscle wasting and weakness. No fasciculation
	Confirmed by: nerve conduction studies and abnormal EMG and muscle biopsy
Cerebellar disease	*Suggested by:* unilateral brisk reflexes in upper and lower limb
	Confirmed by: CT and MRI of brain posterior fossa
Posterior root lesion in C7/C8	*Suggested by:* loss of *triceps* jerk
	Confirmed by: MRI of disc space
Posterior root lesion in C5/C6	*Suggested by:* Loss of *biceps* jerk.
	Confirmed by: MRI of disc space
Posterior root lesion in L3/L4	*Suggested by:* Loss of *knee* jerk
	Confirmed by: MRI of disc space
Posterior root lesion in S1/S2	*Suggested by:* Loss of *ankle* jerk
	Confirmed by: MRI of disc space

Gait abnormality

Some differential diagnoses and typical outline evidence

Somatization 'functional' cause	*Suggested by:* **bizarre gait with exaggerated delay on affected limb**. No other physical signs of a lesion
	Confirmed by: patience and careful follow-up
Contralateral pyramidal tract lesion (in cerebral hemisphere, internal capsule, brain stem, or spinal cord)	*Suggested by:* **stiff leg swung in arc**. Other motor (± sensory) localizing signs indicating level of lesion
	Confirmed by: CT scan or MRI of probable site
Parkinsonism	*Suggested by:* **shuffling gait**, paucity of facial expression and movement, stiffness, tremor, etc.
	Confirmed by: response to treatment by dopamine agonist drugs, etc.
Cerebellar lesion (tumor, ischemia, etc.)	*Suggested by:* **wide-based gait**, inability to stand with feet together, falling to one side (truncal ataxia). Loss of tone and reflexes on same side as lesion
	Confirmed by: MRI of posterior fossa of brain
Dorsal column loss or peripheral neuropathy (due to vitamin B_{12} deficiency, etc.)	*Suggested by:* **bilateral stamping, high-stepping gait**, unsteadiness made worse by closing eyes (positive Romberg's sign)
	Confirmed by: nerve conduction studies and response to treatment of cause (if found)
Bilateral upper motor neuron lesion (usually in spinal cord)	*Suggested by:* **"scissors" or "wading-through-mud" gait**. Bilateral leg weakness and brisk reflexes
	Confirmed by: MRI of clinically probable site of lesion

Pelvic girdle and proximal muscle weakness (e.g., due to hereditary muscular dystrophy	*Suggested by:* **waddling gait (hip tilts down when leg lifted)**. Hypotonic limb weakness and poor reflexes *Confirmed by:* EMG
Joint, bone or muscle lesion	*Suggested by:* **hobbling with minimal time spent on affected limb**. Tenderness and limited range of movement *Confirmed by:* X-rays and response to treatment or resolution of cause
Lateral popliteal nerve palsy	*Suggested by:* **unilateral stamping, high-stepping gait** with foot drop. Flaccid weakness around ankle. Loss of sensation of lateral lower leg *Confirmed by:* nerve conduction studies
Drug effect	*Suggested by:* wide-based gait, nystagmus, past pointing. History of alcohol intake or other drug *Confirmed by:* raised alcohol or other drug level, improvement with withdrawal

Difficulty in rising from chair or squatting position

Some differential diagnoses and typical outline evidence

Polymyositis	*Suggested by:* muscle wasting, weakness, and poor reflexes
	Confirmed by: EMG and muscle biopsy
Carcinomatous neuromyopathy	*Suggested by:* muscle wasting, weakness, and poor reflexes. Evidence of cancer (usually late stage)
	Confirmed by: EMG and evidence of carcinomatosis
Thyrotoxicosis	*Suggested by:* weight loss, tremor, sweating, anxiety, loose bowels. ↑T3 or T4 and ↓↓TSH
	Confirmed by: response to treatment of thyrotoxicosis
Diabetic amyotrophy	*Suggested by:* long history of diabetes mellitus
	Confirmed by: nerve conduction studies and muscle biopsy
Cushing's syndrome	*Suggested by:* facial and truncal obesity with limb wasting
	Confirmed by: high midnight cortisol, etc., and response to treatment
Osteomalacia	*Suggested by:* ↓calcium and ↑alkaline phosphatase
	Confirmed by: response to treatment with calcium and vitamin D
Hereditary dystrophy	*Suggested by:* evidence of primary muscle disease and family history
	Confirmed by: muscle biopsy

GU symptoms

Urinary frequency ± dysuria

Some differential diagnoses and typical outline evidence

Urinary tract infection (UTI)	*Suggested by:* vomiting, fever, abdominal pain, ↑nitirites, white cells, and blood on urine dipstick
	Confirmed by: Mid-stream urine (MSU) microscopy and culture. Ultrasound scan for possible anatomical abnormality
Bladder or urethral calculus	*Suggested by:* suprapubic pain, macroscopic or microscopic hematuria
	Confirmed by: ultrasound of bladder, plain X-ray, intravenous urogram (IVU)
Uterine prolapse	*Suggested by:* incontinent of urine, cervix observed in lower vagina
	Confirmed by: pelvic examination
Prostatic hypertrophy	*Suggested by:* hesitancy, poor stream, large prostate on rectal examination
	Confirmed by: prostate-specific antigen (PSA)↑, ultrasound of prostate gland, and response to transurethral resection of the prostate (TURP)
Spastic bladder due to upper motor neuron lesion	*Suggested by:* weakness, increased tone and reflexes in lower limbs
	Confirmed by: small bladder on ultrasound

Incontinence of urine alone (not feces)

Some differential diagnoses and typical outline evidence

Prostatism	*Suggested by:* hesitancy, dribbling, poor stream, frequency
	Confirmed by: ↑PSA, ultrasound of prostate gland
Uterine prolapse	*Suggested by:* low-volume urinary frequency
	Confirmed by: pelvic examination
Urinary tract infection (UTI)	*Suggested by:* dysuria, frequency, fever, vomiting, ↑nitrites, white cells, and blood on dipstick
	Confirmed by: MSU microscopy and culture. Ultrasound scan for possible anatomical abnormality
Weakness of pelvic floor muscles	*Suggested by:* incontinence during coughing, sneezing, laughing
	Confirmed by: **Urodynamic studies**

Incontinence of urine and feces

Some differential diagnoses and typical outline evidence

Neurogenic bladder	*Suggested by:* paresis, low tone and diminished reflexes in lower limbs, sensory loss in anal region
	Confirmed by: small and spastic bladder (upper motor neuron) or large and hypotonic bladder (lower motor neuron) on **ultrasound scan**
Seizures	*Suggested by:* history of loss of consciousness, tongue biting, jerking movements
	Confirmed by: clinical history, EEG
Dementia	*Suggested by:* chronic worsening confusion, elderly, previous strokes
	Confirmed by: low mental scores, cerebral atrophy on **CT head scan**
Severe depression	*Suggested by:* severe lack of motivation
	Confirmed by: response to treatment of depression
Fecal impaction with overflow	*Suggested by:* hard, rock-like feces in rectum
	Confirmed by: response to evacuation of feces

Painful hematuria (with dysuria)

Some differential diagnoses and typical outline evidence

Urinary tract infection	*Suggested by:* dysuria, frequency, ± low-grade fever ± abdominal pain, ↑ nitrites, white cells, and blood on urine dipstick
	Confirmed by: MSU microscopy and culture. Ultrasound scan for possible anatomical abnormality
Renal calculus	*Suggested by:* dysuria, spasmodic loin-to-groin pain, no fever
	Confirmed by: urinalysis, renal ultrasound, IVU
Trauma	*Suggested by:* dysuria, urethral catheterization, or recent painful sexual intercourse ("honeymoon cystitis")
	Confirmed by: history, normal MSU renal ultrasound, IVU

Painless hematuria

False positives include vaginal or anorectal bleeding.

Some differential diagnoses and typical outline evidence

Renal tumor	*Suggested by:* palpable mass, fever (often previously of unknown origin)
	Confirmed by: ultrasound or CT of abdomen/kidney, IVU
Ureteral tumor	*Suggested by:* colicky pain if obstructed
	Confirmed by: ultrasound or CT abdomen/kidney, IVU
Bladder tumor	*Suggested by:* pelvic pain, pelvic mass
	Confirmed by: cystoscopy, IVU shows filling defects of bladder
Bleeding diathesis	*Suggested by:* anticoagulant therapy, easy bruising, or other bleeding sites
	Confirmed by: abnormal clotting screen ± low platelets
Urinary tract infection (UTI)	*Suggested by:* frequency, ± low-grade fever, ↑ nitrites, white cells, blood on dipstick
	Confirmed by: MSU microscopy and culture. Ultrasound scan for possible anatomical abnormality

Secondary amenorrhea

This is absence of menstruation for ≥3 months.

Some differential diagnoses and typical outline evidence

Pregnancy	*Suggested by:* presentation during childbearing age
	Confirmed by: positive pregnancy test, pelvic ultrasound
Normal menopause	*Suggested by:* >40 years of age, hot flashes
	Confirmed by: FSH high
Premature ovarian failure	*Suggested by:* hot flashes <40 years of age and no signs of other endocrine disease (adrenal failure, hypothyroidism, etc.)
	Confirmed by: LH, FSH ↑, estradiol ↓, ovarian biopsy: atrophic
Polycystic ovary syndrome	*Suggested by:* oligo- or amenorrhea, hirsutism, obesity
	Confirmed by: ↓ sex hormone–binding globulin, ↑ testosterone, ↑LH, cystic ovaries on pelvic ultrasound
Hyperprolacti-nemia	*Suggested by:* galactorrhea, ± headache or bitemporal visual-field defect (if due to large prolactinoma)
	Confirmed by: ↑ serum prolactin. Appearance of pituitary fossa on skull X-ray or CT scan
Thyrotoxicosis	*Suggested by:* heat intolerance, tremor, nervousness, palpitation, frequent bowel movements, goiter
	Confirmed by: ↓TSH, ↑FT4, (± ↑FT3)

Excessive menstrual loss: menorrhagia

Menorrhagia can be due to uterine or systemic disorders.

Some differential diagnoses and typical outline evidence

Fibroids (uterine leiomyomas)	*Suggested by:* (sometimes) urinary frequency, constipation, recurrent abortion, infertility
	Confirmed by: pelvic examination, ultrasound or CT
Endometrial carcinoma	*Suggested by:* abnormal uterine bleeding, blood-stained vaginal discharge, postmenopausal bleeding
	Confirmed by: pelvic ultrasound, tissue sampling of endometrium, hysteroscopy
Pelvic endometriosis	*Suggested by:* dysmenorrhea, dyspareunia, infertility, pelvic mass
	Confirmed by: laparoscopy
Chronic pelvic inflammatory disease	*Suggested by:* lower abdominal pain, fever, vaginal discharge, dysuria, ↑ESR and ↑CRP, leukocytosis
	Confirmed by: high vaginal swab, pelvic ultrasound, ± laparoscopy
Intrauterine contraceptive device (IUD)	*Suggested by:* history of its insertion ± dysmenorrhea
	Confirmed by: symptoms subside after removal of IUD
Primary hypothyroidism	*Suggested by:* cold intolerance, tiredness, constipation, bradycardia
	Confirmed by: ↑TSH, ↓FT4
Bleeding diathesis	*Suggested by:* family history, tendency to bleed, easy bruising
	Confirmed by: abnormal clotting screen

Intermenstrual or postcoital bleeding

Expert pelvic examination is required.

Some differential diagnoses and typical outline evidence

Carcinoma of uterus	*Suggested by:* abnormal or intermenstrual uterine bleeding, blood-stained discharge, postmenopausal bleeding
	Confirmed by: pelvic ultrasound, tissue sampling of endometrium, hysteroscopy
Carcinoma of cervix	*Suggested by:* irregular vaginal bleeding, offensive, watery, or blood-stained vaginal discharge, obstructive uropathy and back pain in late stage
	Confirmed by: appearance on vaginal speculum examination, biopsy of cervix
Cervical or intrauterine polyps	*Suggested by:* intermenstrual spotting or postmenstrual staining
	Confirmed by: appearance on vaginal speculum examination, hysteroscopy

GU signs

General examination checklist

Preliminary findings should have been discovered during the general examination. These include jaundice, anemia, clubbing, xanthelasma, gynecomastia, and lip, buccal mucosa, throat, tongue, or supraclavicular lumps.

Scrotal mass

Some differential diagnoses and typical outline evidence

Inguinal hernia descended into scrotum	*Suggested by:* inability to get above it. Does not transilluminate
	Confirmed by: above clinical examination
Testicular torsion	*Suggested by:* exquisitely tender, unilateral mass in the scrotal sac, chord thickened, and opposite testis lies horizontally (bell-clapper testis)
	Confirmed by: above clinical examination, **Doppler ultrasound** reveals ↓ blood flow
Hematocele	*Suggested by:* history of trauma or scrotal surgery. Tenderness
	Confirmed by: above history and examination, Doppler ultrasound
Acute epididymitis	*Suggested by:* diffuse tenderness in the epididymis, marked redness, and edema
	Confirmed by: **urine microscopy and culture** (white cells and organisms)
Acute orchitis	*Suggested by:* large and tender testes fever
	Confirmed by: above history and examination
Chronic epididymitis	*Suggested by:* chronic, diffuse scrotal tenderness
	Confirmed by: identification of infecting organism by **urine cultures or culture of urethral discharge** after prostatic massage
Varicocele (90% on the left)	*Suggested by:* non-tender, unilateral fleshy mass that feels like a bag of worms, and decreases in size with scrotal elevation
	Confirmed by: above clinical examination (patient must be examined while standing)

Hydrocele	*Suggested by:* non-tender, unilateral mass in scrotal sac
Other causes: obesity, incontinence, diabetes mellitus, psoriasis, lichen planus, scabies, pubic lice	*Confirmed by:* above clinical findings and demonstration of transillumination
Spermatocele	*Suggested by:* non-tender, small nodules posterior to the head of the epididymis
	Confirmed by: above clinical examination, may or may not transilluminate
Epididymal cyst	*Suggested by:* non-tender nodule in the head of epididymis, adjacent to inferior pole of testis, and transillumination
	Confirmed by: above clinical examination and demonstration of transillumination
Seminoma	*Suggested by:* firm, non-tender, non-transilluminable nodule or mass adjacent to a testis
	Confirmed by: **ultrasound of scrotal contents** showing a solid testicular mass, **direct surgical examination**, normal **serum α-fetoprotein**
Teratoma	*Suggested by:* firm, non-tender, non-transilluminable nodule or mass adjacent to a testis
	Confirmed by: **ultrasound of scrotal contents** showing a solid testicular mass, **direct surgical examination**, ↑**serum α-fetoprotein**

Enlargement of prostate

The rectal examination continues by feeling for a prostatic protrusion anteriorly and sweeping around for other masses, including impacted feces.

Some differential diagnoses and typical outline evidence

Prostatitis	*Suggested by:* smooth, enlarged, and tender
	Confirmoed by: **positive urine culture, culture of prostatic secretions**
Benign prostatic hypertrophy	*Suggested by:* smooth, enlarged, firm, non-tender, usually with a palpable median groove
	Confirmed by: normal or slightly ↑*serum PSA, prostatic biopsy*
Prostatic carcinoma	*Suggested by:* irregular, hard, sometimes obliteration of median groove, non-tender
	Confirmed by: ↑↑*serum PSA, prostatic biopsy*

Vulval skin abnormalities

Some differential diagnoses and typical outline evidence

Thrush, *Candida albicans* often in pregnancy, contraceptive and steroids, immunodeficiencies, antibiotics, and diabetes mellitus	*Suggested by:* vulva and vagina red, fissured and sore *Confirmed by:* mycelia or spores on **microscopy and culture**
Allergy	*Suggested by:* exacerbation after wearing nylon underwear, using chemicals or soap *Confirmed by:* response to avoidance of precipitants
Lichen sclerosis	*Suggested by:* being intensely itchy. Bruised red, purpuric appearance. Bullae, erosions, and ulcerations. Later, white, flat, and shiny with an hourglass shape around the vulva and anus *Confirmed by:* above clinical appearance and **biopsy**
Leukoplakia	*Suggested by:* itchiness and white vulval patches due to skin thickening and hypertrophy *Confirmed by:* above clinical appearance and **biopsy**
Carcinoma of the vulva	*Suggested by:* an indurated ulcer with an everted edge *Confirmed by:* **biopsy**

Other causes: obesity, incontinence, diabetes mellitus, psoriasis, lichen planus, scabies, pubic lice

Ulcers and lumps of the vulva

Some differential diagnoses and typical outline evidence

Vulval warts (condylomata acuminata) due to human papilloma virus	*Suggested by:* warts on vulva, perineum, anus, vagina, or cervix. Florid in pregnancy or if immunosuppressed *Confirmed by:* above clinical appearance. Managed initially by annual **cervical smears** and observation of the vulva and anus
Urethral caruncle caused by meatal prolapse	*Suggested by:* small, red swelling at the urethral orifice. Tender and pain on micturition *Confirmed by:* above clinical appearance
Bartholin's cyst and abscess caused by blocked duct	*Suggested by:* extreme pain (cannot sit) and a very swollen, hot, red labium *Confirmed by:* above clinical appearance
Herpes simplex (herpes type II)	*Suggested by:* vulva ulcerated and exquisitely painful. Urinary retention may occur. *Confirmed by:* above clinical appearance

Other causes of vulval lumps: local varicose veins; boils; sebaceous cysts; keratoacanthomata, condylomata, latent syphilis; primary chancre; molluscum contagiosum; abscess; uterine prolapse or polyp; inguinal hernia; varicocele; carcinoma

Other causes of vulval ulcers: syphilis, herpes simplex, chancroid; lymphogranuloma venereum; granuloma inguinale; TB, Behçet's syndrome; aphthous ulcers; Crohn's disease

Lumps in the vagina

Some differential diagnoses and typical outline evidence

Cystocele	*Suggested by:* frequency and dysuria. Bulging upper front wall of the vagina
	Confirmed by: **cystogram** showing residual urine within the cystocele
Urethrocele	*Suggested by:* stress incontinence (leaks with laughing, exertion). Bulging of the lower anterior vaginal wall
	Confirmed by: **micturating cystogram** showing displaced urethra and impaired sphincter mechanisms
Rectocele	*Suggested by:* patient may have to reduce herniation prior to defecation by putting a finger in the vagina. Bulging middle posterior wall
	Confirmed by: **barium enema or MRI scan** showing rectum bulging through weak levator ani
Enterocele	*Suggested by:* bulging of the upper posterior vaginal wall
	Confirmed by: **barium enema or MRI scan** showing loops of intestine in the pouch of Douglas
Uterine prolapse	*Suggested by:* "dragging" or "something coming down," is worse by day. Cystitis, frequency, stress incontinence, and difficulty in defecation
	Confirmed by: seeing the cervix well down in the vagina (first-degree prolapse) or cervix protruding from the introitus when standing or straining (second degree), or the uterus lying outside the vagina, which is keratinized, and the cervix ulcerated (third-degree prolapse or procidentia)
Vaginal carcinoma	*Suggested by:* vaginal bleeding. Tumor in the upper third of the vagina
	Confirmed by: squamous cell carcinoma on biopsy

Ulcers and lumps in the cervix

Some differential diagnoses and typical outline evidence

Cervical ectropion ("erosion" innocuous)	*Suggested by:* red ring of soft glandular tissue around cervical opening, often found with puberty, combined contraceptive pill, during pregnancy. May be bleeding, producing excess mucus or infected
	Confirmed by: (in cases of doubt) **histology** showing columnar epithelium
Nabothian cysts	*Suggested by:* smooth spherical (mucus retention)
	Confirmed by: above clinical appearance
Cervical polyps	*Suggested by:* increased mucus discharge or postcoital bleeding. Pedunculated polyp arising from mouth of cervix
	Confirmed by: **histology** showing pedunculated benign tumor arising from endocervical junction
Cervicitis	*Suggested by:* increased mucus discharge or postcoital bleeding. Very red, swollen cervix with overlying mucous and blood
	Confirmed by: histology being follicular or mucopurulent. Vesicles in herpes. **Culture** may produce chlamydia, gonococci, etc.
Cervical intraepithelial neoplasia (CIN)	*Suggested by:* overlying cervicitis, older age, smokers, lower socioeconomic background, prolonged contraceptive pill use, high parity, history of many sexual partners or a partner having many other partners, early first coitus, sexually transmitted diseases
	Confirmed by: **Papanicolaou smear** showing degree of dyskaryosis but no malignancy on **cervical biopsy**
Cervical carcinoma	*Suggested by:* intermenstrual or postcoital bleeding. Firm or friable mass that bleeds on contact
	Confirmed by: **Papanicolaou smear** showing severe dyskaryosis and malignancy on **cervical biopsy**

Tender or bulky mass (uterus, fallopian tubes, or ovary) on pelvic examination

Some differential diagnoses and typical outline evidence

Pregnancy	*Suggested by:* amenorrhea in sexually active woman. Uterus at 6 weeks of pregnancy is like an egg, at 8 weeks like a peach, at 10 weeks it is like a grapefruit, and at 14 weeks it fills the pelvis
	Confirmed by: pregnancy test positive, pregnancy sac seen on abdominal or **transvaginal ultrasound**
Ovarian tumor, benign functional cysts, theca-lutein cysts, epithelial cell tumors (serous and mucinous), cystadenomas, mature teratomas, fibromas malignant cystadenomas, germ cell or sex cord malignancies, secondaries from the uterus or stomach, Krukenberg tumors spreading via the peritoneum	*Suggested by:* painless pelvic mass often to one side. May or may not have amenorrhea
	Confirmed by: **abdominal or transvaginal ultrasound, biopsy**

Endometritis (uterine infection) after abortion and childbirth, ICU insertion, or surgery. May involve fallopian tubes and ovaries. Low-grade infection is often due to Chlamydia	*Suggested by:* lower abdominal pain and fever; uterine tenderness on bimanual palpation *Confirmed by:* **transvaginal ultrasound, cervical swabs and blood cultures**
Endometrial proliferation due to estrogen stimulation	*Suggested by:* heavy menstrual bleeding and irregular bleeding (dysfunctional uterine bleeding) and polyps *Confirmed by:* cystic glandular hyperplasia in specimen after D&C
Pyometra (uterus distended by pus, associated with salpingitis or secondary to outflow blockage)	*Suggested by:* lower abdominal pain and fever; uterine tenderness on bimanual palpation *Confirmed by:* **transvaginal ultrasound, cervical swabs and blood cultures**
Hematometra due to imperforate hymen in the young, carcinoma, iatrogenic cervical stenosis after cone biopsy	*Suggested by:* lower abdominal pain and uterine tenderness on bimanual palpation *Confirmed by:* no evidence of infection. *Transvaginal ultrasound* appearance
Endometrial tuberculosis (also affects the Fallopian tubes with pyosalpinx)	*Suggested by:* infertility, pelvic pain, amenorrhea, oligomenorrhea *Confirmed by:* **transvaginal ultrasound, cervical swabs** and positive smear or **cultures for** AFB

Ectopic pregnancy	*Suggested by:* abdominal pain or bleeding in a sexually active woman. Gradually increasing vaginal bleeding, shoulder-tip pain (diaphragmatic irritation) and pain on defecation and passing water (due to pelvic blood). Sudden severe pain, peritonism, and shock with rupture
	Confirmed by: **hCG** >6000 IU/L and an intrauterine gestational sac not seen on pelvic ultrasound or if **hCG** 1000–1500 IU/L and no sac is seen on **transvaginal ultrasound**
Fibroids (uterine leiomyomata)	*Suggested by:* heavy and prolonged periods, infertility, pain, abdominal swelling, urinary frequency, edematous legs and varicose veins, or cause retention of urine
	Confirmed by: normal **hCG** and **transvaginal ultrasound** showing discrete lumps in the wall of the uterus or bulging out to lie under the peritoneum (subserosal) or under the endometrium (submucosal), pedunculated
Acute salpingitis often associated with endometritis, peritonitis, abscess, and chronic infection	*Suggested by:* being unwell, with pain, fever, spasm of lower-abdominal muscles (more comfortable lying on back with legs flexed). Cervicitis with profuse, purulent, or bloody vaginal discharge. Cervical excitation and tenderness in the fornices bilaterally but worse on one side. Symptoms vague in subacute infection
	Confirmed by: **laparoscopy**
Chronic salpingitis (unresolved, unrecognized, or inadequately treated acute salpingitis) leading to fibrosis and adhesions, pyosalpinx, or hydrosalpinx	*Suggested by:* pelvic pain, menorrhagia, secondary dysmenorrhea, discharge, deep dyspareunia, depression. Palpable tubal masses, tenderness, and fixed retroverted uterus
	Confirmed by: **laparoscopy** to differentiate between infection and endometriosis

Vaginal discharge

Some differential diagnoses and typical outline evidence

Excessive normal secretion	*Suggested by:* women of reproductive age, milky white or mucoid discharge
	Confirmed by: normal investigations
Bacterial vaginosis	*Suggested by:* fishy odor, discharge, itching, irritation
	Confirmed by: **high vaginal swab, wet saline microscopy shows presence of cells**
Cervical erosions (ectropion)	*Suggested by:* no other obvious symptoms
	Confirmed by: **speculum examination**
Endocervicitis (gonococcus, Chlamydia)	*Suggested by:* symptoms in partner of urethritis
	Confirmed by: inflamed cervix on **speculum examination** and **endocervical swab** result
Carcinoma of cervix	*Suggested by:* blood-stained discharge, irregular vaginal bleeding, obstructive uropathy and back pain in late stage
	Confirmed by: **cervical smear, cytology, colposcopy with biopsy**
Foreign body	*Suggested by:* blood-stained discharge, use of ring pessary, IUD, tampon
	Confirmed by: speculum examination or colposcopy or hysteroscopy
Endometrial polyp	*Suggested by:* blood-stained discharge, intermenstrual spotting, postmenstrual staining
	Confirmed by: **hysteroscopy**

Trichomonas vaginitis	*Suggested by:* profuse greenish yellow, frothy discharge, dysuria, dyspareunia
	Confirmed by: protozoa and WBC on **smear**
Gonococcal cervicitis	*Suggested by:* purulent discharge, lower abdominal pain, fever, cervix appears red and bleeds easily
	Confirmed by: **Gram stain of cervical or urethral exudates** shows intracellular gram-negative diplococci
Candida vaginitis	*Suggested by:* purulent discharge, intense pruritus vulvae
	Confirmed by: hyphae or spores on **cervical smear**
Chlamydia cervicitis	*Suggested by:* purulent discharge, lower-abdominal pain, fever, cervix appears red and bleeds easily
	Confirmed by: **endocervical swab**

Musculoskeletal symptoms and signs

Approach to the patient with musculoskeletal complaints

Patients with disorders of nerves, muscle, or the neuromuscular junction can present with a similar constellation of symptoms. Diseases of the nerve (e.g., polyneuropathy), muscle (e.g., myopathy), and neuromuscular junction (e.g., myasthenia gravis) may present with varying degrees of sensory loss and weakness. Nevertheless, specific patterns of sensory and motor disturbances help differentiate between disorders.

Weakness can arise from dysfunction of nerve, neuromuscular junction, or muscle, and may be a difficult symptom for patients to quantify and localize. Frequently, patients will complain of pain and associated weakness. However, since pain may limit the action and mobility of a joint, the finding of weakness in the setting of pain may not indicate true neurological dysfunction.

It is important to distinguish myalgias (muscle pain) from arthralgias (joint pain). Additionally, many musculoskeletal symptoms are part of a systemic illness, so constitutional symptoms are always important to elicit.

For muscular complaints, the pattern of symptoms is important to ascertain: which muscle groups are involved (localized to one extremity, proximal vs. distal, etc.) and whether there is accompanying weakness. Family history may give you a clue (e.g., inherited muscle storage diseases or a family history of autoimmune disease). The degree of impairment of activities of daily living should always be part of a musculoskeletal assessment.

For joint complaints, the pattern of joint involvement is also important and can give clues to the underlying illness. Monoarticular arthritis has a different differential diagnosis than that of polyarticular arthritis. Associated morning stiffness usually suggests inflammatory arthritis.

Muscle weakness + pain

Many patients who complain of weakness are not weak when muscle strength is formally tested. A careful history and physical examination will help in determining the distinction between asthenia (motor impairment due to pain or joint dysfunction) and true weakness.

Patients with a variety of systemic disorders (cardiopulmonary and joint disease, anemia, cachexia, depression) may interpret difficulties in performing certain tasks as weakness. These patients may be functionally limited but not truly weak. True weakness due to a decrease in muscle power must be differentiated from limitation due to dyspnea, chest pain, joint pain, fatigue, poor exercise tolerance, paresthesias, or spasticity. Muscle complaints should be further characterized by the muscle groups involved, exacerbation with exercise, and the presence of fasciculations.

Muscle pain is relatively uncommon in patients with many types of myopathy and true weakness, but is often a problem for patients with overexertion, cramps, or fibromyalgia.

The physical examination should include not only testing of muscle strength but also a careful search for one of the disorders that can cause the perception of weakness.

Some differential diagnoses and typical outline evidence

Primary muscle disorders

Normal response to strenuous exercise	*Suggested by:* fit, healthy, unaccustomed exercise 1–2 days before
	Confirmed by: spontaneous resolution
Primary thyroid disease—both hyper- and hypothryodism	*Suggested by:* onset over weeks to months. Predominant fatigue. Can have proximal muscle weakness. Also cold intolerance, weight loss
	Confirmed by: ↑TSH, ↓FT4
Cushing's syndrome (also steroid myopathy)	*Suggested by:* proximal muscle weakness with atrophy, first affecting the lower extremities and then the upper extremities, signs of Cushing's syndrome
	Confirmed by: normal CPK, muscle biopsy showing atrophy of type II muscle fibers, laboratory evidence of Cushing's syndrome (**↑urinary free cortisol** or non-suppression on **dexamethasone suppression test**)
Hyperparathyroidism	*Suggested by:* proximal weakness (legs involved more than arms), fatigue, musculoskeletal pain, and hyperreflexia, ↑Ca^{2+}
	Confirmed by: ↑PTH (parathyroid hormone)

Inflammatory myositis Polymyositis Dermatomyositis	*Suggested by:* onset over weeks to months. Predominant weakness of proximal muscles; dermatomyositis accompanied by heliotrope rash and Gottren's rash over metacarpophalangeal (MCP) and proximal interphalangeal (PIP) joints and photosensititvity. Associated malignancy can occur.

Confirmed by: CPK ↑; autoantibody, including anti-nuclear antibody (ANA), anti-SRP, anti Jo-1, anti-Mi-2, anti-Ku and anti-PM-Scl, and anti-hPMS-1; electromyography (EMG) and muscle biopsy |
| Inflammatory myositis Inclusion body myositis | *Suggested by:* onset over months. Predominant weakness; proximal > distal

Confirmed by: CPK ↑, EMG and muscle biopsy, with minimal inflammation and characteristic basophilic rimmed vacuoles within muscle sarcoplasm |
| Polymyalgia rheumatica | *Suggested by:* onset over weeks or months, stiff, painful, and tender proximal muscles. Fatigue, fever in elderly person

Confirmed by: ↑↑ESR. **Rheumatoid factor** negative, prompt response to low-dose prednisone, no other cause |
| Glycogen storage disorder (McArdle's disease) | *Suggested by:* familial history, early adulthood with exercise intolerance, fatigue, myalgia, cramps, myoglobinuria, poor endurance, muscle swelling, and fixed weakness; brief rest after development of muscle stiffness, and myalgias can lead to re-sumption of physical activity without significant symptoms

Confirmed by: low venous lactate after ischemic response to exercise, muscle biopsy, genetic testing |
| Phosphofructokinase (PFK) deficiency (glycogen storage disease VII, Tarui disease) | *Suggested by:* childhood onset with fatigue, muscle cramps, and exercise intolerance. A high carbohy-drate meal or administration of glucose prior to exercise aggravates symptoms, due to decreased availability of free fatty acids and ketones.

Confirmed by: serum creatine kinase ↑. Red blood cell PFK activity reduced to one-half normal. Sometimes mild hemolytic anemia, mild hyper-bilirubinemia, hyperuricemia, due to increased degradation of purine nucleotides in muscle. The ischemic forearm exercise test shows no rise in lactate levels; muscle biopsy |

Myotonic dystrophy	*Suggested by:* skeletal muscle weakness and myotonia, cardiac conduction abnormalities, cataracts, testicular failure, hypogammaglobulinemia, and insulin resistance.
	Muscles involved: facial muscles, levator palpebrae superficialis, temporalis, sternomastoids, distal muscles of the forearm, hand intrinsic muscles (leading to compromised finger dexterity), and ankle dorsiflexors (causing bilateral foot drop)
	Confirmed by: EMG, genetic testing

Neuromuscular dysfunction

Myasthenia gravis	*Suggested by:* onset over weeks or months. Fluctuating skeletal muscle weakness, often with true muscle fatigue. Ptosis or diplopia, bulbar muscle weakness manifests as hoarseness, expressionless face if facial muscles involved, drooped-head syndrome if neck muscles involved
	Confirmed by: bedside tests (Tensilon test and ice pack test). Acetylcholine receptor antibody (AChR-Ab) or against a receptor-associated protein, muscle-specific tyrosine kinase (MuSK-Ab)
Eaton Lambert syndrome	*Suggested by:* slowly progressive proximal muscle weakness, frequently associated with autonomic dysfunction; weakness may improve with repetitive movement. Frequently early manifestation of occult malignancy, especially small cell lung cancer
	Confirmed by: EMG and antibodies to voltage-gated calcium channel (VGCC)

Primary neurological disorders

Multiple sclerosis (MS)	*Suggested by:* relapses and remissions of CNS dysfunction. Onset between 15 and 50 years of age, associated optic neuritis, L'hermitte's sign, internuclear ophthalmoplegia, fatigue, Uhthoff's phenomenon
	Confirmed by: MRI, CSF analysis, evoked potentials
Amyotrophic lateral sclerosis (ALS)	*Suggested by:* combination of upper motor neuron (weakness, hyperreflexia, and spasticity) and lower motor neuron (atrophy and fasciculations) signs and symptoms. Asymmetric limb weakness is the most common presentation.
	Confirmed by: clinical picture and EMG
Primary motor sensory neuropathies, including Charcot–Marie–Tooth disease	*Suggested by:* distal calf muscle atrophy, atrophy of hand and foot muscles, loss of reflexes, pes cavus foot deformity, hammer toes
	Confirmed by: EMG and sural nerve biopsy

Other

Fibromyalgia	*Suggested by:* variable onset—weeks to years. Diffuse pain and stiffness and sleep disturbance (nonrestorative sleep). Important to exclude sleep apnea
	Confirmed by: absence of another condition, tender points
Celiac disease and other malabsorption states	*Suggested by:* arthralgias, myalgias, iron-deficiency anemia, osteoporosis
	Confirmed by: small bowel biopsy, *IgA anti-tissue transglutaminase, IgA endomysial antibody,* or *anti-gliadin antibody*

Monoarthritis

One joint is affected by pain, swelling, overlying redness, stiffness, and local heat (±fever).

Some differential diagnoses and typical outline evidence

Acute septic arthritis	*Suggested by:* extremely painful, hot, red joint, high fever
	Confirmed by: ↑↑WBC. **Joint aspiration:** synovial fluid turbid. **Culture** growing *Staphylococcus, Streptococcus,* gram-negative organisms (rare), gonococci, or TB
Gout	*Suggested by:* one acutely inflamed joint (frequently the first MTP joint) at a time, but other joints in hands, arms, legs, and feet can be involved. Tophi on ears and along extensor tendon sheaths
	Confirmed by: urate crystals (negatively birefringent in plane-polarized light) present on **joint aspiration**. Elevated serum uric acid insufficient for diagnosis
Pseudogout (Ca²⁺ pyrophosphate arthropathy/ chondrocalcinosis)	*Suggested by:* one painful joint (usually knee), especially in elderly *or* history of hyperparathyroidism *or* hypothyroidism *or* osteoarthritis *or* hemochromatosis
	Confirmed by: **joint aspiration:** synovial crystal deposits positively birefringent in plane-polarized light. Chondrocalcinosis on X-ray
Reactive arthritis	*Suggested by:* asymmetric mono- or oligoarthritis, urethritis, conjunctivitis, especially in a young man, with a history of diarrhea or urethritis that occurred 2–6 weeks previously. Also suggested by associated plantar fasciitis, achilles tendonitis
	Confirmed by: **rheumatoid factor** negative (i.e., seronegative). **Urinalysis:** first glass of a 2-glass urine test shows debris in urethritis
Osteoarthritis	*Suggested by:* monoarthritis of weight-bearing joint, especially in joint with a history of remote trauma or in an obese patient
	Confirmed by: joint aspiration:non-inflammatory fluid, joint space narrowing and osteophytes on X-ray

Traumatic hemarthrosis	*Suggested by:* acutely inflamed joint after trauma
	Confirmed by: ***joint aspiration:*** aspiration of blood from joint
Psoriatic arthritis	*Suggested by:* inflamed joint or sausage digit, pitting and thickening of fingernails
	Confirmed by: psoriatic plaques on elbows and extensor surfaces of limbs, scalp, behind ears and around navel. ***Rheumatoid factor*** negative (i.e., seronegative).
Leukemic joint deposits	*Suggested by:* acutely inflamed joint, diagnosis of leukemia
	Confirmed by: exclusion of other diagnoses, particularly septic arthritis; in patient without known leukemia, ***peripheral blood smear*** and/or ***bone marrow consistent with leukemia***

Polyarthritis

Several joints are affected by pain, swelling, overlying redness, stiffness, and local heat (±fever).

Some differential diagnoses and typical outline evidence

Viruses	*Suggested by:* recent-onset inflamed joints. Usually small joints of the hands. Common viruses include parvovirus, Epstein–Barr virus, hepatitis B and C
	Confirmed by: ↑*viral titers*, rheumatoid factor negative (seronegative)
Rheumatoid arthritis	*Suggested by:* Painful and stiff joints for >6 weeks with morning stiffness lasting ≥1 hour. Usually symmetric involvement of small joints of hands, wrists
	Confirmed by: **rheumatoid factor** positive, anti-CCP Ab. X-rays showing periarticular osteopenia or erosions, rheumatoid nodules on extensor surfaces
Gout	*Suggested by:* polyarticular presentation more common in chronic tophaceous gout; all joints can be involved. Tophi on ears and tendon sheaths
	Confirmed by: urate crystals (negatively birefringent in plane-polarized light) present on **joint aspiration**. Elevated serum uric acid insufficient for diagnosis
Pseudogout (Ca^{2+} pyrophosphate arthropathy/ chondro-calcinosis)	*Suggested by:* polyarticular presentation unusual, but can occur; more common in elderly *or* history of hyperparathyroidism *or* hypothyroidism *or* osteoarthritis *or* hemochromatosis
	Confirmed by: **joint aspiration:** synovial crystal deposits positively birefringent in plane-polarized light. Chondrocalcinosis on X-ray
Osteoarthritis	*Suggested by:* bony enlargement of distal interphalangeal (DIP) and PIP joints (Heberden's and Bouchard nodes), decreased flexibility, can have angulation deformities. Morning stiffness ≤30 minutes
	Confirmed by: **rheumatoid factor** negative; frequently family history
Sjögren's syndrome	*Suggested by:* pattern similar to rheumatoid arthritis, accompanied by diminished lacrimation causing dry eyes, and diminished salivation causing dry mouth
	Confirmed by: **rheumatoid factor** positive (low titer) and ANA positive **anti-Ro** (SSA) and **anti-La** (SSB) antibodies present (not always)

Rheumatic fever (reactive arthritis to earlier infection with Lancefield group A β-hemolytic streptococci)	*Suggested by:* migratory joint pain and swelling (a major Jones criterion) *Confirmed by:* evidence of recent streptococcal infection plus 1 more major revised Jones criteria or 2 more minor criteria *Evidence of streptococcal infection* = scarlet fever or positive **throat swab** or increase in **ASOT** >200 or ↑**DNase B titer** *Major criteria:* carditis or migratory polyarthritis or subcutaneous nodules or erythema marginatum or Sydenham's chorea *Minor criteria:* fever or ↑ESR/CRP, arthralgia (but not if arthritis is one of the major criteria), prolonged P–R interval on ECG (but not if carditis is major criterion), previous rheumatic fever. **Rheumatoid factor** negative
Systemic lupus erythematosus (SLE)	*Suggested by:* pattern similar to rheumatoid arthritis, accompanied by other signs and symptoms suggestive of lupus (malar rash, photosensitivity, serositis, etc.) *Confirmed by:* **ANA** positive and **rheumatoid factor** negative, **and fulfillment of 4 or more criteria for diagnosis of lupus: ANA, double-stranded DNA, other autoantibodies, seizure, psychosis, cytopenias, proteinuria or red cell casts, serositis,** malar rash, discoid rash, photosensitivity, oral ulcers
Ulcerative colitis	*Suggested by:* large- or small-joint polyarthritis, with sacroiliitis, occasionally spondylitis, with a background of diarrhea with blood and mucus and crampy abdominal discomfort *Confirmed by:* **rheumatoid factor** negative. Inflamed, friable mucosa on **sigmoidoscopy,** and biopsy shows inflammatory infiltrate, goblet cell depletion, etc.
Crohn's disease	*Suggested by:* large- or small-joint polyarthritis, with sacroiliitis, occasionally spondylitis, with a background of diarrhea with blood and mucus and crampy abdominal discomfort, weight loss *Confirmed by:* **rheumatoid factor** negative. **Small bowel films** showing ileal strictures, proximal dilatation, inflammatory mass or fistula. **Barium enema:** "cobblestoning," "rose thorn" ulcers, colonic strictures with rectal sparing

Drug reaction (immune complex mediated)	*Suggested by:* polyarticular small-joint arthritis. History of suspicious drug
	Confirmed by: **rheumatoid factor** negative and improvement on withdrawing of drug
Psoriatic arthritis	*Suggested by:* polyarticular arthritis can resemble rheumatoid arthritis, can involve DIP joints (associated with sacroiliitis and, occasionally, spondylitis); can have pitting and thickening of fingernails
	Confirmed by: psoriatic plaques on elbows and extensor surfaces of limbs, scalp, behind ears, and around navel. **Rheumatoid factor** negative

Pain or limitation of movement in the hand and wrist

Most of the arthritides listed previously can involve the hand. The most common of these include osteoarthritis, rheumatoid arthritis, psoriatic arthritis, crystals (gout and pseudogout), viral, and systemic lupus erythematosus (SLE). Other nonarthritic conditions are listed below.

Ask patient to flex and extend fingers and then wrists. Observe patient fastening buttons. Note degree of movement and any limitation or pain.

Some differential diagnoses and typical outline evidence

Dupuytren's contracture usually familial or associated with alcohol or anti-epileptic therapy	*Suggested by:* progressive flexion deformity of base ring and little fingers, mainly with palmar fibrosis. Often bilateral. Family history
	Confirmed by: fixed flexion at MCP joints first, then interphalyngeal joints (inability to place hand on flat surface is severe)
Ganglion cyst	*Suggested by:* painless, spherical swelling at wrist
	Confirmed by: fluctuant, soft sphere. Disappears spontaneously or after a blow (e.g., from a book)
Carpal tunnel syndrome	*Suggested by:* pain and parasthesia of the thumb, index and radial side of the ring finger
	Confirmed by: EMG
Trigger finger due to nodule sticking in tendon sheath	*Suggested by:* fixed flexion at the ring or little finger with no fibrosis in palm. Patient unable to extend finger spontaneously due to pain
	Confirmed by: "click" as fingers passively extended. Nodule palpable on flexor surface of finger
De Quervain's syndrome— stenosing tenosynovitis	*Suggested by:* pain at wrist, e.g., when lifting teapot. History of forceful hand-use, e.g., wringing clothes
	Confirmed by: pain over radial styloid process, made worse by forced adduction and flexion of thumb into palm
Volkmann's ischemic contracture due to ischemia flexor muscles of thumb and fingers (supplied by brachial artery)	*Suggested by:* flexion deformity at thumb, fingers, wrist, and elbow with forearm pronation. History of trauma or surgery near to brachial artery, or plaster of Paris applied too tightly to forearm
	Confirmed by: cold, dark, ischemic arm, no pulse at the wrist, and pain when fingers extended
Recent trauma	*Suggested by:* history of recent impact and acute deformity
	Confirmed by: acute pain and deformity clinically and on X-ray

Pain or limitation of movement at the elbow

Many of the arthritides listed previously can involve the elbow. The most common of these include osteoarthritis, rheumatoid arthritis, psoriatic arthritis, and crystal-induced arthritides (gout and pseudogout), Other nonarthritic conditions are listed below.

Ask the patient to straighten the arms, and compare them for deformity and deviation from the normal valgus angle. Most patients hyperextend the elbow between 5° and 15°. Ask the patient to flex the elbow and to supinate and rotate normally over 90°. Note the degree of movement, and any limitation or pain.

Some differential diagnoses and typical outline evidence

Epicondylitis: tennis elbow (tenoperiostitis)	*Suggested by:* preceding repetitive strain, e.g., use of screwdriver, tennis racket. Pain worse when patient asked to flex fingers and wrist and pronate hand against resistance
	Confirmed by: absence of any evidence of swelling or loss of range of motion. Improvement after avoidance of repetitive movement
Old trauma	*Suggested by:* history of past impact or fracture and deformity
	Confirmed by: deformity on clinical examination and **elbow X-ray**
Recent trauma	*Suggested by:* history of recent impact and acute deformity
	Confirmed by: acute pain and deformity clinically and on **elbow X-ray**

Pain or limitation of movement at the shoulder

Many of the arthritides listed previously can involve the shoulder. The most common of these include osteoarthritis and rheumatoid arthritis. Other nonarthritic conditions are listed below.

Ask patients to put their arms behind their head, and behind their back and note the angle at which any restriction and pain occurs.

Some differential diagnoses and typical outline evidence

Rotator cuff tears of the supraspinatus tendon or adjacent subsapularis or infraspinatus tendons	*Suggested by:* limitation and/or pain on abduction at the shoulder to the first 60° range (achieved by scapular rotation). Age >40 years, participation in sports (common sports injury) *Confirmed by:* passive movement is pain-free and spontaneous above 90°. **MRI** showing communication between joint capsule and subacromial bursa
Supraspinatus tendinopathy (due to partial tear)	*Suggested by:* limitation and/or pain on abduction at the shoulder in the final 60° to 90° range. Age 35–60 years *Confirmed by:* some active movement up to 90°. Movement is pain-free and spontaneous above 90°.
Chronic supraspinatus inflammation, calcification	*Suggested by:* past history of acute limitation and continued limitation and/or pain on abduction at the shoulder in the final 60° to 90° range. Age 35–60 years *Confirmed by:* clinically or calcification in muscle on **shoulder X-ray** sometimes
Biceps tendonitis	*Suggested by:* pain in front of the shoulder aggravated by contraction of the biceps. *Confirmed by:* above clinical findings.
Rupture of long head of biceps	*Suggested by:* pain in front of the shoulder *Confirmed by:* pain aggravated by contraction of the biceps and lump (contracting muscle belly) appears.
Frozen shoulder— adhesive capsulitis	*Suggested by:* marked reduction in active and passive movement with <90° abduction *Confirmed by:* above clinical findings and normal **shoulder X-ray**

Pain or limitation of movement at the neck

Many of the arthritides listed previously can involve the neck. The most common of these include osteoarthritis and rheumatoid arthritis. Other nonarthritic conditions are listed below.

Look at the patient from the side to see if there is normal cervical (and lumbar) lordosis. Ask the patient to 1) flex and extend the neck, 2) tilt the head, moving the ear toward the shoulder, and 3) rotate the neck by looking over the shoulders. Note the angle at which any restriction and pain occur.

Some differential diagnoses and typical outline evidence

Spasmodic torticollis/ cervical dystonia due to trapezius and sternomastoid spasm	*Suggested by:* recurrent onset of sudden painful, stiff neck with torticollis, from age 10 to 30. Family history or minor injury *Confirmed by:* history and absence of root compression pattern pain or paresis
Infantile torticollis due to birth damage of steromastoid	*Suggested by:* onset in early childhood (up to age 3 years). Head tilted to shoulder and retarded facial growth on affected muscle side *Confirmed by:* palpable nodule in muscle on affected side. **Biopsy of nodule**: fibrous only, no gangliocytoma
Cervical rib with compression of lower brachial plexus affecting median and ulnar nerves and brachial artery	*Suggested by:* weakness, pain, and numbness in forearm and hand, usually on ulnar side *Confirmed by:* wasting and weakness of thenar and hypothenar muscles. Loss of sensation medially in hand and arm. Arm cyanosis and absent pulse. Cervical rib may not be visible on **neck X-ray** (fibrous band instead)
Posterior prolapsed cervical disc usually C5/C6 disc and C6/C7 disc effect on nerve roots	*Suggested by:* torticollis, stiffness and pain in neck over side of disc lesion. Pain, numbness in arm and tip of little or middle finger or thumb *Confirmed by:* loss of biceps or supinator reflexes. Loss of sensation in medial or lateral borders of hand. **MRI scan** shows posterior protrusion.
Anterior prolapsed cervical disc usually C5/C6 disc and C6/C7 disc affect spinal cord	*Suggested by:* torticollis, stiffness & pain in neck over side of disc lesion. Numbness and weakness in leg *Confirmed by:* flaccid first, then spastic paresis of leg. Loss of knee, ankle reflexes, and extensor plantar response. Loss of vibration sense, touch and pain with sensory level. **MRI scan** shows protrusion

Pain or limitation of movement of the back: with sudden onset over seconds to hours originally

Evaluation may be limited because of significant pain. Look from the side to see if there is normal lumbar lordosis. Ask the patient to touch the toes and watch for movement of the spine (rounded?) and hips. Ask the patient to arch backward, bend to each side, and rotate the trunk from side to side. Have the patient lie down and measure the length of the legs. Raise each straight leg for any restriction before 45°.

Some differential diagnoses and typical outline evidence

Mechanical pain Strains, tears, or crushing of ligaments, discs, vertebrae with normal healing	*Suggested by:* recent onset over minutes of pain and restriction of movement in the lower back
	Confirmed by: recovery with minimal loss of function over days or weeks
Posterior lumbar disc prolapse	*Suggested by:* onset over seconds of severe back pain on coughing, sneezing, or twisting after earlier strain. Radiation to buttock, thigh, or calf if prolapse compresses posterior root
	Confirmed by: back flexed and extension restricted. Straight-leg raising stops before 45° by pain. Loss of sensation in lateral foot (L4/5). Loss of ankle jerk and sensation in sole of foot (S1)
Anterior lumbar disc prolapse	*Suggested by:* onset over seconds of severe back pain on coughing, sneezing, or twisting after earlier strain. If large, prolapse compresses cauda equina, with leg weakness, incontinence, and numbness around perineum
	Confirmed by: flaccid paresis of leg(s). Loss of knee and ankle reflexes and extensor plantar response. Loss of vibration sense, touch and pain with sensory level. *MRI scan* shows protrusion
Spondylolisthesis due to spondylolysis, congenital malformation of articular process, osteoarthritis of posterior facet joints	*Suggested by:* sudden onset over minutes of back pain with or without sciatica in adolescence
	Confirmed by: *plain back X-ray* shows forward displacement of vertebra over the one below

Acute vertebral fracture secondary to osteoporosis	*Suggested by:* severe pain with history of osteoporosis or previous vertebral fracture. Spinal kyphosis can be present. Lumbar vertebral fractures can produce pain radiating to abdomen
	Confirmed by: X-ray appearance suggestive of wedge fracture
Central disc protrusion	*Suggested by:* sudden onset over minutes or hours with bilateral sciatica, disturbance of bladder or bowel function. Saddle or perineal anesthesia
	Confirmed by: history and compression of cord visible on *MRI scan*

Pain or limitation of movement of the back: with onset over days to months originally

Many of the arthritides listed previously can involve the back. The most common of these are osteoarthritis and the spondyloarthropathies, including ankylosing spondylitis and psoriatic arthritis. Other nonarthritic conditions are listed below.

Look at the patient from the side to see if there is normal lumbar lordosis. Ask the patient to touch the toes, and watch for movement of the spine (rounded?) and hips. Ask the patient to arch backward, bend to each side, and rotate the trunk from side to side. Lay the patient down and measure the length of the legs. Raise each straight leg for any restriction before 45°.

Perform modified Schober test

With the patient standing straight and feet together, mark a line on the spine at the level of the top of the iliac crest (approximately L5), then measure and mark 10 cm above and 5 cm below that line. Ask the patient to bend over and touch the toes, bending the knees if necessary. The excursion of the lumbar spine should be at least 20 cm.

Some differential diagnoses and typical outline evidence

Lumbar spinal stenosis due to facet joint osteoarthrosis	*Suggested by:* onset of pain over months worse on standing or walking with radiation down the legs. Pain improved with flexing forward, or walking with the aid of a grocery cart
	Confirmed by: pain on extension of back. Straight-leg raising normal. Distinguished from vascular claudication by precipitation with standing as well as walking
Spinal tumors Primary arising in spinal cord, meninges, nerve roots Secondary usually from lung, breast, prostate, thyroid, kidney, lymphoma, myeloma	*Suggested by:* onset of back pain over months, with progressive pain or paresis in one or both legs. Physical signs depend on the part of cord or nerve roots affected.
	Confirmed by: "hot spot" on bone scan with erosion or sclerosis on plain X-ray of hot spot. Space-occupying lesion on **MRI** or **CT scan** and **histology on biopsy**

Pyogenic spinal infection usually of disc space due to *Staphylococcus*, *Salmonella typhi*, etc.	*Suggested by:* onset of pain over days or weeks. Little or no fever, tenderness or raised WBC. ESR is raised. Background of debilitation, surgery, or diabetes
	Confirmed by: bone rarefaction or erosion with joint space narrowing on ***back X-ray***. "Hot spot" on ***isotope bone scan*** and space-occupying lesion on ***MRI*** or ***CT scan***
Spinal TB with abscesses and cord compression (Pott's para-plegia), psoas abscess	*Suggested by:* onset of weeks or months. Little fever, tenderness, or ↑WBC. ESR ↑. Background of debilitation, diabetes
	Confirmed by: bone rarefaction or erosion with joint space narrowing, then wedging of vertebrae. Space-occupying lesion on ***MRI and CT scan***. Tubercle bacilli on stains or ***culture of drainage material***
Spondylitis (ankylosing spondylitis and associated disorders)	*Suggested by:* onset over months. Usually presenting in young adult, with morning stiffness of ≥1 hour. ↑CRP or ESR; HLA-B27 positive
	Confirmed by: early disease may only be evident by sacroiliitis confirmed by X-ray or MRI. Late disease confirmed by abnormal Schober, decreased thoracic expansion, on X-ray: sacroiliac erosion or fusion with bridging syndesmophytes leading to bamboo spine
Idiopathic scoliosis of thoracic or lumbar spine	*Suggested by:* progressive loss over years of horizontal alignment of shoulders and hips with age, usually in adolescent girls more than boys
	Confirmed by: absence of evidence of specific or treatable cause. Increased scoliosis with growth
Kyphotic pain	*Suggested by:* history of previous vertebral fractures with "Dowager's hump" for years, with associated protuberant abdomen and height loss
	Confirmed by: X-ray appearance suggestive of congenital deformity, Scheurmann's or Calve's osteochondritis, wedge fracture from osteoporosis or carcinoma
Scoliotic pain	*Suggested by:* lateral curvature visible from the back and associated rib prominence apparent from the front
	Confirmed by: history and X-ray appearance of bony congenital anomaly, past poliomyelitis, syringomyelia, torsion dystonia, spinal tumors, spondylolisthesis, arthrogryphosis, enchondromatosis, osteogenesis imperfecta, neurofibromatosis, Chiari malformation, Duchenne muscular dystrophy, Freiderich's ataxia, Marfan syndrome, Pompe's disease

Pain or limitation of movement of the hip

Many of the arthritides listed previously can involve the hip. The most common of these are osteoarthritis, rheumatoid arthritis, and the spondyloarthropathies, including ankylosing spondylitis and psoriatic arthritis. Other nonarthritic conditions are listed below.

Assess the patient's activity. Test flexion (normal >120°) by grasping ankle in one hand and iliac crest in the other to eliminate pelvic rotation. Test abduction (normal 30°–40°) preventing pelvic tilt. Test abduction in flexion (normal >70°) and adduction (normal >30°) by moving one foot over the other, internal and external rotation (normal >30°). Measure the true length of the legs from the anterior superior iliac spine to medial malleoli. The Trendelenburg test is positive if the hip drops when the foot on that same side is lifted from the ground. Look for a leg length discrepancy that can exacerbate hip pain (usually on the shorter leg).

Some differential diagnoses and typical outline evidence

Osteoarthritis	*Suggested by:* onset over months or years. Pain, stiffness, and limitation of movement, initially of internal rotation. Frequently unilateral
	Confirmed by: **A-P and lateral X-ray of hips** shows loss of joint space, deformity of head and acetabulum with osteophytes and sclerosis
Inflammatory arthritis	*Suggested by:* onset over months or years. Pain, stiffness, and limitation of movement, initially of internal rotation, more commonly bilateral in patients with systemic inflammatory arthritis
	Confirmed by: **A-P and lateral X-ray of hips** shows loss of joint space, deformity of head and acetabulum, eventually with secondary osteoarthritic changes
Osteonecrosis, *aka* avascular necrosis	*Suggested by:* onset over days to months. Pain, stiffness, and limitation of movement, initially of internal rotation. History of corticosteroid use or excessive alcohol intake
	Confirmed by: **A-P and lateral X-ray of hips:** early disease may only be evident on **MRI scan** of hips; within months, a crescent lucency within the superior edge of femoral head will be evident, and eventually, collapse of the femoral head and secondary osteoarthritic changes

Coxa vara (angle between neck and femur <125°) caused by congenital slipped upper femoral epiphyses, fracture with malunion or non-union, osteomalacia, or Paget's disease	*Suggested by:* limp with Trendelenburg "dip" to affected side. True shortening of leg *Confirmed by:* angle between neck and femur <125° on *X-ray*
Perthes' disease Idiopathic osteonecrosis of the hip	*Suggested by:* pain in hip or knee with limp, with onset over months from 3 to 11 years of age. Limitation of hip movement in all ranges *Confirmed by: A-P and lateral X-ray* of hips shows widening of joint space and decrease in size of femoral head, patchy density, and later collapse
Slipped femoral epiphysis	*Suggested by:* pain in groin, front of thigh, or knee and limping with onset over minutes if acute, or weeks to months. Limitation of flexion, abduction, and medial rotation *Confirmed by:* displacement of growth plate visible on *lateral view of hip* (not A-P)
Tuberculous arthritis	*Suggested by:* pain and limp in a 2- to 5-year old, especially in endemic areas. Pain and spasm in all directions of movement *Confirmed by:* rarefaction of bone on *X-ray* then fuzziness of joint margin, then erosions. AFB in *biopsy ± culture of synovial membrane*
Developmental dysplasia with dislocation leading to osteoarthritis	*Suggested by:* pain, stiffness, and restricted movement in childhood or adolescence if undiagnosed (or noisy reduction of dislocation in neonatal click test) *Confirmed by:* shallow acetabulum with or without current dislocation on *A-P and lateral X-ray of hips* (or ultrasound in neonate)

Pain or limitation of movement of the knee

Many of the arthritides listed previously can involve the knee. The most common of these are osteoarthritis, gout, pseudogout, rheumatoid arthritis, and the spondyloarthropathies, including ankylosing spondylitis and psoriatic arthritis.

Look for quadriceps wasting, deformity of the knee, or swelling. Compare flexion and extension on both sides. Abduct and adduct tibia with the knee flexed at 30° to test medial and lateral ligaments. With the knee flexed at 90° pull and push tibia to test anterior and posterior cruciate ligaments.

Feel for warmth over the knee (the knee should be cooler than the anterior lower leg). A small knee effusion can be detected by "milking" the fluid into the superior patellar pouch medially, and then pressing on the lateral patella to see a fluid wave. Look for leg length discrepancy that can exacerbate pain in the shorter leg.

Some differential diagnoses and typical outline evidence

Osteoarthritis	*Suggested by:* onset of months or years, worse in cold and damp. Deformity (can be varus, bow-legged, or valgus, knock-kneed) and swelling. Crepitus on passive movement. More common in obese patients or if there is a history of previous trauma to that joint *Confirmed by:* above history and examination. Loss of joint space on X-ray with deformity (usually medial compartment), osteophytes, and sclerosis
Chondromalacia patellae	*Suggested by:* patella aching after sitting in young adults. Patellar tenderness *Confirmed by:* above history and examination or softening or fibrillation of patellar cartilage on arthroscopy or *MRI scan*
Recurrent patellar subluxation	*Suggested by:* knee often giving way (especially in knock-kneed girls) *Confirmed by:* above increased lateral movement of patella
Patella tendinopathy (jumper's knee)	*Suggested by:* pain on forceful movement of knee in sport *Confirmed by:* tenderness over patellar tendon
Ileotibial tract syndrome	*Suggested by:* pain when running *Confirmed by:* tenderness over lateral femoral condyle.
Medial shelf syndrome	*Suggested by:* brief locking of knee *Confirmed by:* inflamed synovial fold above medial meniscus on arthroscopy
Hoffa's fat pad syndrome	Suggested by: brief locking of knee and pain under patella, more common in obese woman with valgus knee deformities *Confirmed by:* hypertrophic pad between articular surfaces on *MRI scan* or arthroscopy

Acute arthritis due to sepsis, crystal-induced arthritis	*Suggested by:* onset over hours or days of pain, swelling, warmth
	Confirmed by: aspiration, microscopy and culture. Urate ↑ in gout
Meniscal cyst	*Suggested by:* variable swelling, worse when knee flexed to 60°, less when flexed further. Knee clicking and giving way
	Confirmed by: cyst present on **MRI scan**
Ligament tears	*Suggested by:* sudden pain and swelling after forceful abduction or adduction at knee
	Confirmed by: above history, tenderness on examination, appearance on **MRI scan**
Anterior cruciate tears	*Suggested by:* history of posterior blow or rotational force when foot fixed to ground
	Confirmed by: tibia moves forward when pulled (after effective analgesia or anesthesia), appearance on **MRI scan**
Meniscal tear	*Suggested by:* history of forceful twisting to a flexed knee. Knee locks when extension attempted
	Confirmed by: tear visible on **MRI scan**
Osgood-Schlatter disease Osteochondritis	*Suggested by:* 11- to 12-year-old girl or 13- to 14-year-old boy after rapid growth spurt, with pain and swelling of the tibial tubercle, can occur after exercise, occasionally locking
	Confirmed by: tenderness and soft tissue or bony prominence of the tibial tubercle
Osteoid osteoma	*Suggested by:* pain and after exercise, intermittent knee swelling and locking
	Confirmed by: defect on articular surface on X-ray
Loose bodies due to osteochondritis dessicans, osteoarthritis, chip fractures, synovial chondromatosis	*Suggested by:* locking of knee during extension and flexion. Swelling and effusion
	Confirmed by: seeing loose bodies on arthoscopy
Bursitis (with or without infection) due to prepatellar bursitis (housemaid's knee), etc.	*Suggested by:* localized pain and swelling over site of bursa (e.g., below patella)
	Confirmed by: localized pain and swelling over site of bursa. With infection, aspiration of the bursal fluid and microscopy and culture. For repetitive injury, improvement with rest, analgesia, and physiotherapy

Pain or limitation of movement of the foot and ankle

Many of the arthritides listed previously can involve the feet. The most common of these are osteoarthritis, gout, rheumatoid arthritis, and the spondyloarthropathies, including ankylosing spondylitis and psoriatic arthritis.

Watch the patient's gait and examine wear on the shoe sole and the print on the floor from their damp foot. Ask the patient to extend or dorsiflex (normal >25°), flex (normal 30°), evert and invert. Ask the patient to extend the toes (normal >60°) and stand on tiptoe.

Some differential diagnoses and typical outline evidence

Hallux valgus Associated with bunion and osteoarthritis	*Suggested by:* big toe deviated laterally. Frequently causes pain especially with tight shoes *Confirmed by:* above clinical appearance
Pes planus	*Suggested by:* loss of medial foot arch (appearance of damp surface in contact with floor, normal in early childhood). Pain if foot and heel everted in some *Confirmed by:* above clinical appearance and response to exercises and medial heel shoe wedges in some cases
Pes cavus idiopathic, due to spina bifida, past polio	*Suggested by:* accentuated foot arches and other neurological disorders, e.g., spina bifida *Confirmed by:* above clinical appearance
Posterior ankle tendinopathy	*Suggested by:* pain and/or swelling of the tendon *Confirmed by:* MRI
Achilles tendon rupture	*Suggested by:* audible snap with pain in the calf; has been associated with fluoroquinolone antibiotics especially combined with corticosteroids *Confirmed by:* inability to stand on toes, MRI
Hammer toes	*Suggested by:* tip of toe points downward *Confirmed by:* toe extended at the metatarsophalangeal (MTP) joint, flexed at the proximal interphalangeal (PIP) joint, but extended at the DIP joint
Claw toes	*Suggested by:* tip of toe points down and back *Confirmed by:* toe extended at the MTP joint, flexed at the proximal (PIP) and distal (DIP) joints
Hallux rigidus	*Suggested by:* pain localized proximal to big toe *Confirmed by:* tenderness and swelling of first MTP joint. X-ray may show a distal ring of osteophytes

Metatarsalgia due to shoe pressure, previous trauma, rheumatoid arthritis, sesamoid fracture, synovitis	*Suggested by:* pain in forefoot
	Confirmed by: tenderness of heads of metatarsals
Morton's metatarsalgia due to interdigital neuroma	*Suggested by:* localized sharp pain on dorsum of foot, with radiation between 2 metatarsals down to toes
	Confirmed by: tenderness on compression of site of neuroma between metatarsals
March fracture	*Suggested by:* localized foot pain after excessive walking
	Confirmed by: tenderness of second or third metatarsal. X-ray showing fracture
Calcaneum disease; arthritis of subtalar joint; tear of calcaneal tendon; post-calcaneal bursitis; plantar fasciitis; etc.	*Suggested by:* localized heel pain
	Confirmed by: **MRI scan** appearance

Chapter 17

Psychiatric symptoms and signs

Psychiatric signs

Psychiatric symptoms and signs are noted to a large extent during the history and examination. The patient may have complained of anxiety or depression, but in order for these diagnoses to be accepted by others, specific features should be present, some of which are observed, rather than reported by the patient.

General excessive anxiety

Some differential diagnoses and typical outline evidence

Generalized anxiety disorder	*Suggested by:* long history of fearful anticipation, irritability, sensitivity to noise, restlessness, poor concentration, worrying thoughts, insomnia, nightmares, depression, obsessions, depersonalization, dry mouth, difficulty swallowing, tremor, dizziness, headache, parasthesias, tinnitus, epigastric discomfort, frequent or loose motions, constriction or discomfort in the chest, difficulty breathing or hyperventilation, palpitations and awareness of missed beats, frequency or urgency of micturition, erectile dysfunction, menstrual problems. Panic attacks, depression, and alcohol dependence *Confirmed by:* no evidence of thyrotoxicosis, hypoglycemia, Cushing's disease, or pheochromocytoma
Panic disorder	*Suggested by:* intense feeling of apprehension or impending disaster. Develops quickly and unexpectedly without a recognizable trigger. Shortness of breath and smothering, nausea, abdominal pain, depersonalization, choking, numbness, tingling, palpitations, flushes, trembling, shaking, chest discomfort, fear of dying, sweating, dizziness, faintness *Confirmed by:* Four symptoms of panic attack in one episode and four attacks in a month, or a persistent fear of attacks
Alcohol withdrawal	*Suggested by:* recent decrease in alcohol intake, usually superimposed on habitually high intake. Visual and/or tactile hallucinations suggest delirium tremens. *Confirmed by:* subsequent episodes in similar circumstances
Thyrotoxicosis	*Suggested by:* heat intolerance, tremor, nervousness, palpitation, frequent bowel movements, goiter *Confirmed by:* ↓TSH, ↑FT4
Hypoglycemia	*Suggested by:* preceded by seconds or minutes by anxiety, fear, chest tightness, sweating, hunger, and darkening of vision. Usually in diabetic, usually on insulin *Confirmed by:* ↓ blood glucose (<40 mg/dL)
Pheochromocytoma	*Suggested by:* abrupt episodes of anxiety, fear, chest tightness, sweating, headaches, and marked rises in BP *Confirmed by:* catecholamines (↑VMA, ↑HMMA) or free metanephrine ↑ in urine and blood soon after episode

Anxiety in response to specific issues

Some differential diagnoses and typical outline evidence

Anorexia nervosa	*Suggested by:* intense fear of gaining weight, though underweight. Amenorrhea in women for ≥3 months and diminished sexual interest. Bingeing and vomiting, purging or excessive exercise. Depression and social withdrawal, sensitivity to cold, delayed gastric emptying, constipation, low blood pressure, bradycardia, hypothermia
	Confirmed by: BMI <17.5 kg/m² and many of above clinical features
Bulimia nervosa	*Suggested by:* fear of gaining weight, recurrent episodes of binge eating, far beyond normally accepted amounts of food. Vomiting, use of laxatives, diuretics ± appetite suppressants
	Confirmed by: normal menses and normal weight
Somatization or hysteria alone or with depression, anxiety, schizophrenia, and substance abuse	*Suggested by:* physical symptoms with preoccupation with bodily sensations combined with a fear of physical illness
Somatization disorder (Briquet's syndrome)	*Suggested by:* long history of numerous unsubstantiated physical complaints with no adequate physical explanation and refusal to be reassured
Simple phobia	*Suggested by:* symptoms and signs of generalized anxiety disorder
	Confirmed by: inappropriate anxiety in the presence of particular circumstances, e.g., enclosed spaces (claustrophobia), spiders (arachnophobia)
Social phobia	*Suggested by:* intense and persistent fear of being scrutinized or negatively evaluated by others, resulting in fear and avoidance of social situations (e.g., meeting people in authority, using a telephone, speaking in front of a group). May fear most or specific social situations

Agoraphobia	*Suggested by:* panic attacks in crowds or situations where escape is difficult. Staying at home, will not visit doctors. Also depression, depersonalization, and obsessional thoughts
Post-traumatic stress disorder caused by experiencing or witnessing a traumatic event, e.g., major accident, fire, assault, military combat	*Suggested by:* memories, nightmares (up to years after event), flashbacks, numbing of emotions, anxiety and irritability, insomnia, poor concentration, hypervigilance. Accompanying depression, anxiety, and drug or alcohol abuse or dependence

Depression

Some differential diagnoses and typical outline evidence

Major depression	*Suggested by:* depressed mood ± loss of interest in pleasure
	Confirmed by: for example, the additional presence of ≥5 of the following 7 symptoms: (1) change in appetite or weight, (2) psychomotor agitation or retardation, (3) insomnia or hypersomnia, (4) sense of worthlessness or guilt, (5) fatigue or loss of energy, (6) recurrent thoughts of death, (7) poor concentration
Mild to moderate depression	*Suggested by:* depressed mood ± loss of interest in pleasure
	Confirmed by: for example, the additional presence of <5 of the following 7 symptoms: (1) change in appetite or weight, (2) psychomotor agitation or retardation, (3) insomnia or hypersomnia, (4) sense of worthlessness or guilt, (5) fatigue or loss of energy, (6) recurrent thoughts of death, (7) poor concentration
Depression secondary or partly due to other conditions	*Suggested by:* history of any other illness that undermines self-confidence but especially anxiety disorders, alcohol abuse, substance abuse
	Confirmed by: improvement when underlying condition alleviated
Depression secondary or partly due to medication	*Suggested by:* history of taking beta blockers, alpha blockers, anticonvulsants, calcium channel blockers, corticosteroids, oral contraceptives, antipsychotic drugs, drugs used for Parkinson's disease (e.g., levodopa)
	Confirmed by: improvement when drug stopped or changed
Seasonal affective disorder	*Suggested by:* "winter blues": depression of mood + ↑ sleep, ↑ food intake (with carbohydrate craving), and weight gain, sometimes with opposite mood swings in summer

Hallucinations, delusions, or thought disorder

Hallucinations are visions, voices, and sounds not apparent to others present. *Delusion* is the holding of a belief despite evidence to the contrary. In *thought disorder*, thoughts jump from one idea to another in a bizarre way.

Some differential diagnoses and typical outline evidence

Mania and hypomania	*Suggested by:* persistent high or euphoric mood out of keeping with circumstances
	Confirmed by: pressure of speech, no insight, over-assertiveness, increased energy and activity, grandiose delusions, spending sprees, increased appetite, hallucinations, disinhibition, increased sexual desire, labile mood, elation, self-important ideas, diminished pain threshold, irritability, poor concentration, hostility when thwarted, diminished desire or need for sleep
Bipolar disorder or manic depression	*Suggested by:* consists of episodes when the patient has mania (bipolar I) or hypomania (bipolar II) against a background of depression
Acute schizophrenia	*Suggested by:* sufferer's apparent inability to distinguish between imaginary and external world
	Confirmed by: at least one of the following Schneider first-rank symptoms: somatic hallucinations, thought insertion ± withdrawal, thought broadcasting, primary delusions (in addition to thought delusions, passivity feelings, thought echo, or hearing voices referring to the patient in the third person)
Chronic schizophrenia	*Suggested by:* sufferer appearing unable to relate to external world, with blunting of affect
	Confirmed by: thought disorder and poverty of thought, apathy, inactivity, lack of volition, social withdrawal, and loss of affect

Confusion (global cognitive deficit)

This condition may be acute or chronic.

Some differential diagnoses and typical outline evidence

Acute confusional state (delirium) caused by infection, drugs, metabolic, alcohol or drug withdrawal, hypoxia, cardiovascular disease, intracranial lesion, thyrotoxicosis or hypothyroidism, carcinomatosis, epilepsy, nutritional deficiency	*Suggested by:* global cognitive deficit with onset over hours or days, fluctuating conscious level (typically worse at night), impaired memory (on recovery amnsia of the events is usual), disorientation in time and place, odd behavior (may be underactive, drowsy ± withdrawn or hyperactive and agitated), disordered thinking, often slow and muddled ± delusions (e.g., accuse relatives of taking things), disturbed perceptions, hallucinations (particularly visual), mood swings *Confirmed by:* outcome consistent with underlying cause and treatment
Chronic confusion due to Alzheimer's disease (60%), vascular (multi-infarct) dementia, dementia with Lewy bodies	*Suggested by:* patient admitting to "being a bit forgetful," but relatives complain of loss of short-term memory and inability to perform normally simple tasks, failure to cope at home, or self-neglect *Confirmed by:* no impairment of consciousness, clear history of progressive impairment of memory and cognition ± personality change, ± cerebral atrophy on CT brain scan
Alzheimer's disease	*Suggested by:* features of dementia *Confirmed by:* absence of features of vascular (multi-infarct) dementia or Parkinsonism
Vascular (multi-infarct) dementia	*Suggested by:* tends to occur with a stepwise progression of dementia with each subsequent infarct and pseudobulbar palsy *Confirmed by:* by multiple lacunar infarcts or larger stroke's cause on CT scan
Lewy body dementia	*Suggested by:* fluctuating but persistent dementia with Parkinsonism and hallucinations *Confirmed by:* histology at postmortem
Other neurodegenerative diseases: Huntington's chorea, bovine spongiform encephalopathy	*Suggested by:* other neuromuscular signs, e.g., seizures, abnormal posture, etc. *Confirmed by:* clinical and postmortem brain specimens

Laboratory tests

Asymptomatic microscopic hematuria

This is detected on routine urine dipstick testing.

Some differential diagnoses and typical outline evidence

Menstruation	*Suggested by:* history of current, recent, or imminent periods and no urinary symptoms
	Confirmed by: negative on repeating in mid-cycle
Urinary tract infection (UTI)	*Suggested by:* fever, frequency or dysuria, Nitrites ↑, leukocytes ↑ on dipstick
	Confirmed by: urine microscopy and culture, response to antibiotics. Ultrasound scan for possible anatomical abnormality
Recent urethral trauma	*Suggested by:* recent urethral catheterization
	Confirmed by: history, no infection in urine
Bleeding diathesis	*Suggested by:* bruising, anticoagulant therapy
	Confirmed by: abnormal platelet and clotting screen
Calculus or tumor anywhere in renal tract	*Suggested by:* persistent ×3 microscopic hematuria
	Confirmed by: urinalysis, renal ultrasound, CT scan, then cystoscopy by urologist
Glomerulonephritis primary or secondary to systemic lupus erythematosus (SLE), subacute bacterial endocarditis (SBE), etc.	*Suggested by:* persistent ×3 microscopic hematuria, associated proteinuria, hypertension
	Confirmed by: urine microscopy, renal ultrasound, immunoglobulins (Igs), complement, anti-nuclear antibody (ANA), anti-neutrophil cytoplasmic antibody (ANCA)-positive blood cultures or response to antibiotics
Nephritis secondary to NSAIDs, etc.	*Suggested by:* persistent ×3 microscopic hematuria, taking NSAID or other suspicious drug
	Confirmed by: urine microscopy, renal ultrasound, improvement on stopping suspected drug

Asymptomatic proteinuria

Total protein excretion is usually <50 mg/24 hours, of which albumin alone is normally <30 mg/24 hours. Abnormal proteinuria is regarded as >150 mg/24 hours.

Some differential diagnoses and typical outline evidence

Postural or orthostatic proteinuria	*Suggested by:* specimen from an ambulatory person <40 years of age
	Confirmed by: protein testing negative on early morning urine specimen
Nonspecific febrile illness	*Suggested by:* known febrile illness
	Confirmed by: normal when illness resolved
Urinary tract infection (UTI)	*Suggested by:* fever. Presence of nitrites, leukocytes, and blood on urine dipstick test
	Confirmed by: Urine microscopy and culture. Ultrasound scan of abdomen for possible anatomical abnormality
Glomerulonephritis primary or secondary to SLE, etc.	*Suggested by:* proteinuria >1 g/24 hours, persistent x3 microscopic hematuria, hypertension
	Confirmed by: urine microscopy, renal ultrasound, and serum immunoglobulins, complement, ANA, ANCA, etc.
Nephritis secondary to NSAIDs, etc.	*Suggested by:* proteinuria >1 g/24 hours, taking NSAID or other suspicious drug
	Confirmed by: urine microscopy, renal ultrasound, improvement on stopping suspected drug
Nephrotic syndrome due to minimal-change disease, diabetes mellitus, etc.	*Suggested by:* proteinuria >3 g/24 hours
	Confirmed by: serum albumin low (<3 g/dL), edema and ↑ cholesterol and ↑ triglycerides

Glycosuria

This almost always indicates diabetes, and the blood glucose should be tested, but consider other possibilities.

Some differential diagnoses and typical outline evidence

Diabetes mellitus	*Suggested by:* fatigue or other unexplained symptoms, thirst, polydipsia, polyuria
	Confirmed by: fasting blood glucose ≥126 mg/dL on two occasions OR fasting; random or glucose tolerance test (GTT) glucose ≥200 mg/dL once only with symptoms
Renal glycosuria	*Suggested by:* patient well or renal disease
	Confirmed by: glycosuria with normal blood sugar on GTT

Raised urine or serum bilirubin

Some differential diagnoses and typical outline evidence

Hepatocellular jaundice (due to hepatitis or very severe liver failure) (see p. 422)	*Suggested by:* jaundice with *dark* stools and dark urine. Also raised urine urobilinogen (you can check this immediately)
	Confirmed by: raised serum bilirubin and raised urine urobilinogen. Highly abnormal liver function tests. Normal bile ducts but abnormal liver parenchyma on ultrasound scan
Obstructive jaundice due to intrahepatic causes (drugs, hepatitis, etc.) or extrahepatic (stones, tumors, etc.) (see p. 423)	*Suggested by:* jaundice with *pale* stools and dark urine. Also NO raised urinary urobilinogen
	Confirmed by: raised plasma bilirubin, markedly raised alkaline phosphatase; otherwise, slightly abnormal liver function tests. Dilated bile ducts on ultrasound scan

Hepatocellular jaundice

This condition is *suggested by* jaundice with *dark* stools and dark urine. It is *confirmed by* raised serum bilirubin and raised urine urobilinogen. There are highly abnormal liver function tests. Normal bile ducts appear on ultrasound scan.

Some differential diagnoses and typical outline evidence

Acute (viral) hepatitis A	*Suggested by:* tender hepatomegaly
	Confirmed by: presence of hepatitis A IgM antibody suggests acute infection
Acute hepatitis B	*Suggested by:* history of IV drug use, blood transfusion, needle punctures, tattoos, tender hepatomegaly
	Confirmed by: presence of HBsAg in serum
Acute hepatitis C	*Suggested by:* history of transfusion or other blood products. Tender hepatomegaly
	Confirmed by: presence of anti-HCV antibody and antigen
Alcoholic hepatitis	*Suggested by:* history of drinking, presence of spider nevi and other signs of chronic liver disease
	Confirmed by: AST:ALT ratio >2, liver biopsy
Drug-induced hepatitis, e.g., acetaminophen (dose dependent), halothane (independent)	*Suggested by:* drug history, recent surgery
	Confirmed by: improvement after stopping the offending drug
Primary hepatoma	*Suggested by:* weight loss, abdominal pain, RUQ mass
	Confirmed by: ultrasound/CT liver, liver biopsy, ↑α-fetoprotein
Right heart failure	*Suggested by:* ↑JVP, hepatomegaly, ankle edema
	Confirmed by: CXR, echocardiogram

Obstructive jaundice

This condition is *suggested by* jaundice with *pale* stools and dark urine. It is *confirmed by* raised urine and serum bilirubin but NO raised urobilinogen in urine. Markedly raised alkaline phosphatase occurs, with otherwise slightly abnormal liver function tests. Dilated bile ducts appear on ultrasound scan.

Some differential diagnoses and typical outline evidence

Common bile duct stones	*Suggested by:* pain in RUQ ± Murphy's sign
	Confirmed by: ultrasound liver/biliary ducts
Cancer of head of pancreas	*Suggested by:* painless jaundice, palpable gallbladder (Courvoisier's law), weight loss
	Confirmed by: CT pancreas, ERCP or MRCP
Sclerosing cholangitis	*Suggested by:* progressive fatigue, pruritus
	Confirmed by: serum alkaline phosphatase, no gallstones, ERCP (beading of the intra- and extrahepatic biliary ducts)
Primary biliary cirrhosis	*Suggested by:* scratch marks, non-tender hepatomegaly, ± splenomegaly, xanthelasmata and xanthomas, arthralgia
	Confirmed by: positive antimitochondrial antibody, ↑↑serum IgM, liver biopsy
Drug induced, e.g., oral contraceptives, phenothiazines, anabolic steroids, erythromycin	*Suggested by:* drug history
	Confirmed by: symptoms recede when offending drug is discontinued
Pregnancy (last trimester)	*Suggested by:* jaundice during pregnancy and severe itching
	Confirmed by: resolution following delivery
Alcoholic hepatitis or cirrhosis	*Suggested by:* history of drinking, presence of spider nevi and other signs of chronic liver disease
	Confirmed by: liver biopsy
Dubin–Johnson syndrome	*Suggested by:* intermittent jaundice and associated RUQ pain. No hepatomegaly
	Confirmed by: normal alkaline phosphatase, normal liver function tests. Urinary bilirubin is raised. Pigment granules on liver biopsy

Hypernatremia

Some differential diagnoses and typical outline evidence

Hypertonic plasma with hypervolemia (e.g., excess IV saline) or hypovolemia (e.g., diabetic polyuria or diabetes insipidus)	*Suggested by:* little hypotonic fluid orally or intravenously and thirsty, high volume of urine with low sodium content (e.g., in diabetic polyuria) *Confirmed by:* plasma osmolality high and urine osmolality higher (unless diabetes insipidus)
Diabetes inspidus with hypovolemia	*Suggested by:* drinking excessively and passing large volumes of urine (polydipsia and polyuria). Thirst *Confirmed by:* plasma osmolality high and urine osmolality low
Primary hyper-aldosteronism due to adrenal hyperplasia or Conn's syndrome with adrenal tumor	*Suggested by:* normal fluid intake, blood pressure elevated. Serum potassium ↓ *Confirmed by:* plasma renin activity low and aldosterone levels high. CT or MRI scan appearance

Hyponatremia

This also usually indicates hypotonicity—low plasma osmolality.

Some differential diagnoses and typical outline evidence

Hypotonic with hypovolemia due to excess renal or nonrenal loss	*Suggested by:* excessive diuretic therapy, history of renal tubular disease, diarrhea, vomit, fistula, burns, small bowel obstruction, blood loss
	Confirmed by: response to removal or treating of cause, IV saline with careful monitoring of electrolytes in severe cases
Hypotonic with normovolemia	*Suggested by:* history of severe hypothyroidism or glucocorticoid deficiency
	Confirmed by: response to treating cause, balancing fluid intake
Hypotonic with hypervolemia	*Suggested by:* history of water overload, cardiac failure, cirrhosis, renal failure, glucocorticoid deficiency, inappropriate antidiuretic hormone (ADH) secretion
	Confirmed by: response to treating cause, reducing fluid intake
Syndrome of inappropriate ADH secretion (SIADH)	*Suggested by:* serum sodium usually <120 mmol/L. Confusion, progressing to coma, mild edema
	Confirmed by: urine osmolality > serum osmolality despite serum osmolality being low (<270 mmol/L). Urine sodium >20 mmol/L usually

Hyperkalemia

Some differential diagnoses and typical outline evidence

Drug effect: potassium administration or other drug effect	*Suggested by:* potassium supplements, blood transfusion, ACE inhibitor, spironolactone, amilioride, triamterene, etc.
	Confirmed by: normal potassium when drug reduced or stopped
Metabolic acidosis, renal failure, diabetic ketoacidosis	*Suggested by:* usually obvious illness and severe metabolic disturbance, pH↓ and plasma HCO_3↓
	Confirmed by: response to treatment of metabolic disturbance
Addison's disease	*Suggested by:* fatigue, blood pressure low, pigmented buccal mucosa and palmar creases, Na↓, K↑
	Confirmed by: random and 9 A.M. cortisol ↓, ACTH↑, and poor response to corticotropin stimulation. Response to IV hydrocortisone and normal saline
Recent blood transfusion	*Suggested by:* history
	Confirmed by: fall in potassium after a few hours
Spurious result due to hemolysis in specimen bottle	*Suggested by:* laboratory reporting hemolysis in specimen bottle
	Confirmed by: normal potassium when repeated with no delay in delivery to lab

Hypokalemia

Some differential diagnoses and typical outline evidence

Diuretic therapy	*Suggested by:* taking thiazide or loop diuretic
	Confirmed by: normal potassium after stopping diuretic
Beta-agonist treatment	*Suggested by:* taking high doses of beta-agonist, usually in nebulizer for acute asthmatic attack in hospital
	Confirmed by: normal potassium after stopping drug
Vomiting, e.g., pyloric stenosis	*Suggested by:* history of severe vomiting with poor fluid intake
	Confirmed by: normal potassium without subsequent need for replacement when cause of vomiting treated
Chronic diarrhea, purgative abuse, intestinal fistula, villous adenoma of rectum	*Suggested by:* history of severe diarrhea or mucous loss
	Confirmed by: normal potassium without need for further replacement when cause treated subsequently
Primary hyperaldosteronism due to adrenal hyperplasia or Conn's syndrome with adrenal tumor	*Suggested by:* normal fluid intake, blood pressure ↑. Serum potassium ↓
	Confirmed by: plasma renin activity low and aldosterone levels high. CT or MRI scan appearance
Renal tubular defect	*Suggested by:* recovery phase from renal failure, recent pyelonephritis, associated myeloma, heavy metal poisoning
	Confirmed by: test for renal concentrating ability

Hypercalcemia

Present when specimen taken without a venous cuff and calcium result was corrected for albumin concentration.

Some differential diagnoses and typical outline evidence

Bone metastases from carcinoma of breast, bronchus, kidney, thyroid, ovary, colon	*Suggested by:* normal phosphate and high alkaline phosphatase
	Confirmed by: metastases on X-rays, CT or nuclear bone scan
Thiazide diuretics	*Suggested by:* mild hypercalcemia, drug history, normal phosphate and alkaline phosphatase.
	Confirmed by: normal calcium when drug stopped
Primary (or tertiary) hyperparathyroidism	*Suggested by:* low phosphate and high alkaline phosphatase (tertiary after years of secondary hyperparathyroidism)
	Confirmed by: plasma parathyroid levels high with high calcium
Myeloma	*Suggested by:* normal phosphate and alkaline phosphatase
	Confirmed by: Bence–Jones protein in urine. Protein electrophoresis. Lesions on X-ray, CT, or bone scan
Sarcoidosis	*Suggested by:* high phosphate and alkaline phosphatase. Bilateral hilar shadows on chest X-ray
	Confirmed by: noncaseating granulomata on biopsy, ↑ vitamin D levels and ↑ ACE levels
Vitamin D excess	*Suggested by:* drug history and ↑ phosphate
	Confirmed by: normal calcium when drug stopped
Thyrotoxicosis	*Suggested by:* mildly ↑ calcium, T4 ↑ or T3 ↑ and TSH very ↓. Normal phosphate and alkaline phosphatase
	Confirmed by: response to treatment of thyrotoxicosis
Ectopic parathyroid hormone due to lung cancer, usually	*Suggested by:* ↓ phosphate and ↑ alkaline phosphatase
	Confirmed by: plasma parathyroid levels ↑ with high calcium, presence of underlying neoplasm

Hypocalcemia

Present when specimen taken without a venous cuff and corrected for albumin concentration.

Some differential diagnoses and typical outline evidence

Vitamin D deficiency—due to dietary deficiency or 1, 25(OH)2D abnormality	*Suggested by:* diet history, ↓ phosphate and ± ↑alkaline phosphatase
	Confirmed by: decreased 1, 25(OH)$_2$ vitamin D, normal calcium after adequate treatment with vitamin D
Hypoparathyroidism (transient or permanent after thyroid surgery, autoimmune disease, radiations)	*Suggested by:* recent neck surgery ± ↑phosphate
	Confirmed by: parathyroid hormone ↓ or normal in presence of calcium ↓
Chronic renal failure	*Suggested by:* ± ↑phosphate, ± ↑creatinine, ± ↑alkaline phosphatase, normochromic anemia
	Confirmed by: improvement with control of renal failure and phosphate levels
Pseudohypo-parathyroidism	*Suggested by:* short stature, obesity, round face, short metacarpals, ± ↑phosphate
	Confirmed by: plasma parathyroid levels ↑ with calcium ↓ or normal
Pancreatitis	*Suggested by:* abdominal pain and tenderness, phosphate normal or ↓ normal alkaline phosphatase
	Confirmed by: ↑↑ serum amylase and ultrasound scan of abdomen
Fluid overload	*Suggested by:* history and ↓ phosphate and normal alkaline phosphatase
	Confirmed by: normalization with correction of fluid balance
Rhabdomyolysis	*Suggested by:* muscle pains, phosphate ↑
	Confirmed by: CPK↑↑, ± creatinine ↑

Raised alkaline phosphatase

Some differential diagnoses and typical outline evidence

Paget's disease	*Suggested by:* deformity of skull or tibia typically, ↑↑alkaline phosphatase
	Confirmed by: bone deformity, especially of skull and tibia, and urinary hydroxyproline ↑
Vitamin D deficiency due to dietary deficiency	*Suggested by:* diet history, ↓ phosphate and ↑alkaline phosphatase
	Confirmed by: 1,25 (OH)$_2$ vitamin D level ↓ and normal calcium after oral vitamin D and calcium supplement
Bone metastases from breast, bronchus, kidney, thyroid, ovary, colon	*Suggested by:* normal phosphate, ↑ calcium, and ↑alkaline phosphatase
	Confirmed by: evidence of metastases on X-ray, CT, or bone scan
Primary or tertiary hyperparathyroidism	*Suggested by:* low phosphate and ↑ alkaline phosphatase after years of secondary hyperparathyroidism
	Confirmed by: plasma parathyroid levels high with high calcium
Cholestasis	*Suggested by:* jaundice with *pale* stools and *dark* urine. Bilirubin conjugated and thus soluble in urine
	Confirmed by: ↑ urine and serum bilirubin but NO ↑ urobilinogen in urine. ↑↑ alkaline phosphatase, otherwise slightly abnormal liver function tests

Raised blood urea nitrogen (BUN) and creatinine (azotemia)

Some differential diagnoses and typical outline evidence

High protein load due to GI bleed, catabolism, sepsis, etc.	*Suggested by:* ↑BUN and near-normal creatinine, suggestive history and clinical signs *Confirmed by:* recovery when catabolism or GI bleeding stops
Prerenal azotemia due to hypovolemia from low fluid intake or high fluid loss of any cause	*Suggested by:* ↑BUN and creatinine with BUN/creatinine ratio >20. Low urine Na (<20 mEq/L) or fractional excretion of Na (<1). History of fluid imbalance with fluid loss exceeding intake. *Confirmed by:* improvement with restoration of fluid volume
Chronic renal failure (CKD, CRF) due to pyelonephritis, glomerulonephritis, interstitial nephritis, diabetes mellitus, renovascular disease, analgesic nephropathy, hypertension	*Suggested by:* ↑BUN and creatinine and not rising rapidly over days. ↓Hb, small renal size on ultrasound scan, etc. *Confirmed by:* renal biopsy appearance
Acute tubular necrosis, severe hypotension, nephrotoxins (NSAIDs aminoglycosides, amphoteracin B, etc.)	*Suggested by:* raised BUN and creatinine and rising rapidly over days. Hb normal. Recent acute illness with hypotension and oliguria (fall in urine output <1 mL/kg/hr). ↑K+, etc. Ultrasound scan: normal kidney size and no obstructive uropathy *Confirmed by:* no improvement when euvolemic and renal biopsy
Obstructive (or "postobstructive") renal failure	*Suggested by:* raised BUN and creatinine and rising further. Hb normal. Fall in urine output *Confirmed by:* Ultrasound scan showing dilatation of renal calyces or ureters. Improvement in renal function with bladder or ureteral catheterization or nephrostomy

Low hemoglobin

Some differential diagnoses and typical outline evidence

Microcytic anemia (see p. 433)	*Suggested by:* history of blood loss or familial microcytic anemias (especially in patients of Mediterranean origin)
	Confirmed by: ↓Hb and ↓MCV
Macrocytic anemia (see p. 434)	*Suggested by:* FH of pernicious anemia, medication or alcohol use
	Confirmed by: ↓Hb and ↑MCV
Normocytic anemia (see p. 435)	*Suggested by:* history of chronic intercurrent illness, e.g., pancytopenia, chronic renal failure
	Confirmed by: ↓Hb and MCV normal

Microcytic anemia

This is usually accompanied by low mean corpuscular hemoglobin concentration

Some differential diagnoses and typical outline evidence

Iron-deficiency anemia	*Suggested by:* history of blood loss (e.g., history of heavy periods, passing blood rectally) or poor diet
	Confirmed by: ↓ serum iron, ↓ ferritin, and total iron binding capacity ↑
Thalassemia: α, β, intermedia, and variants	*Suggested by:* FH, Mediterranean origin. MCV very low for degree of anemia
	Confirmed by: blood film: target and nucleated cells. Hb electrophoresis shows ↑HbF or ↑HbA2
Sideroblastic anemia, rarely congenital or acquired, due to alcohol, lead poisoning, etc.	*Suggested by:* history of chronic intercurrent illness e.g., chronic renal failure
	Confirmed by: ↑ serum iron, ↑ ferritin, and total iron binding capacity normal

Macrocytic anemia

Some differential diagnoses and typical outline evidence

B_{12} deficiency: pernicious anemia (PA), intestinal malabsorption	*Suggested by:* associated autoimmune disease, e.g., primary hypothyroidism, vitilgo, etc. Hb ↓, WBC and platelets low
	Confirmed by: ↓ serum B_{12} (folate often ↓ too, due to anorexia) but PA diagnosed in absence of general malabsorption
Folate deficiency	*Suggested by:* poor diet, pregnancy, lactation, general malabsorption
	Confirmed by: ↓ folate but serum B_{12} normal
Anti-folate drugs	*Suggested by:* phenytoin typically, barbiturates and similar, methotrexate and similar
	Confirmed by: response to high-dose folic acid treatment or stopping drug (serum folate may be normal)
Alcohol abuse	*Suggested by:* history of abuse and poor diet
	Confirmed by: response to abstention (serum folate may be normal)
Hepatitis and liver disease	*Suggested by:* abnormal liver enzymes
	Confirmed by: normal (or high) B_{12} and poor response to folic acid
Hypothyroidism	*Suggested by:* ↓T4 and ↑TSH
	Confirmed by: normal B_{12} and response to treatment with thyroxin
Hemolysis (due to reticulosis)	*Suggested by:* urobilinogen in urine
	Confirmed by: reticulocytes on blood film
Myelodysplasia	*Suggested by:* hepato- or splenomegaly
	Confirmed by: bone marrow examination, normal B_{12} and folate

Normocytic anemia

Some differential diagnoses and typical outline evidence

Anemia of chronic disease (e.g., rheumatoid arthritis, hypogonadism, etc.)	*Suggested by:* associated chronic disease *Confirmed by:* iron, B_{12}, normal. Folate often ↓, ferritin often ↑ from inflammation
Chronic renal failure (CKD, CRF)	*Suggested by:* azotemia, history of renal disease *Confirmed by:* response to erythropoietin treatment only
Anemia of pregnancy	*Suggested by:* pregnant state *Confirmed by:* persistence despite folic acid and iron supplements, resolution after birth
Hypothyroidism	*Suggested by:* ↓T4 and ↑TSH *Confirmed by:* normal B_{12} and response to treatment with thyroxin
Hemolysis	*Suggested by:* urobilinogen in urine *Confirmed by:* reticulocytes on blood film
Bone marrow failure	*Suggested by:* pancytopenia *Confirmed by:* bone marrow examination

Very high ESR or CRP

An ESR (erythrocyte sedimentation rate) or CRP (C-reactive protein) level that is just above normal is nonspecific, as it may be associated with any cause of inflammation, including infection. An ESR near 100 or above, however, is a good lead.

Some differential diagnoses and typical outline evidence

Severe bacterial infection, e.g., osteomyelitis, empyema, peritonitis	*Suggested by:* high fever, leukocytes ↑↑
	Confirmed by: positive bacterial culture from blood and/or site of infection and response to antibiotics and/or surgical drainage
Giant cell arteritis	*Suggested by:* localized headache, especially over temple, late loss of vision, ± muscle pain and stiffness in shoulder area
	Confirmed by: vessel wall inflammation on biopsy
Bacterial endocarditis	*Suggested by:* fever, changing heart murmur, splinter hemorrhages of nail beds
	Confirmed by: bacterial growth from several blood cultures, echocardiogram showing vegetations
Myeloma	*Suggested by:* bone pain or fractures. Bence–Jones protein in urine and monoclonal protein band on electrophoresis
	Confirmed by: myeloma cells on bone marrow examination
Prostatic carcinoma	*Suggested by:* bone pain, few urinary symptoms
	Confirmed by: sclerotic bone lesions and raised prostate-specific antigen (PSA) and/or prostatic biopsy

Chest X-ray appearances

The general approach

1. Use optimal viewing conditions, preferably recessed lighting to avoid monitor glare.

2. Check the patient's name, gender, age, and medical record number to ensure correct identity.

3. Check if the film is labeled PA (X-rays passing from posterior to anterior in a standard way) or AP (X-rays passing from anterior to posterior). AP views are commonly performed when the patient is ill, using a portable X-ray tube. These views will often be semi-erect films with suboptimal exposure factors. X-rays passing through the body from anterior to posterior magnify the mediastinum; therefore AP films should not be used to assess cardiac size or hilar configuration.

4. Check which sides are labeled left and right and whether the cardiac apex is on the left (if not, the patient may have dextrocardia).

5. Check the patient's positioning. Are the sternoclavicular joints equidistant from the spinous processes of the vertebral column? If not, then the patient was rotated. Rotation causes asymmetry of shoulder girdle muscles projected over the lung fields. Consequently, the side that has the less space between the end of the clavicle and spinous process has more muscle projected over the lung fields and is whiter than the other side. Be cautious in the interpretation of a rotated chest radiograph.

6. Check to see if the vertebral column is visible through the heart shadow. If not, then it is "under-penetrated" (the X-ray beam was too weak); normal lung tissue will look abnormally opaque (white).

7. Check to see if the lung fields appear dark. If they are, and the vertebral column can be seen very clearly, and the heart shadow is vague, the film is "over-penetrated," and abnormalities may be missed.

8. Check to ensure the diaphragm is between the fifth and sixth anterior rib ends. If it is higher, then the patient did not take a deep breath, and interpretation of the appearance of the lungs and mediastinum will be suboptimal. If the diaphragmatic domes are flattened, then emphysematous changes are likely.

9. After addressing the basic technical issues, are there objects in the X-ray that strike you immediately? Check for foreign bodies, e.g., endotracheal tubes, catheters, chest drains, etc. A striking radio-opaque (white) or lucent (dark) area is likely to be a good lead.

10. Assess the X-ray systematically for subtle abnormalities by:
    a. initially looking at the film without considering the clinical scenario. There is often a tendency to miss obvious things that do not fit with the differential diagnosis. Afterwards, review the X-ray again with the clinical information in mind.
    b. looking at each lung separately, starting at the base and progressing to the apex, carefully looking for abnormalities. Compare the left to the right lung by starting at the lung bases and progressing to the apices, scanning from the lateral border or the right lung to the lateral border of the left lung and back to the opposite side and repeating until the apices are reached. Look "behind" the heart and below the diaphragm.

    c. looking at the superior mediastinum, the hilum, the heart, the
       cardiophrenic angles, the diaphragm, and the costophrenic angles.
    d. lastly, looking at the ribs, the shoulders, and the overlying soft
       tissue from the neck down to the upper abdomen. Note artifacts
       from skin folds, hair, clothing, and buttons.
11. Remember to compare any abnormal chest film with the patient's
    prior studies. Progression over time will often hold the key to the
    correct diagnosis.

This chapter briefly describes common X-ray features of frequently
encountered clinical chest diseases. Have the X-rays formally reviewed
by a radiologist if you do not recognize a sign.

Abnormal chest X-ray appearances

Many chest X-ray appearances will be immediately recognizable as indicat-
ing a specific diagnosis. If not, classify an appearance into one of the head-
ers on the following pages, and then approach the differential diagnosis
systematically. A selection of representative chest X-ray images follows
each section in this chapter and contains images discussed here and cited
in the text.

Area of uniform lung opacification with a well-defined border

This typically occurs when there is an abnormal substance (e.g., water, pus, blood, cells) in the alveolar spaces next to an anatomic border such as a fissure, resulting in a sharp border. The "silhouette sign" consists of loss of normal demarcation between opaque (white) tissue and the normally darker (lucent) lung due to abnormal opacification of the lung.

The position of this sign can help localize an affected lobe as follows: loss of a diaphragm silhouette → (implies) lower lobe consolidation; loss of right (R) heart border silhouette → R middle lobe consolidation; loss of left (L) heart border silhouette → lingular segment consolidation; loss of upper R mediastinal border silhouette → R upper lobe consolidation. A veil-like shadow over the whole L hemithorax → L upper lobe consolidation.

Some differential diagnoses and typical outline evidence

Consolidation due to lobar pneumonia Figures 19.1a, 19.1b	*Suggested by:* well-demarcated uniform whiteness, with a straight border (due to containment by fissural pleura) **with no volume loss** ± air bronchograms. History of bronchial breathing, fever, neutrophils, productive cough
	Confirmed by: resolution on antibiotics and clearing of opacification after 6 weeks
Collapsed (atelectatic) lobe due to bronchial obstruction from carcinoma, mucus plug, foreign body, misplaced endo-tracheal tube, right middle lobe syndrome, endobronchial granuloma Figure 19.2	*Suggested by:* dense, well-demarcated whiteness with straight borders (due to containment by fissures **with volume loss**). History suggestive of cause (e.g., cachexia, monophonic wheeze, and central soft tissue opacity in carcinoma or inhalation of foreign body, or recent endotracheal intubation)
	Confirmed by: resolution following appropriate treatment for intraluminal cause, bronchoscopy, and biopsy for carcinoma
Pulmonary infarction	*Suggested by:* wedge-shaped regions of opacification peripherally ± atelectasis and pleural effusion. History of pleuritic chest pain, hemoptysis, cough, dyspnea.
	Confirmed by: Pulmonary embolism on CT angiogram

Dense pulmonary fibrosis Figure 19.3	*Suggested by:* parenchymal opacification (i.e., reticulonodular shadowing), usually with volume loss, often shrunken against apical pleura. History of TB exposure, radiation, hypersensitivity pneumonitis, chronic sarcoid, ankylosing spondylitis, or pneumoconiosis
	Confirmed by: no change on long-term follow-up
Pleural effusion: transudate (CHF, atelectasis, nephrosis, cirrhosis) or exudate (long differential) Figure 19.4	*Suggested by:* homogeneous dense area of opacification with blunting of the costophrenic angles ± obscuring of the hemidiaphragm in erect position, less dense superiorly with concave meniscus. No air bronchogram. Shift with change of position ± interfissural or subpulmonary loculation. Dullness to percussion. Decreased breath sounds
	Confirmed by: thoracentesis, ± ultrasound to differentiate from consolidation
Empyema	*Suggested by:* large, lentiform pleural opacification. Typically from direct spread of pneumonia. History of spiking temperature
	Confirmed by: thoracentesis (pus or high WBC, pH↓, bacteria present)
Pneumonectomy Figure 19.5	*Suggested by:* dense white area over entire lung with ipsilateral displacement of mediastinal structures, evidence of surgery
	Confirmed by: history of pneumonectomy
Complete lung collapse	*Suggested by:* dense white area over entire lung, mediastinum shifted to affected side, dullness to percussion, increased tactile vocal fremitus, absent breath sounds
	Confirmed by: CT thorax and complete obstruction of main bronchus or bronchoscopy

Area of uniform lung opacification

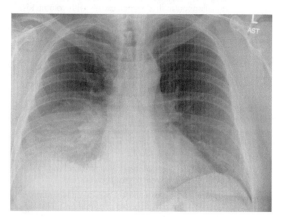

Figure 19.1a Right lower lobe pneumonia, silhouetting the right hemidiaphragm (frontal image).

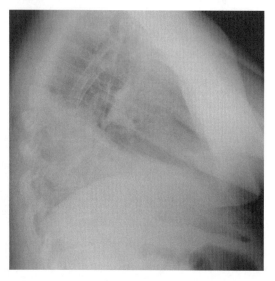

Figure 19.1b Right lower lobe pneumonia, silhouetting the right hemidiaphragm (lateral image).

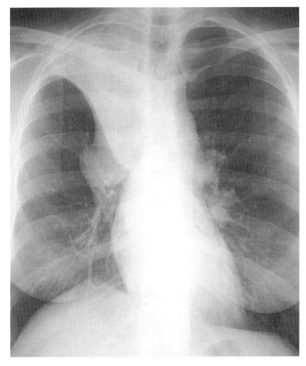

Figure 19.2 Right upper lobe atelectasis resulting from a large right hilar cancer forming the classic "Golden's S sign".

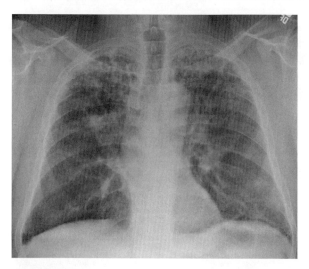

Figure 19.3 Apical fibrosis and bilateral hilar retraction due to stage 4 sarcoidosis.

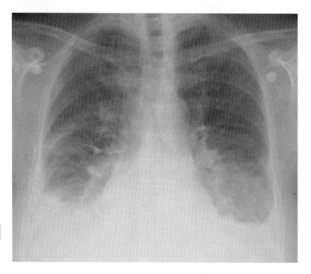

Figure 19.4 Bilateral pleural effusions due to congestive heart failure (CHF). Note that there is a pulmonary linear septal pattern with Kerley B lines.

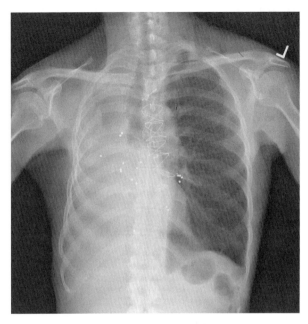

Figure 19.5 Pneumonectomy resulting in mediastinal shift to the right. Note multiple BB pellets in the chest and median strenotomy wires.

Round opacity (or opacities) >5 mm in diameter

Beware of skin or rib lesions or artifacts from hair or clothing that can mimic intrathoracic pathology.

Some differential diagnoses and typical outline evidence

Bronchogenic carcinoma (adenocarcinoma, large cell: commonly peripheral; small cell, squamous: commonly central) Figures 19.2, 19.6	*Suggested by:* solitary opacity with irregular, lobulated, or spiculated border ± hilar enlargement, destructive bone changes in ribs, and other features of metastases. Background cough, hemoptysis, cachexia. High probability of carcinoma if >3 cm (e.g., a mass) *Confirmed by:* tissue diagnosis via bronchoscopy or CT-guided biopsy
Pulmonary metastasis	*Suggested by:* multiple rounded opacities ± background history of neoplasia or lymphoma *Confirmed by:* CT scan appearance ± biopsy
Rounded pneumonia or lung abscess	*Suggested by:* round opacity in child, cavitating thick-rimmed lesion in adult. Background of raised inflammatory markers, neutrophilia and cough, pyrexia, spiking fevers (in abscess) *Confirmed by:* sputum microscopy, culture, and sensitivity resolution following appropriate antibiotic therapy
TB granuloma Figure 19.7	*Suggested by:* coin lesion ± cavitation in upper lobe. Background history of TB exposure, lymphadenopathy *Confirmed by:* CT scan appearance. AFB on smear or culture
Rheumatoid nodule	*Suggested by:* peripherally positioned, ± cavitatation and frequently changed appearance over time. Background history of rheumatoid arthritis with multiple soft tissue nodules *Confirmed by:* CT scan appearance and positive rheumatoid serology

Histoplasmosis	*Suggested by:* coin lesion ± cavitation in upper lobe. Patient from appropriate geographical area (Midwest, Ohio and Mississippi River Valleys, Africa) or HIV-positive
	Confirmed by: CT scan appearance. Yeast-like organisms in sputum. Positive complement fixation test
Wegener's granulomatosis Figure 19.8	*Suggested by:* multiple rounded opacities ± cavitatation with background of proteinuria, skin lesions, etc.
	Confirmed by: serum anti-neutrophil cytoplasmic antigen (ANCA) positivity, biopsy of lung lesion or kidney
Klebsiella pneumonia	*Suggested by:* multi-lobar cavitating opacities in an elderly patient
	Confirmed by: growth on blood or respiratory cultures and response to appropriate antibiotics
Hydatid cyst	*Suggested by:* Water lily sign, which is an opacity in a lower lobe with dark cavity ± daughter cysts within large cyst. History of contact with sheep, dogs, etc.
	Confirmed by: CT scan appearance, positive complement fixation test, or enzyme-linked immunosorbent assay (ELISA)
Pulmonary AV malformation	*Suggested by:* occasional hemoptysis
	Confirmed by: CT thorax showing feeding blood vessel on contrast-enhanced scan
Benign tumors	*Suggested by:* lesion with no change over period of at least a year and <1 cm with no symptoms
	Confirmed by: fat in the lesion by CT (hamartoma), excision and histopathology

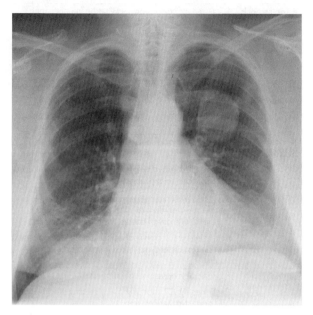

Figure 19.6 Left upper lobe primary bronchogenic carcinoma on frontal image of the chest.

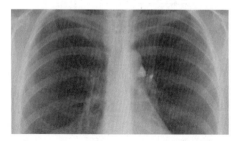

Figure 19.7 Small, calcified nodule in the left upper lobe laterally with a calcified mediastinal lymph node, a result of granulomatous disease. This particular radiologic appearance is known as a "Ghon" or "Ranke Complex."

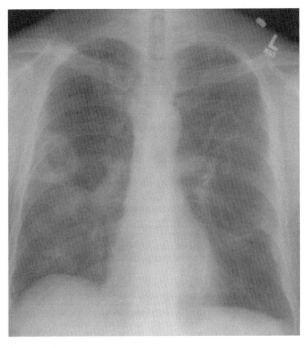

Figure 19.8 Wegener's granulomatosis with large bilateral cavitary masses.

Multiple nodules and miliary pattern

These are round lesions 2–5 mm in diameter of variable density, ranging from small and soft in the miliary (<2 mm) pattern to larger and calcified persistent pulmonary nodules seen after recovery from chickenpox.

Some differential diagnoses and typical outline evidence

Metastases Figure 19.9	*Suggested by:* low-density nodules more profuse in the lower lung zones ± mediastinal widening and other manifestations of malignancy, e.g., lytic lesions in ribs. History of malignancy, e.g., thyroid or renal cell carcinoma. Anorexia and weight loss *Confirmed by:* imaging, tissue diagnosis
Miliary tuberculosis Figure 19.10	*Suggested by:* innumerable grain-like, low-density discrete nodules with history of TB contact *Confirmed by:* AFB on sputum, culture of bone marrow or biopsy specimens from pleura, lung, liver, or lymph nodes
Sarcoidosis Figure 19.11	*Suggested by:* low-density nodules more profuse in the perihilar and mid-lung zones. Bilateral hilar ± paratracheal lymph node enlargement. History of rash or uveitis *Confirmed by:* histology showing noncaseating granuloma with no acid-fast bacilli, ↑serum ACE
Persistent pulmonary nodules of chicken pox	*Suggested by:* dense opacities suggesting calcification. No current symptoms. History of adult-onset chickenpox. Now rare in the United States *Confirmed by:* no change over months on serial X-rays
Pulmonary hemosiderosis from mitral stenosis with pulmonary hypertension Figure 19.12	*Suggested by:* dense opacities due to calcification. History of tapping left ventricular impulse (palpable first heart sound) *Confirmed by:* other clinical findings, ECG findings, echocardiogram, and cardiac catheterization
Pneumoconiosis	*Suggested by:* discrete opacities, mainly in upper lobes, that eventually coalesce into mass-like regions (progressive massive fibrosis) with hilar retraction. History of >10 years working in coal mining, metal mining, or quarrying *Confirmed by:* comparison with previous CXR. HR-CT scan

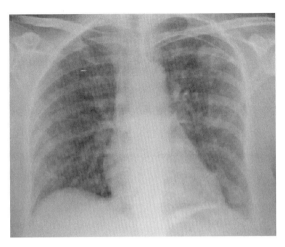

Figure 19.9 Multiple micronodular lung cancer metastasis with left PICC (peripherally inserted central catheter) line

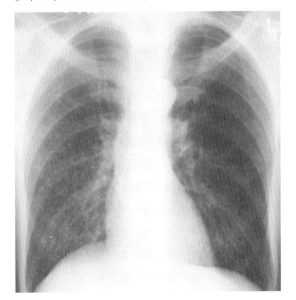

Figure 19.10 Miliary tuberculosis with multiple bilateral micronodules.

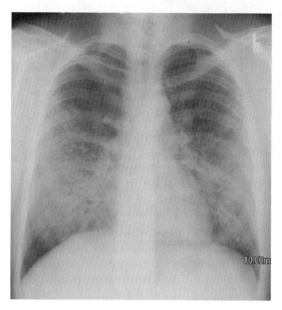

Figure 19.11 Sarcoidosis with airspace disease showing the typical pattern of midlung involvement; in this particular case there is no adenopathy (stage 3).

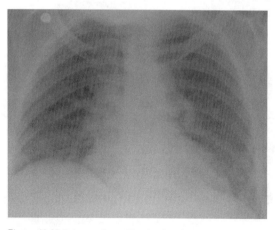

Figure 19.12 Pulmonary hemosiderosis at lung bases as a result of mitral valve stenosis.

Diffuse poorly defined, hazy opacification

Some differential diagnoses and typical outline evidence

Pulmonary edema (cardiogenic, or fluid overload, or both) Figure 19.13 (severe cases may resemble 19.14)	*Suggested by:* symmetrical haziness more florid in a perihilar distribution, fluffy alveolar opacities ± confluence, (if fluid is in airspaces), Kerley B lines or peribronchial cuffing (if in interstitium), or effusion (if in pleural space). History of fluid overload ± heart disease, fine crackles in lung bases
	Confirmed by: ventricular dysfunction on echocardiogram if cardiogenic and response to diuretics or vasodilators
Acute respiratory distress syndrome (ARDS) Figure 19.14	*Suggested by:* symmetrical diffuse, poorly defined opacities that become confluent. History of acute illness and severe hypoxia. Normal heart size, no signs of left ventricular failure (LVF). History of precipitating cause (e.g., septic shock, trauma, transfusion, aspiration, drug exposure, fat/amniotic fluid emboli, viral infection)
	Confirmed by: acute onset, bilateral infiltrates, pulmonary capillary wedge pressure (PCWP) <19 mmHg or no CHF, PaO_2/FiO_2 <200, in the presence of good LV function
Infective infiltration due to viral pneumonia, PCP, bacterial pneumonia Figure 19.15	*Suggested by:* region of patchy pulmonary infiltrate ± air bronchogram ± pleural effusion. If diffuse, more likely to be viral or *Pneumocystis* pneumonia (PCP). History of cough, sputum, raised inflammatory markers, neutropenia (viral), or neutrophilia (bacterial)
	Confirmed by: positive cultures or resolution following appropriate antibiotics
Alveolar cell carcinoma	*Suggested by:* region of poorly defined opacification that may contain air bronchogram. History of progressive breathlessness, copious watery, productive cough. No resolution with antibiotic therapy
	Confirmed by: sputum cytology, lung biopsy
Pulmonary hemorrhage Figure 19.16	*Suggested by:* region of poorly defined opacification (can be diffuse) ± air bronchogram. History of cocaine use, Goodpasture's syndrome, SLE, Wegener's granulomatosis, or coagulopathy
	Confirmed by: Bronchoscopy, CT appearance, renal biopsy (for Goodpasture's syndrome), evidence of SLE, lung biopsy or serum ANCA positivity (for Wegener's)

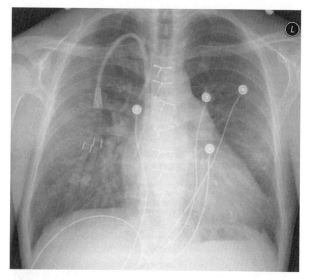

Figure 19.13 Pulmonary edema and Kerley B lines in a patient on hemodialysis.

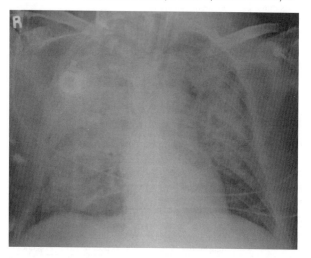

Figure 19.14 ARDS, showing patchy opacificaton in an intubated patient.

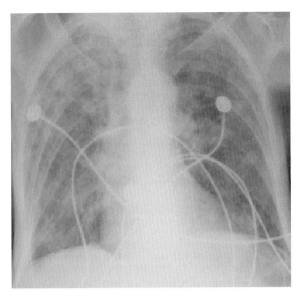

Figure 19.15 Herpes simplex virus (HSV) pneumonia with diffuse infiltrates.

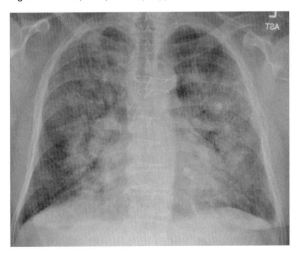

Figure 19.16 Diffuse pulmonary hemorrhage of uncertain etiology.

Increased linear markings

This indicates thickening of the interstitial tissues.

Some differential diagnoses and typical outline evidence

Pulmonary fibrosis Figure 19.17	*Suggested by:* increased interstitial markings with history of asbestosis exposure, pneumoconiosis due to coal, silica, or beryllium, or medical history of collagen vascular disease, sarcoidosis, or hypersensitivity (extrinsic allergic alveolitis)
	Confirmed by: increased reticular markings, traction bronchiectasis, or honeycombing on HR-CT. Lung biopsy
Interstitial fluid = pulmonary edema Figures 19.4, 19.13	*Suggested by:* smooth thickening of the interlobular septa (Kerley B lines) with background lung crackles
	Confirmed by: rapid resolution following diuretic therapy or correct fluid balance or dialysis
Metastatic cells = lymphangitic carcinomatosis	*Suggested by:* smooth thickening of the interlobular septa with background of other features of malignancy
	Confirmed by: HR-CT, lung biopsy, or progressive malignant disease
Bronchiectasis Figure 19.18	*Suggested by:* tram lines and rings with background of cough with high volume of sputum (± foul and purulent (if super-added infection) *Confirmed by:* HR-CT

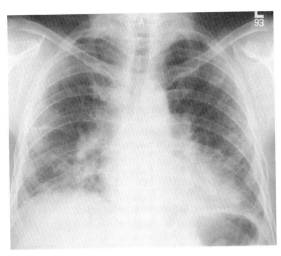

Figure 19.17 Idiopathic pulmonary fibrosis with a peripheral and basilar predominance.

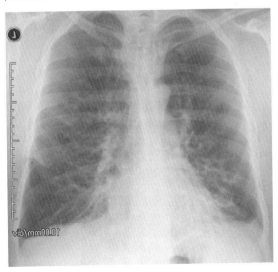

Figure 19.18 Extensive bronchiectasis with cylindrical and cystic features in this 34 year old male with cystic fibrosis (note that markings on film are reversed).

Symmetrically dark lungs (no or decreased lung markings)

Some differential diagnoses and typical outline evidence

Chronic obstructive pulmonary disease (COPD) Figure 19.19a, 19.19b	*Suggested by:* long, narrow heart and chest, flat diaphragm, horizontal ribs with the seventh rib visible anteriorly and eleventh rib visible posteriorly. Prominent pulmonary arteries with peripheral pruning (in pulmonary hypertension). Large, thin-rimmed dark areas with no lung markings—bullae. Long history of smoking
	Confirmed by: Lung function tests showing fixed obstructive deficit, FEV_1 <80%, FEV_1/FVC <70%
Asthma	*Suggested by:* hyperexpanded lungs. No loss of lung markings. Background history of asthma
	Confirmed by: spirometric improvement following appropriate treatment

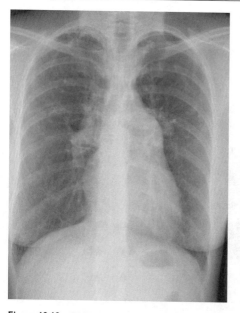

Figure 19.19a COPD with pulmonary hypertension as evidenced by enlarged central pulmonary arteries and peripheral arterial pruning (frontal image).

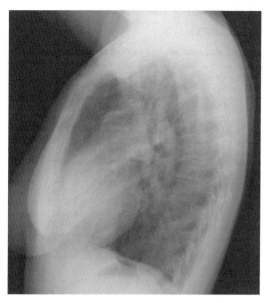

Figure 19.19b COPD with pulmonary hypertension (lateral image) as evidenced by enlarged pulmonary arteries and flattening of the diaphragms.

Area of dark lung (no or decreased lung markings)

Some differential diagnoses and typical outline evidence

Pneumothorax Figure 19.20	*Suggested by:* visible lung edge with absence of lung markings peripheral to this; mediastinal shift may occur in severe cases. Beware of skin folds that may mimic a lung edge. History of sudden onset of breathlessness
	Confirmed by: more definitive appearance on expiratory film or CT scan.
Tension pneumothorax (medical emergency)	*Suggested by:* visible lung edge with absence of lung markings peripheral to this, mediastinal shift away from the collapsed lung. History of acute, progressive dyspnea, tachycardia, low BP
	Confirmed by: relief when a needle or catheter is inserted, the lung re-expands, and vital signs normalize
Bulla Figure 19.21	*Suggested by:* loss of lung markings inside lucent, thin-rimmed circular region. History of COPD
	Confirmed by: comparison with previous CXR, CT thorax
Mastectomy	*Suggested by:* no breast shadow
	Confirmed by: history of mastectomy

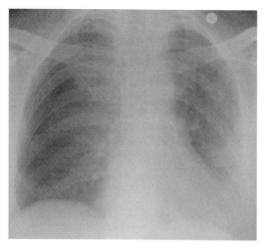

Figure 19.20 Right lateral pneumothorax with loss of lung markings and visible lung edge.

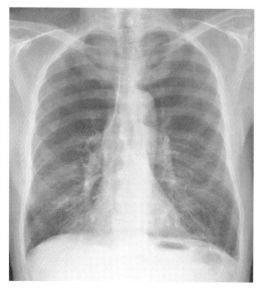

Figure 19.21 Emphysema with large bilateral apical bullae and vascular distortion.

Enlarged hila

Check that the X-ray is not rotated. Rotation of the chest can result in a falsely enlarged hilum or unequal hila. If prior X-rays or studies are available, compare to determine the duration of the abnormality.

Some differential diagnoses and typical outline evidence

Metastatic lymphadenopathy or primary bronchogenic carcinoma Figure 19.22	*Suggested by:* unilateral hilar opacity ± lung opacity or bilateral hilar opacity ± evidence of metastatic deposits, e.g., lytic rib lesions. Prior history of neoplasia
	Confirmed by: bronchoscopy ± CT staging. Sputum cytology showing cancer cells
Hodgkin's or non-Hodgkin's lymphoma Figure 19.23	*Suggested by:* bilateral hilar shadows, ± parenchymal opacification. History of anemia, lymph node enlargement
	Confirmed by: histology with Reed–Sternberg cells in Hodgkin's, specific histology, tumor markers, flow cytometry in non-Hodgkin's
Primary tuberculosis with hilar node (primary complex)	*Suggested by:* unilateral hilar mass (lymphadenopathy) and poorly defined opacificaiton in peripheral lung field, often with paratracheal nodal enlargement. History of TB
	Confirmed by: CT scan showing no tumor. Acid-fast bacilli on ZN stain and culture growth from sputum after up to 12 weeks for TB. Resolution on specific anti-TB therapy
Prominent pulmonary artery due to embolus	*Suggested by:* smooth, nonlobular appearance tapering off peripherally with dark peripheral lung fields
	Confirmed by: CT-pulmonary angiogram
Prominent pulmonary arteries due to pulmonary hypertension	*Suggested by:* bulky bilateral hila with outline suggestive of prominent pulmonary arteries, tapering off peripherally with dark peripheral lung fields ± widening of upper mediastinum (SVC) ± bulging right heart border
	Confirmed by: CT-pulmonary angiogram, echocardiographic or right heart catheterization evidence of pulmonary hypertension
Sarcoidosis Figure 19.24	*Suggested by:* bilateral hilar convex shadows, possibly with other lung changes of sarcoid. History of rash, uveitis, etc.
	Confirmed by: histology showing noncaseating granuloma with no acid-fast bacilli

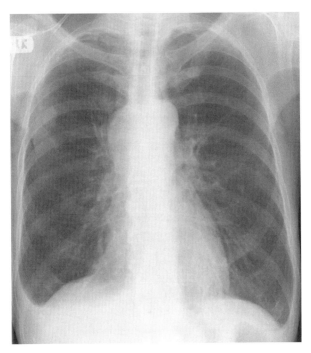

Figure 19.22 Right upper lobe primary lung cancer with metastasis to the right side of the mediastinum and right hilum (note right hilar fullness and small right pleural effusion).

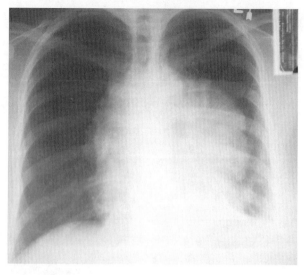

Figure 19.23 Left hilar mass in a patient with non-Hodgkin's lymphoma.

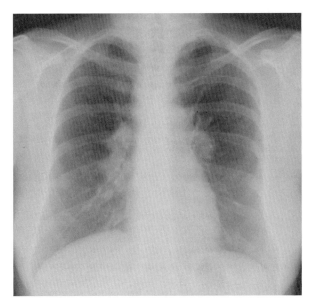

Figure 19.24 Bilateral hilar and right paratracheal lymphadenopathy in patient with sarcoidosis (stage 2), This pattern is known as the "1,2,3 sign."

Upper mediastinal widening

Some differential diagnoses and typical outline evidence

Retrosternal goiter Figure 19.25	*Suggested by:* superior mediastinal mass shadow extending from the neck
	Confirmed by: clinical examination, ultrasound, or radioisotope scan
Hodgkin's or non-Hodgkin's lymphoma or metastatic lymphadenopathy	*Suggested by:* dense, often multinodular masses causing mediastinal widening *Confirmed by:* correlated CT scan appearance, mediastinoscopy, or surgical removal showing histology
Thymoma Figure 19.26a, 19.26b	*Suggested by:* clearly outlined opacity (calcification in 20% of cases). History of myasthenia gravis in 30%
	Confirmed by: correlated CT scan appearance and histology from mediastinoscopy or surgical removal and histology from mediastinoscopy or surgical removal
Teratoma: benign or malignant	*Suggested by:* anterior mediastinal opacification, rarely with calcification, e.g., in teeth *Confirmed by:* correlated CT scan appearance ± fat, hair, teeth, and histology from mediastinoscopy or surgical removal
Aortic aneurysm Figure 19.27	*Suggested by:* opacification continuous with descending aorta shadow *Confirmed by:* correlated CT scan appearance
Mediastinal lymphadenopathy from primary bronchogenic carcinoma Figure 19.22	*Suggested by:* pulmonary nodule or mass, not always visualized especially in small cell lung cancer *Confirmed by:* correlated CT scan appearance, mediastinoscopy, or surgical biopsy or removal

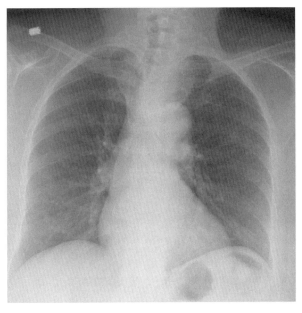

Figure 19.25 Substernal goiter with tracheal deviation to the right.

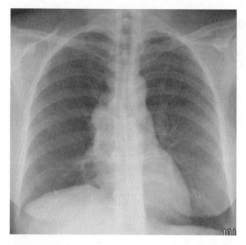

Figure 19.26a Anterior mediastinal mass; differential includes thymoma, teratoma, lymphoma and thyroid gland. (This case was a partially calcified thymoma; frontal image.)

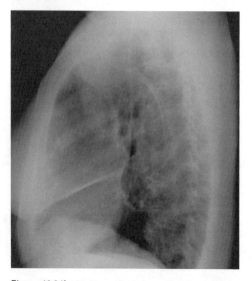

Figure 19.26b Anterior mediastinal mass (partially calcified thymoma; lateral image).

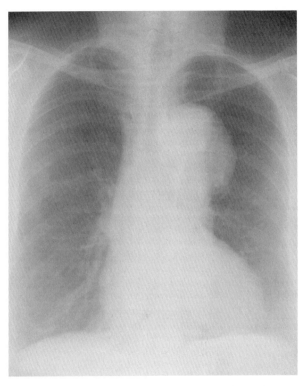

Figure 19.27 Aortic aneurysm involving the arch and proximal descending thoracic aorta.

Abnormal cardiac silhouette

Some differential diagnoses and typical outline evidence

Left ventricular failure (LVF) Figure 19.28	*Suggested by:* large heart to the left of midline (with central trachea), enlarged upper lobe pulmonary vasculature (cephalization), fluffy lung opacities centrally more than peripherally
	Confirmed by: echocardiogram showing poor contraction of left ventricle
Pulmonary hypertension	*Suggested by:* prominent right heart border (right ventricle), upwardly rounded apex, and bilateral prominence of hila. Loud pulmonary valve closure. Possible history of pulmonary embolism (PE)
	Confirmed by: tall R waves in V1 to V3 on ECG and right axis deviation
Cardiomyopathy	*Suggested by:* globally enlarged heart with clear borders (indicating poor contraction). History of predisposing condition, e.g., chronic alcohol abuse, amyloid, leukemia, or rheumatoid arthritis
	Confirmed by: echocardiogram showing low ejection fraction
Pericardial effusion	*Suggested by:* large, globular cardiac outline and clear borders (indicating little or no contraction)
	Confirmed by: echocardiogram showing effusions
Atrial septal defect	*Suggested by:* unusually convex right heart border, upwardly rounded cardiac apex, and bilateral prominence of hila
	Confirmed by: echocardiogram showing a jet of blood from the left atrium to the right atrium and/or positive bubble study
Mitral stenosis	*Suggested by:* large heart, enlarged left atrium (rounded opacity behind the heart which 'splays' the carinal angle) ± calcification in position of mitral valve and dense nodules due to hemosiderosis. History of rheumatic heart disease
	Confirmed by: echocardiogram and cardiac catheterization

Left ventricular aneurysm, pseudoaneurysm Figure 19.29a, 19.29b	*Suggested by:* bulge in left ventricular border ± calcification. History of ischemic heart disease ± myocardial infarction *Confirmed by:* echocardiogram
Mediastinal emphysema	*Suggested by:* gas around the mediastinal contour, ± surgical emphysema. History of acute asthma, recent esophagogastroduodenoscopy (EGD), esophageal rupture, etc., signs of surgical emphysema *Confirmed by:* CT thorax
Hiatal hernia	*Suggested by:* circular shadow behind the heart, ± air-fluid level, absent gastric bubble. Intermittent appearance on previous CXR *Confirmed by:* barium swallow, endoscopy

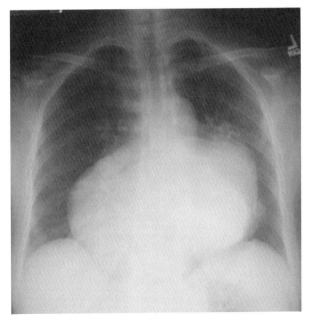

Figure 19.28 Cardiomegaly involving all four cardiac chambers due to tricuspid and mitral regurgitation.

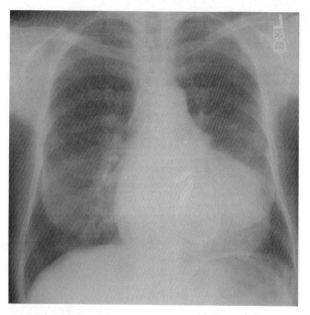

Figure 19.29a Left ventricular aneurysm, partially calcified, due to an MI after cardiac valve replacement (frontal image).

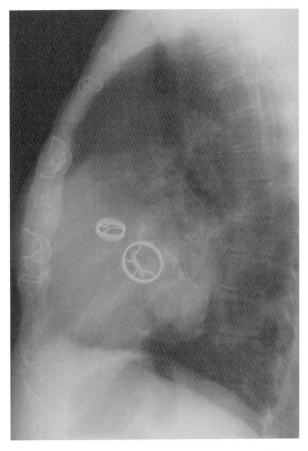

Figure 19.29b Left ventricular aneurysm, partially calcified, due to an MI after cardiac valve replacement. Note *in situ* valve rings (lateral image).

Index